Postgraduate Vascular Surgery

A Candidate's Guide to the FRCS and Board Exams

Second Edition

D1581770

CLINICAL TALK

ISSN: 1756-7793

Series Editors: Andrew Goldberg *(University College London and the Royal National Orthopaedic Hospital NHS Trust, Stanmore, UK)*

Gerard Stansby *(University of Newcastle and Freeman Hospital, Newcastle Hospitals NHS Trust, UK)*

CLINICAL TALK

Postgraduate Vascular Surgery

A Candidate's Guide to the FRCS and Board Exams

Second Edition

Editors

Vish Bhattacharya
Newcastle University and Queen Elizabeth Hospital, UK

Gerard Stansby
Newcastle University and Freeman Hospital, UK

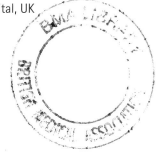

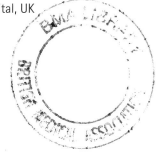**World Scientific**

NEW JERSEY · LONDON · SINGAPORE · BEIJING · SHANGHAI · HONG KONG · TAIPEI · CHENNAI · TOKYO

Published by

World Scientific Publishing Europe Ltd.

57 Shelton Street, Covent Garden, London WC2H 9HE

Head office: 5 Toh Tuck Link, Singapore 596224

USA office: 27 Warren Street, Suite 401-402, Hackensack, NJ 07601

Library of Congress Cataloging-in-Publication Data

Names: Bhattacharya, Vish, editor. | Stansby, Gerard, editor.
Title: Postgraduate vascular surgery : a candidate's guide to the FRCS and board exams /
    [edited by] Vish Bhattacharya (Newcastle University and Queen Elizabeth Hospital, UK),
    Gerard Stansby (Newcastle University and Freeman Hospital, UK).
Other titles: Clinical talk series.
Description: 2nd edition. | New Jersey : World Scientific, 2018. |
    Series: Clinical talk | Includes bibliographical references and index.
Identifiers: LCCN 2017054278 | ISBN 9781786344939 (hc : alk. paper) |
    ISBN 9781786346018 (pbk : alk. paper).
Subjects: | MESH: Vascular Surgical Procedures | Vascular Diseases--surgery | Handbooks
Classification: LCC RD598.5 | NLM WG 39 | DDC 617.4/13--dc23
LC record available at https://lccn.loc.gov/2017054278

British Library Cataloguing-in-Publication Data
A catalogue record for this book is available from the British Library.

For any available supplementary material, please visit
http://www.worldscientific.com/worldscibooks/10.1142/Q0144#t=suppl

Desk Editors: Suraj Kumar/Jennifer Brough/Shi Ying Koe

Typeset by Stallion Press
Email: enquiries@stallionpress.com

Printed in Singapore

Preface

Welcome to the second edition of *Postgraduate Vascular Surgery*. After the huge success of our first edition, we decided to update all the chapters and add some new ones for the second edition.

All the chapters have been written by experts in their field and co-authored by vascular, anaesthetic, or radiology trainees. The majority of authors have successfully taken the Intercollegiate Speciality Board exams in Surgery over the last two decades.

This is a 'high-stake' exam and comes at a critical stage in a young surgeon's career when he or she is nearing the end of Specialist Registrar training. This book provides a quick, 'easy-to-read' reference for candidates already under pressure to cover a vast array of subjects. The first edition also proved to be very popular among trainees writing the European Board of Vascular Surgery exams as well the postgraduate exams in vascular surgery in other countries.

This book has been divided into two sections.

The first section covers an introduction to the format of the exams and is followed by examples of common clinical cases that keep getting discussed in the exams. The authors have incorporated the views of several trainees to make this section relevant to their needs.

The second section has been written by experts in their respective fields who have provided succinct chapters in a concise format. Key points have been mentioned at the beginning of the chapters to aid quick revision before the examinations. References have been deliberately kept to a minimum so than readers can go back and read the relevant articles in detail, if they wish.

Although this book is targeted towards trainees in vascular surgery, we hope that it will also benefit established vascular surgeons by providing a ready reference in the ever-changing world of vascular surgery.

We thank all the contributors for their hard work and timely submission of manuscripts. We thank the publishers at World Scientific for their dedication and expertise.

Vish Bhattacharya
Gerard Stansby

List of Contributors

Mohamed Abdelhamid
Specialist Registrar in Vascular Surgery
Guy's and St Thomas' NHS Foundation Trust
London SE1 9RT, UK

Omar Ashour
Specialist Registrar in Vascular Surgery
Kent Surrey and Sussex Deanery
Kent

Hassan Badri
Consultant in Vascular and Endovascular Surgery
The Pennine Acute Hospitals NHS Trust
Oldham OL1 2JH, UK

Arun Prakash Balakrishnan
Consultant in Vascular Surgery
Countess of Chester Hospital
Chester CH2 1UL, UK

Vish Bhattacharya
Consultant in Vascular Surgery
Associate Medical Director
Queen Elizabeth Hospital
Gateshead NE9 6SX, UK

Paul Blair
Consultant in Vascular Surgery
Royal Victoria Hospital
Belfast BT12 6BA, UK

Julie Brittenden
Professor of Vascular Surgery
Department of Cardiovascular and Medical Sciences
University of Glasgow
Glasgow G12 8QQ, UK

Jocelyn Brookes
Consultant Endovascular Radiologist
The Royal Free Hospital
London NW3 2QG, UK

Roderick Chalmers
Consultant in Vascular Surgery
University of Edinburgh
Edinburgh EH16 4SB, UK

Mike Clarke
Consultant in Vascular Surgery
Freeman Hospital
Newcastle upon Tyne NE7 7DN, UK

David M. Cressey
Consultant in Anaesthesia
Freeman Hospital
Newcastle upon Tyne NE7 7DN, UK

Saroj Das
Professor of Surgery
Institute of Bioengineering
Director of Clinical Studies, Imperial College London
Consultant Surgeon
The Hillingdon Hospital & London North West Health Care NHS Trust
Uxbridge UB8 3NN, UK

Robert Davies
Consultant in Vascular and Endovascular Surgery
Leicester Royal Infirmary
Leicester LE1 5WW, UK

Jeremy French
Consultant in HPB and Transplantation Surgery
Freeman Hospital
Newcastle upon Tyne NE7 7DN, UK

Katherine Gardner
The Hillingdon Hospital NHS Foundation Trust
Uxbridge UB8 3NN, UK

Bridget Griffiths
Consultant in Rheumatology
Freeman Hospital
Newcastle upon Tyne NE7 7DN, UK

George Hamilton
Professor of Vascular Surgery
The Royal Free Hospital
London NW3 2QG, UK

Monica Hansrani
Consultant in Vascular Surgery
Lead for Vascular Access
James Cook University Hospital
Middlesbrough TS4 3BW, UK

Mark Kay
Consultant in Vascular Surgery
Queen Elizabeth Hospital
Birmingham B15 2TH, UK

Tim Lees
Consultant in Vascular Surgery
King's College London
Dubai

Sebastian Mafeld
Interventional Radiology Fellow
Toronto, Canada

Asif Mahmood
Consultant in Vascular Surgery
University Hospital Coventry
Coventry CV2 2DX, UK

Ragai Makar
Consultant in Vascular Surgery
Countess of Chester Hospital
Chester CH2 1UL, UK

Derek Manas
Professor of HPB and Transplantation Surgery
Freeman Hospital
Newcastle upon Tyne NE7 7DN, UK

Colette Marshall
Consultant in Vascular Surgery
Executive Medical Director
Bedford Hospital NHS Trust
Bedford MK42 9DJ, UK

James McCaslin
Consultant in Vascular and Endovascular Surgery
Freeman Hospital
Newcastle upon Tyne NE7 7DN, UK

Abigail H. M. Morbi
Vascular Research Fellow
University Hospital Southampton NHS Foundation Trust
Southampton SO16 6YD, UK

A. Ross Naylor
Professor of Vascular Surgery
Leicester Vascular Institute
Glenfield Hospital
Leicester LE3 9QP, UK

Craig Nesbitt
Registrar in Vascular Surgery
Freeman Hospital
Newcastle upon Tyne NE7 7DN, UK

Ian D. Nesbitt
Consultant in Anaesthesia
Freeman Hospital
Newcastle upon Tyne NE7 7DN, UK

Colin Nice
Consultant in Interventional Radiology
Freeman Hospital
Newcastle upon Tyne NE7 7DN, UK

Catherine Pye
Core Trainee in Oncology
Guys & St Thomas's Hospital
London SE1 7EH, UK

Ahmad Rafizi Hariz Bin Ramli
Consultant Vascular and Endovascular Surgeon
University Malaya Medical Centre
59100 Kuala Lumpur, Malaysia

Jennifer Robson
Clinical Lecturer in Vascular Surgery
University of Edinburgh
Edinburgh EH16 4SA, UK

Muhammed Anees Sharif
Consultant in Vascular and Endovascular Surgery
Abertawe Bro Morgannwg University Health Board
Port Talbot SA12 7BR, UK

Cliff Shearman
Emeritus Professor of Vascular Surgery
Southampton University Hospitals NHS Trust
Southampton SO16 6YD, UK

Jonathan Smout
Consultant in Vascular Surgery
Aintree University Hospital
Liverpool L9 7AL, UK

Gerard Stansby
Professor of Vascular Surgery
Freeman Hospital
Newcastle upon Tyne NE7 7DN, UK

Theo Tsiris
Senior Fellow in HPB and Transplantation Surgery
Freeman Hospital
Newcastle upon Tyne NE7 7DN, UK

Arunagiri Viruthagiri
Senior Fellow in Vascular Surgery
Queen Elizabeth Hospital
Birmingham B15 2TH, UK

Rajiv Vohra
Professor of Surgery
Consultant in Vascular Surgery
Selly Oak Hospital
University Hospital Birmingham
Birmingham B15 2TH, UK

Rob Williams
Consultant in Interventional Radiology
Freeman Hospital
Newcastle upon Tyne NE7 7DN, UK

Peng Wong
Consultant in Vascular Surgery
James Cook University Hospital
Middlesbrough TS4 3BW, UK

Contents

Section 1

Final FRCS Vascular: Introduction

Chapter 1

Clinicals — Introduction to the Examination and Clinical Cases

James McCaslin, Jonathan Smout and Asif Mahmood

Key Points

- One long and three short cases in the FRCS clinical exam in 30 minutes.
- Previous practice to examine in a systematic manner with a senior colleague in an outpatient setting is useful.
- The initial starter question may lead to more complex issues.
- Patients usually stable elderly mobile patients.
- Short cases usually a pool of cases with venous ulcers, KTS or carotid tumours.

The format of the Final FRCS clinical examination for vascular candidates used to consist of both general surgery and vascular 'clinicals'. However, with speciality recognition, the new vascular exam will have increased emphasis on vascular problems, with little or no general surgery cases. It is anticipated that the new vascular examination will consist of a long case and three short cases taken in succession, with two examiners who will take turns in questioning and marking the candidate. The cases are either a patient encounter, or interpreting an investigation. With the Final examination being directed at ascertaining competence to become a consultant, the questions tend to relate to management issues rather that testing your ability to perform a head-to-toe clinical assessment. However, as senior trainees it is expected that you should know how to examine a patient in an orderly and effective fashion. Failure to demonstrate this in the clinical encounters will ring alarm bells with the examiners.

The short case format of the 'clinicals' should not be viewed as a hurdle, but rather an opportunity for you to impart your fundamental knowledge on a broad range of topics. The examination process is an efficient way of assessing a wide range of subjects in a limited period of time and in a systematic manner. Candidates who have gone through the 'clinicals' are often left stunned by the number of topics that have been discussed in a blur of 30 min. Candidates should therefore see the benefits of this system where a poor performance for one case becomes a small part of the whole marking scheme. It is essential that candidates who feel that they have done badly at one station don't dwell on their misfortune, but compose themselves and get on with the rest of the assessment believing they can still pass.

It is important that as the candidate you listen carefully to the examiner's questions. The instructions will often be extremely focussed, and initially seem quite a minor request. The initial 'starter' question will then lead on to more complex issues. The questions are generally not intended to catch you out, so do what you are asked to do. It is essential that you appear comfortable dealing with patients. Although observed examination practice with colleagues is very useful, it can also be helpful to get into a habit of examining patients in outpatient clinics in the same systematic manner as you would use in the examination. Your actions will then become effortless and automatic in the high-adrenaline situation of the exam. It is important to get over the 'pass/fail' information and common conditions before moving on to rarities. As the clinical examinations and vivas all depend on verbal interaction to impart your knowledge, it is vitally important to practice viva questioning with colleagues. This will help you formulate a structure to your answers in an orderly fashion, and you should quickly notice an improvement in your performance.

When anticipating cases for your clinical examination, common conditions in mobile patients will appear most frequently. If you have ever been in the situation of organising patients for a clinical examination, you realise that the mobile elderly and those with stable chronic disease are easiest to recruit. There will always be a small pool of rarities such as Klippel–Trénaunay syndrome (KTS) or CBTs that are willing to turn up for exams. It would be extremely unusual for an acute life- or limb-threatening problem to turn up in an examination. On the day, try to smile when introducing yourself to the patients and thank them following the encounter (the same applies to thanking the examiners!). The examination day can actually become quite repetitive for the patients and examiners alike. Try hard to make them feel that their participation is valued, and demonstrate that you can put patients at ease.

Last minute revision can be helpful as topics recently read have a habit of turning up in exams. Despite this, turning up to the exam sleep deprived will not help your performance; hence, a sensible balance must be met. Research has demonstrated that moderate sleep deprivation produces impaired cognitive and motor performance similar to alcohol intoxication. You would not expect to pass an exam whilst intoxicated!

Clinical Case Examples

Popliteal aneurysm

The basics

Popliteal aneurysms (PAs) are the commonest peripheral aneurysm (Fig. 1). Approximately half are bilateral and half are associated with an abdominal aortic aneurysm (AAA). Conversely, 5–10% of patients with an AAA have a PA. The majority of PAs present with distal ischaemic complications in either the acute or chronic situation. The prevalence of a PA is thought to be around 1% for those in their eighth decade. When presenting acutely with distal limb ischaemia, limb loss occurs in up to 50% of cases. PAs almost exclusively occur in males. When treatment is indicated PAs are generally treated by surgical exclusion, although endovascular management is a newer development in selected cases. Occasionally, patients with patent PAs and very diseased run-off may be

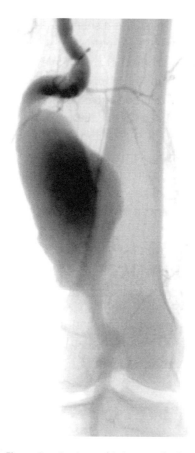

Figure 1.   Angiographic image of a PA.

managed long-term with anticoagulation to reduce the risk of aneurysm thrombosis.

The case

PAs are usually easy to identify as an expansile, or prominent, pulsation in the popliteal fossa. The artery is best palpated against the tibia in the midline of the popliteal fossa, with the knee in the extended position (or with a few degrees of flexion). The artery can also be palpated with the knee flexed to 130°, in this position, the popliteal fascia loosens to aid palpation. However, in doing so the manoeuvre deepens the artery from the skin surface. When thrombosed, PAs may be more difficult to diagnose clinically. It is important to assess the distal circulation for evidence of embolisation into the foot or calf vessels. Other posterior knee swellings include a Baker's cyst, or a semimembranosus bursa. Remember, a PA can exist at any point along the course of the popliteal artery and include the lower SFA as well. In contrast, Baker's cyst originates below the level of the knee joint as it extends beneath the gastrocnemius muscle. A Baker's cyst will often be associated with symptoms and signs suggestive of degenerative arthritis of the knee joint. When present, an enlarged semimembranosus bursa will be located medially under the popliteal edge of the semimembranosus muscle.

Questions

How do PAs present?

In the acute situation, PAs usually present with distal ischaemia as a consequence of acute thrombosis or distal embolisation. In the chronic situation, they present with intermittent claudication as a result of chronic embolisation to the tibial vessels. Asymptomatic PAs are often identified when screening patients with known aortic aneurysms. In contrast to aortic aneurysms, rupture of a PA is a relatively rare occurrence (<5%). Other rarer presentations result from local pressure on surrounding nerves and/or popliteal vein, and they can be the cause of a DVT.

Tell me about the anatomy of the popliteal artery?

The popliteal artery commences when the superficial femoral artery passes through the adductor hiatus in the thigh. The popliteal artery terminates by dividing at the tibioperoneal trunk at the lower border of popliteus muscle. It also gives off the anterior tibial artery, which may have a high take-off in some. The popliteal artery also gives off genicular branches at several levels to form a large collateral network about the knee joint. The artery is the deepest major structure in the popliteal fossa, and sits beneath the popliteal vein(s). The tibial nerve lies superficial to the popliteal vein. This organisation is not in the classical vein/artery/nerve configuration.

How would you approach the popliteal artery?

Although the popliteal artery can be approached via a lateral incision, the most common routes of proximal and distal access are via either a medial, or a posterior approach.

In the medial approach, the suprageniculate artery is accessed via an incision in the distal third of thigh along the anterior border of the sartorius muscle. This muscle is mobilised posterior and the artery is identified between the medial intra-muscular septum anteriorly and semimembranosus muscle posteriorly. The infrageniculate popliteal artery is exposed medially via a longitudinal incision, 1 cm behind the posterior/medial border of the tibia. The long saphenous vein (LSV) is usually located posterior to the incision, and care must be taken not to damage it! If an LSV bypass is planned, it may be best to have marked it with Duplex. A tissue plane is bluntly created between the soleus and gastrocnemius muscles. The tendons of sartorius, gracilis and semitendinosus often require division for more proximal access. The popliteal vein(s) must be carefully mobilised, as this sits in front of the artery from the medial approach. The nerves should be preserved. The sciatic nerve divides into the tibial and common peroneal nerve about 5–12 cm proximal to the popliteal crease. At the popliteal crease, the nerves are midway between skin and bone. They are lateral and superficial to the popliteal artery and vein in a separate sheath.

In a posterior approach, a lazy-S incision is made in the popliteal fossa with the patient positioned prone. The aneurysm is opened and any back-bleeding vessels oversewn. This has advantages such as being able to decompress the aneurysm (especially useful if large), anatomical reconstruction of the popliteal artery with a shorter graft and, most importantly, better control of branch vessels into the PA (thereby eliminating ongoing growth, which occurs in around 20% of medial repairs). The trade-off to this is the perceived potential to injure the tibial nerves and popliteal vein, along with a more limited exposure, which has led some authors to question if this may lead to poorer graft patency. Neither of these concerns have definitively shown a posterior approach to be worse than medial repair, however.

What are your indications for elective repair?

In contrast to AAAs, where there is clear consensus on indications for intervention in terms of size, this is not the case for PAs. Most surgeons would treat PAs exceeding 2 cm in diameter, although patient factors may influence the decision for intervention. These factors may include patient fitness, the anatomical configuration of the PA, evidence of distal embolisation and poor run-off or the presence of critical ischaemia. Most surgeons would view distal embolisation as a strong indicator for treatment, irrespective of aneurysm size. The presence of mural thrombus on duplex scanning and significant distortion of the aneurysm should be viewed as concerning signs. Prevention of aneurysm thrombosis is critical as limb loss is markedly worse in the acute setting than for elective surgery.

When is thrombolysis utilised?

It has been observed that catheter-based thrombolysis is associated with higher risks of ischaemic complications when used to manage acute PAs, in comparison to treating an acute graft occlusion. During the lysis process, a large volume of thromboembolic material is destabilised and inevitably embolised distally. Studies have demonstrated that in at least 10% of patients the limb deteriorates acutely during the lysis process. The main role of thrombolysis is 'on table' to clear thrombus from the run-off vessels during the process of surgical revascularisation. Thrombolysis can sometimes be used where no distal target vessels are seen for surgical bypass on initial angiography and the limb is only in the 'marginally' threatened category.

What major problem faces endovascular treatment of PAs?

There is little doubt that covered endovascular stents can effectively exclude PAs and provide an adequate conduit to supply blood to the lower leg. The main concerns regarding popliteal stent grafts relate to their long-term durability. With the constant flexing of the knee joint, the physical stresses challenge the integrity and positioning of popliteal stent grafts. Endovascular exclusion was first described in 1994, and most of the literature reports come from institutional case series. Endovascular treatment was mainly being performed in asymptomatic patients, and initial results were poor. With the development of newer, more flexible devices, these results have improved, with 5-year patency rates of >75% being published. A recent Cochrane review [1] concluded that insufficient data were available to make a firm decision on stent-graft repair of PAs, even though the one included study showed equivalence with open repair.

Carotid body tumour (CBT)

The basics

CBTs are a paragangliomas derived from the neural crest ectoderm. Paragangliomas are a rare neoplasm that can be found in the abdomen, thorax, and head and neck region. They are usually considered benign and complete surgical removal results in cure. The rule of '5%' is often quoted as 5% are bilateral, 5% familial, 5% systemically malignant and 5% locally reoccur. In reality, nearer 10% are familial and in these patients a third have bilateral tumours. In contrast to retroperitoneal paragangliomas, where the majority are hormonally active, <5% of CBTs are hormonally active. In the neck, paragangliomas can also arise from the vagus nerve (glomus vagale) and jugular bulb (glomus jugulare). There are three distinct groups of patients: sporadic (majority), familial and hyperplastic (associated with chronic hypoxia).

The case

The thought of a CBT in your final examination might overwhelm you with fear, but it shouldn't! With their management being a relatively specialised subject, you will not be expected to know a large amount about CBTs or to have treated one. Twenty minutes reading will provide you with all the knowledge you need to impress the examiners. The examination case will take the form of either a neck mass, post-operative case, and/or a CT/MR scan to review. The mass will be palpated at the level of (or above) the hyoid bone, along the anterior border of sternocleidomastoid. The CBT is firm in consistency and hence often referred to as a 'potato tumour', the mass is laterally mobile but vertically fixed. The tumour is itself not pulsatile, although a transmitted pulsation may be present, or a pulsation may be palpable from an overlying external carotid artery. Differential diagnoses to consider are cervical lymphade-nopathy (are there nodes elsewhere?), branchial cyst, carotid artery aneurysm (expansile mass), carotid artery tortuosity, or other cervical paragangliomas. Due to the anatomical distortion and intra-operative bleeding, cranial nerve injury is more common when treating CBTs than during CEA (glossopharyngeal, vagus [including laryngeal branches], hypoglossal, accessory).

Questions

How do CBTs usually present?

CBTs usually present as a painless neck mass (>50%), and can also pre-sent with compression of local structures or pain. The most common nerves to be compressed are the glossopharyngeal, vagus and hypoglos-sal nerves. CBTs rarely present with symptoms of cerebral ischaemia.

What are the typical CT/MR findings?

Due to the location of the CBT, they typically splay the carotid bifurcation on angiography (arterial/CT or MR) (Fig. 2). If the tumour does not dis-play this feature, it is more likely to be another type of paraganglioma. The tumour derives its blood supply from the external carotid artery. The tumours are usually well defined, and when large can encase the carotid vessels.

What is the preop assessment?

All patients should have had a Duplex scan and neurological examination as part of their initial investigations. Further investigations include laryn-goscopy (vocal cord assessment), plus urinary catecholamine testing in patients experiencing hypertensive episodes or those with other neu-roendocrine tumours (and contralateral CBTs on imaging). MIBG scanning may also be used if a functional tumour is suspected. MRI scanning is

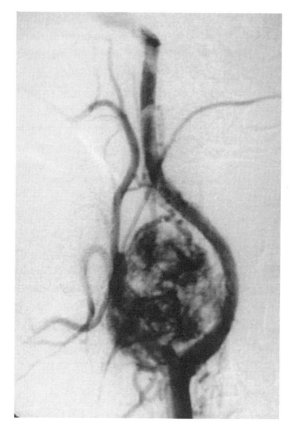

Figure 2.   Intra-arterial angiography of CBT. Note splaying of the carotid bifurcation and high vascularity of the tumour.

valuable for diagnostic purposes, and to identify the cranial limits of the tumour. Angiography is useful with larger tumours to identify their blood supply. Genetic testing for mutations in succinate dehydrogenase (SDH) subunit genes can identify familial tumours (approximately 1:4) and help delineate those patients at risk of having multiple tumours.

What classification system is used for CBTs?

The Shamblin classification (I–III) is used to stratify CBTs. Shamblin I tumours are small and easily dissected from the vessel wall, Shamblin II tumours are of medium size and partially encircle the carotid vessels. Shamblin III tumours are large (>4 cm) and more completely encircle the carotid vessels. The Shamblin class III tumours classically require excision and a vascular reconstruction with an interposition graft.

What endovascular interventions can be helpful in managing large tumours?

CBTs have a rich blood supply, and can be associated with a significant peri-operative blood loss. In addition, operative bleeding can make a safe dissection more difficult. The tumours derive their blood supply from external carotid artery branches. Pre-operative tumour embolisation, or covered stent placement over the external carotid artery feeding vessels have both been advocated to reduce bleeding, for particularly large tumours. Both of these options remain controversial as they both pose a small risk of cerebral embolisation.

Femoral anastomotic pseudoaneurysms

The basics

Femoral anastomotic pseudoaneurysms (FAPs) often occur as a conse-quence of previous aortobifemoral bypass surgery (Figs. 3(a) and 3(b)). The relationship of the anastomosis to a constantly moving hip joint may be a contributory factor in the degeneration of the arterial wall at the site of the anastomosis. Compliance may also be an issue in the pathogenesis of FAPs at the junction between the elastic artery and an inelastic pros-thetic material. Their incidence at 5 years is around 5–10%; studies with longer-term follow up naturally demonstrate higher occurrence for FAPs. Continued smoking and wound infection at the time of the original operation are thought to be risk factors for FAP development. In the case of aortobifemoral surgery, the aneurysms are often bilateral.

The case

FAPs are an ideal examination case with their chronic nature and obvious clinical signs. On clinical examination, femoral anastomotic

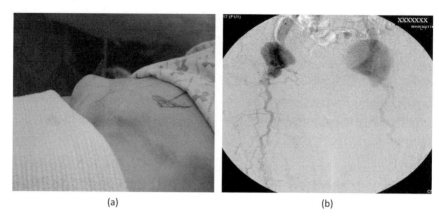

(a)	(b)

Figure 3.   (a) Femoral anastomotic pseudoaneurysms. Visible on bilateral groin inspection as late consequence of aortobifemoral surgery. (b) Femoral anastomotic pseudoaneurysms. Angiogram of same patient, demonstrating bilateral femoral artery aneurysms. Note full length bilateral superficial femoral artery occlusions.

pseudoaneurysms are easy to palpate due to their superficial location. The leg and abdomen should be inspected for scars from the previous surgery. The main differential diagnoses are of other aneurysms of the femoral artery, including atherosclerotic, mycotic, traumatic (including iatrogenic) and aneurysms related to connective tissue disorders.

Questions

How do FAPs present?

FAPs usually present with a visible or palpable pulsatile groin lump. Due to local pressure effects, the patient can experience pain from peripheral nerve irritation (mass effect). Patients may also present less frequently with distal embolisation, rupture and aneurysm thrombosis.

What factors predispose to FAP formation?

Factors that may predispose to FAP formation include infection (early and late), poor surgical techniques (i.e., inadequate tissue bites, undue graft tension), concomitant endarterectomy, and the continued processes of arterial degeneration from atherosclerosis (hence promoted by continued smoking).

What are your indications for surgery?

Larger aneurysms >2–3 cm (debatable) in diameter or those that have become symptomatic with pain should be considered for surgery. Patient factors and rate of growth may influence the size for intervention. The presence of distal embolisation should lower the threshold for repair.

What is your approach to surgical repair?

The approach to surgical repair will be influenced by evidence of an infective process in the aneurysm or groin. For chronic FAPs where infection is not suspected, the aneurysm can be repaired by placement of an interposition graft between graft and normal native artery. The aneurysm should be controlled proximally and distally and the aneurysm should be opened throughout its length. The anastomosis should be tension free and good bites of healthy arterial wall should be taken. Fogarty occlusion balloons may be useful for controlling back-bleeding side branches, as scarring in the groin may have made the initial dissection difficult. For cases where infection is evident, the surgery should include local debridement and removal of infected graft material. The revascularisation should be performed through healthy tissue using an autologous conduit where possible. In all cases, tissue should be sent for culture. The lab should be made aware that slow growing bacteria such as staph. epidermidis may be implicated. Antibiotic therapy should be discussed with the microbiologists and reflect the likely causative organisms in your local area.

Vascular access

The basics

Dialysis utilising arteriovenous fistulae has been practiced since the 1960s. The classical Cimino-Brescia fistula connects the radial artery to the cephalic vein at the wrist level. For use as a dialysis conduit, flow rates of at least 200 mL/min are required and there needs to be a suitable length of vein for needle access. Pre-operative duplex scanning should be performed to assess the arterial inflow and run-off; diseased run-off in particular will predispose to steal syndrome. Venous imaging is also important to evaluate the most appropriate vein for anastomosis and to look for evidence of outflow stenosis. Outflow stenosis is more frequent where central venous catheters have been employed and for revision fistulae.

The case

The autologous arteriovenous (AV) fistula is the preferred method of dialysis in patients with long-term, end-stage renal failure. In the examination you may be presented with an arm to examine in a patient with an AV fistula. On inspection, the arm should be examined for dilated superficial veins and scars from a current (or previous) fistula. The arm should be inspected for scarring consistent with current needle punctures for dialysis. It is also important to examine the arm for evidence of distal ischaemia, particularly in the digits. On palpation, the fistula should have a palpable 'thrill', or if occluded a thrombosed vein may be palpable. The distal pulses should be assessed. On auscultation, a strong bruit will be audible if the flow is sufficient. Proximal to the fistula there should be a sufficient length of vein for two-needle dialysis.

Questions

What is the preferred location for a primary AV fistula?

The preferred location for an AV fistula is as distal as possible (artery and veins permitting) in the non-dominant arm. Although many surgeons utilise the radial artery and cephalic vein at the wrist for primary fistulae, some surgeons have demonstrated good results with fistulae made with these vessels in the anatomical snuff box. Distal sites are utilised to allow new fistulae to be created at more proximal locations in the case of fistula failure, plus a lower risk of distal ischaemia. The non-dominant arm is preferred to allow the recipient to perform activities during the lengthy dialysis process. Use of the non-dominant arm also means that if any complications occur as a consequence of the intervention, they will have a lesser impact on the patient's function.

What findings on palpation can suggest that a fistula is at risk?

In a functioning fistula, a strong thrill will be easily palpable in the majority of cases. The presence of a weak thrill suggests the presence of inflow disease or narrowing at the site of the anastomosis. Pulsatility in the fistula suggests the presence of a stenosis or occlusion in the venous runoff. Look for dilated veins on the shoulder and chest wall to corroborate your diagnosis. If a thrill is unclear in the examination, you should also listen with a stethoscope for a bruit or use a Doppler.

Why is cardiac failure problematic in patients with AV fistulae?

Most fistulae used for dialysis have a blood flow of 500–1000 mL/min. In patients with more proximal fistulae such as those in the antecubital fossa, the flow rates may be ever higher than this. These high-flow rates can be demanding on patients with existing cardiac failure. High-output cardiac failure can be diagnosed by observing a fall in pulse rate on manual occlusion of the fistula (Branham's sign). Patients with poor cardiac output will also be at risk of fistula occlusion or insufficient flow for effective dialysis from poor flow.

What are the complications of an AV fistula?

- **Bleeding** — Some degree of haematoma or bleeding is commonplace due to the soft tissue dissection, normal antithrombotic therapy and the natural early mobility of the arm. Exploration is advocated if there is any concern that the pressure effects from the haematoma could compromise the fistula, if there is a large symptomatic haematoma, or if there is nerve injury due to compression.
- **Thrombosis** — Early thrombosis can occur due to technical problems with the anastomosis or underlying arterial or venous disease. Re-exploration has been advocated to correct these technical issues unless there is evidence of non-correctible arterial or venous problems at the time of the operation. This view has been challenged by others with the observation that re-explored fistulae often rethrombosis, hence, the creation of a new fistula at a more proximal location may be a better option. Thrombolysis has also been employed to salvage thrombosed fistulae, and can be combined with angioplasty of a stricture if present.
- **Failure to mature** — An autologous AV fistula requires time for remodelling and venous dilatation prior to commencement of dialysis. This should be at least 4–6 weeks. In fistulae that remain small

and have poor flow, investigations should be performed to look for an underlying reversible cause.

- **Steal** — Steal occurs more commonly in proximal than distal fistulae. Treatment can involve surgical narrowing of the fistula or ligation or ligation of the retrograde blood flow into the fistula from the distal limb. In some situations, the fistula must be ligated. More complex interventions such as the distal revascularisation-interval ligation (DRIL) procedure have been successfully performed, whereby the artery is ligated just distal to the anastomosis. A distal bypass is then performed from a more proximal to a more distal arterial location to reperfuse the distal arm. All the treatment methods described for steal syndrome have associated technical and therapeutic challenges. One of the more recent alternatives developed for brachiocephalic fistula, steal is disconnecting the anastomosis and extending the fistula onto the proximal radial artery; hence, providing a better blood flow into the ulnar artery feeding the forearm. Look for signs of an AVF in any patient presented to you in the exam with digital ischaemia.
- **Infection** — Superficial sepsis usually respond to antibiotics. Severe infection may present with a major haemorrhage requiring fistula ligation.
- **Aneurysm formation** — Although aneurysmal dilatation of the fistula is common, it does not usually require surgical intervention. When aneurysms do occur, it is important to investigate for proximal venous stenosis that may be causing hypertension in the fistula.
- **Ischaemic monomelic neuropathy (IMN)** — This occurs almost exclusively in diabetic patients with some pre-existing peripheral neuropathy and usually presents within hours of surgery. It is important to be vigilant to this rare condition as left untreated permanent neurological damage can occur. This condition will not correct unless the fistula is reversed. An alternative (more distal) AVF can be formed, as IMN never occurs with an AVF distal to the brachial artery.

Lymphoedema

The basics

Lymphoedema occurs when the circulation of lymph from the peripheral tissues back to the central system is impaired. The majority of cases are due to obliteration of the lymphatics (80%), although proximal obstruction and lymphatic valvular dysfunction are also causes. Lymphoedema is generally classified into primary and secondary causes. Primary causes are subclassified by the age of onset into 'Congenital' (<1 year), 'Praecox' (<35 years) and 'Tarda' (>35 years).

The case

Lymphoedema of the lower limbs is a regular vascular examination case (lymphoedema of the arm following treatment for breast cancer treatment is also commonly seen in the vascular or general surgical exams). The clinical findings are of leg swelling that does not easily pit. The skin and subcutaneous tissues become fibrosed and less compliant with time, hence the ability to 'pit' the skin is lost. The skin can also become thickened and hyperkeratotic in appearance. Typical features of lymphoedema include a tree-trunk appearance of the lower leg (NB step for the trunk at the ankle), 'buffalo' hump on the dorsum of the foot and squared-off toes (in cross section) (Fig. 4). 'Stemmer's' sign occurs when it is no longer possible to pinch the skin on the dorsum of the second toe. Chylous vesicles may appear on the shins. It is important to examine the patient for other causes of leg swelling and evidence of secondary cause of lymphoedema.

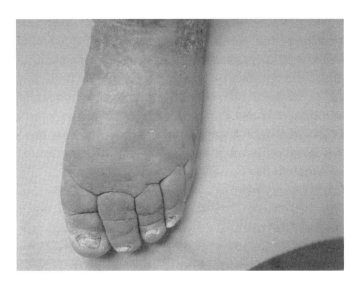

Figure 4.   Lymphoedema of the foot.

Questions

What are the secondary causes of lymphoedema?

Secondary lymphoedema mainly falls into three categories: infective, malignancy and iatrogenic. The commonest cause worldwide is from the parasitic infestation filariasis. In UK, the commonest cause for lymphoedema is malignancy; either due to the disease process itself, or as a consequence of its treatment. Recurrent minor infections can cause lymphoedema by chronic lymphangitis and progressive damage to the lymphatic system.

(1) Infective — Parasitic (filariasis), bacterial (staphylococcus, streptococcus, TB).
(2) Malignancy — Infiltration or compression of lymphatic vessels and nodes.
(3) Iatrogenic — Radiotherapy, surgery (either direct surgery on the lymph nodes, via 'collateral' damage during vascular surgical procedures, or by major surgery obliterating lymphatic routes).

How is lymphangioscintigraphy performed?

The colloid of a radioactive isotope (Technetium) is injected bilaterally into the interdigital spaces between the second and third toes. The proximal progression of the isotope is assessed using a high-resolution collimator, which takes images at regular intervals. Bilateral ilioinguinal node visualisation with isotope should occur within 1 h in the normal individual. The images demonstrate the progression (or hold up) of lymphatic flow. Abnormalities that may be seen include an interruption of lymphatic flow, collateral lymph vessels, dermal backflow, delayed flow, delayed visualisation or non-visualisation of lymph nodes, a reduced number of lymph nodes and dilated lymphatics.

What findings on MRI are suggestive of lymphoedema?

On MRI scanning there is generalised subcutaneous oedema with a honeycomb pattern. The latter is a result of the subcutaneous fibrosis. MRI can also demonstrate anatomical detail of lymphatics and is complementary to scintigraphy.

What surgical procedures are performed to manage lymphoedema?

Surgery is infrequently performed to manage lymphoedema. The mainstay of management is with complex decongestive therapy. Surgery is confined to severe cases where conventional measures have failed. Surgery is divided into debulking procedures and lymphatic bypass surgery. The classic 'Homan's' procedure involves incisions along the affected portion of the limb. The lymphoedematous subcutaneous tissue is excised with preservation of the skin flaps. The skin flaps are cut to size and closed. Several procedures may be necessary to manage severe disease. The 'Charles' procedure is a slightly more aggressive procedure whereby the affected subcutaneous tissue is resected down to muscle fascia and then covered with a skin graft (Charles never actually performed this procedure on the leg!). Although the results from the operation can be good in selected cases, there can also be significant morbidity including delayed wound healing, infection and nerve injury.

Diabetic foot

The basics

Ischaemia is an underlying feature in around half of patients with diabetes and foot ulceration. The remaining cases will predominantly be neuropathic in their aetiology. Limb loss is 15 times more frequent in diabetic than non-diabetic patients, and it is commonly preceded by foot ulceration. The diabetic foot is prone to ulceration for a number of key factors, including neuropathy, impaired vascularity at a micro- and macrovascular level, deformity and immune effects. Diabetes is frequently complicated by renal impairment, and this accelerates the development of vascular disease. Diabetic retinopathy also makes wound care all the more difficult.

The case

Patients with chronic diabetic foot disease are in plentiful supply and often more than willing to attend hospital for an examination. No matter where the foot lesion is located the same basic assessment of the foot must be performed. During the examination, you must assess the vascularity, look for evidence of neuropathy, presence of callus, assess foot deformity, look for signs of infection and comment on the wound condition. Where bone can be probed at the base of an ulcer, the likelihood of osteomyelitis is greatly increased. It is probably easiest to perform a general inspection of the foot and then assess each aspect in turn.

Questions

How does diabetic neuropathy influence foot disease?

To describe the changes, it is best to split them up into motor, sensory and autonomic. The motor changes are thought to predominantly affect the small muscles of the foot with preservation of the long flexors and extensors. This leads to clawing of the toes with prominence of the plantar metatarsal heads. Patients are often unaware of their sensory neuropathy, and its presence impedes their ability to avoid injuries and protect healing wounds. Autonomic neuropathy has several effects: firstly, it reduces sweating and causes dryness and fissuring of the skin; secondly, it alters foot microcirculation, causing shunting blood from the skin circulation.

How is neuropathy tested?

The simplest and most practical method for testing for neuropathy utilises pressure perception with 10-g nylon monofilament (Fig. 5). Buckling of the monofilament with pressure indicates a skin pressure of 10-g. The skin is tested in a standardised pattern at several points on the foot. Impaired sensation demonstrated by this method has been shown to correlate with the risk of ulceration.

What are the principles in managing acute diabetic foot disease?

- Vascular assessment and revascularisation where necessary.
- *Treating infection* — Draining sepsis, antibiotics.
- *Wound care* — Debridement, wound dressings and 'off loading' of wound.

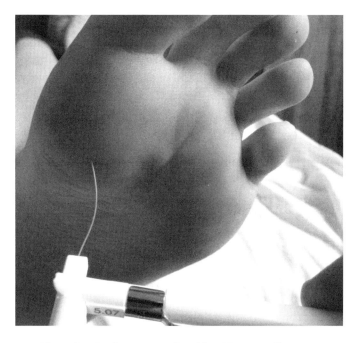

Figure 5.   Testing neuropathy with a 10-g monofilament.

The general principle is to revascularise the limb where necessary before surgery is performed. The exception to this is where spreading sepsis is present and the sepsis should be drained or debrided acutely to stop further soft tissue damage and systemic sepsis. When debridement occurs, the soft tissues should be dissected back until clean and viable.

What is 'Charcot's foot'?

Charcot's neuroarthropathy is a complex condition whereby bone destruction and joint deformity occurs. The changes result from neuropathy, and diabetes is the commonest cause of neuropathy in the western world. Presentation is often delayed due to the impaired sensation of pain. In the acute phase, the foot is warm and swollen, and these changes can be mistaken for cellulitis or sepsis. However, it is normally painless, and this finding should ring alarm bells for Charcot's as a differential. As the condition progresses, the foot becomes structurally deformed with collapse of the medial arch. There is a rocker bottom deformity to the foot with bony prominences. The skin temperature is often several degrees higher in the affected foot. Bone changes will usually be obvious on plain X-rays, although in the initial phase the imaging may be normal. Once the diagnosis is suspected the foot must be immobilised (often in a non-contact cast) until the deformity has stabilised.

What imaging aids the diagnosis of osteomyelitis?

Osteomyelitis is often difficult to diagnose in the diabetic foot. The presence of neuropathy and adjacent ulceration can complicate the situation. In around 70% of cases there will be plain radiographic evidence of bone destruction. Serial plain radiographs in suspected cases are valuable in looking for changes in the bone integrity; the serial radiographs should be taken at 2-week intervals. Three phase bone scans and isotope white cell scans can also be used in combination with plain radiographs to improve accuracy. In combination with plain radiographs, these modalities are sensitive for osteomyelitis in over 90% of case. MRI has now established itself as the investigation of choice in diagnosing osteomyelitis and deep infections in the diabetic foot. MRI findings of osteomyelitis include a decreased bone marrow T1 signal, increased T2 signal and post-gadolinium enhancement. MRI can also identify associated abnormalities such as cellulitis, abscess formation, sinus tracts, and cortical bone destruction.

Complications of carotid endarterectomy

The basics

The main complications of carotid endarterectomy (CEA) include stroke, nerve injury, haemorrhage, cardiac ischaemia and death. Carotid patch infection is fortunately a relatively infrequent complication (<1%), and you are unlikely to see one in the exam, but should be able to talk about it — it is associated with a high stroke and death rate.

The case

In previous examinations, candidates have been introduced to a patient with a visible scar from a CEA. The candidates have been asked about the patient's likely intervention, and then questioned about various aspects of carotid surgery. Pre- or post-operative carotid patients are a common examination case.

Questions

What percentage stenosis do you take as an indication to intervene on symptomatic carotid disease?

The two key trials here are NASCET and ECST. They both used different methods to judge the degree of ICA stenosis (and both used direct angiography — a seldom employed test nowadays!). This means that knowing which method was used to calculate the percentage stenosis is important when deciding upon intervention. NASCET used the distal ICA diameter as the comparator, whilst ECST used the estimated true size of the vessel at the point of the stenosis. Most surgeons now accept the NASCET method as the most accurate (and this is the recommendation of a working group from the Vascular Society GB&I and the Society of Vascular Technology GB&I), and accordingly would consider intervention for a symptomatic stenosis of greater than 50% (all other factors being equal).

Which cranial nerves are at risk during carotid endarterectomy?

The cranial nerves most commonly injured during carotid surgery include the hypoglossal, vagus and laryngeal nerves.

- The hypoglossal nerve is the most commonly injured major nerve during CEA. The Hypoglossal nerve crosses the internal carotid artery and external carotid artery near the upper limit of internal carotid artery dissection. Due to its location it runs the risk of division, diathermy- or traction-injury during surgery. Hypoglossal nerve injury classically presents with tongue deviation towards the side of nerve injury. Injury during CEA occurs in 5–10% of cases and is usually a transient phenomenon. It is more common if the nerve has been mobilised.
- The vagus nerve is usually located posteriorly in the carotid sheath. This posterior location makes it vulnerable to clamp injuries if the

arterial clamp is placed carelessly on the internal or common carotid.

- The superior laryngeal nerve is susceptible to injury where it descends behind the internal carotid artery and then passes posteriorly close to the superior thyroid artery. Injury to the superior laryngeal nerve probably goes unnoticed most of the time.
- The non-recurrent laryngeal nerve, when present, is at particular risk during CEA. Non-recurrent nerves occur in 0.5–1% of people and are commonest on the right-hand side. In its non-recurrent course, the nerve passes transversely from under the carotid sheath and will be at right-angles to the normal position.
- The glossopharyngeal nerve is rarely damaged during a straightforward CEA. The glossopharyngeal nerve is susceptible to injury when a more extensive cranial dissection is performed. The nerve is deep to and courses in a similar direction to the posterior belly of the digastric muscle.
- The spinal accessory nerve exits the skull in a posterior direction just deep to the styloid process. The nerve is susceptible to injury during 'high'-carotid dissections or during the retrojugular approach to the carotid artery. The spinal accessory nerve provides motor innervation to the trapezius and sternocleidomastoid.

Would you use local or general anesthesia?

The GALA trial (CEA under GA or LA) showed no advantage for either LA or GA. It remains a choice between the patient and surgeon concerned. You should have a view on what you should do in your practice and be prepared to justify it.

Does patching reduce the risk of peri-operative stroke?

The Cochrane Stroke Review Group has published a meta-analysis comparing carotid patching to primary closure. The analysis demonstrated a reduction in the ipsilateral stroke rate and restenosis with patching. Many surgeons use a Dacron patch, although some may use vein patches or material such as bovine pericardium. Current best practice is to use a patch on virtually all patients.

What precaution should be taken prior to contralateral carotid surgery in a patient who has already had ipsilateral CEA?

The vocal cords should be checked for evidence of recurrent laryngeal nerve injury from the first procedure. Bilateral nerve injury can cause significant difficulties with voice, swallowing and obstruction of the upper airway — the neutral position of the cords is in the midline.

What is the risk of disabling stroke or death?

The risk of death or *disabling* stroke in both the European and North American CEA trials (NASCET and ECST) is approximately 3%. The combined rate of death and *all* strokes is virtually double this figure. Data from the European and North American asymptomatic CEA trials (ACST and ACAS) the 30-day any stroke or death rates are near 2.5%, suggesting that the asymptomatic patients and/or the surgery is lower risk. Vascular units should strive to audit their own results and present their own complication rates when consenting patients.

What is the frequency of haematoma formation?

Data from randomised trials often identify much higher rates of complication than self-reported case series. In the 'general anaesthetic vs. local anaesthetic (GALA) for carotid surgery' trial haematoma rates were close to 10% and just over one third of these cases required re-exploration for bleeding. Haematoma in the neck can result in airway obstruction and should be considered a serious problem as per thyroid surgery. The mechanism of airway obstruction is through a combination of laryngeal oedema plus direct compression. Reintubation should be considered sooner rather than later where airway compromise is suspected.

When would you use a carotid shunt?

Unless conclusive trial evidence becomes available, controversy will reign over approaches to carotid shunting. Policies include shunting all patients, selective shunting and not-shunting. You should decide on your policy and be able to justify it in the exam. An appropriate policy is to shunt all CEAs under general anaesthetic and selectively shunt those under local anaesthesia, depending upon reaction to clamping.

How is cerebral perfusion monitored during CEA?

Although sophisticated methods exist to measure cerebral perfusion such as xenon washout, infra-red spectroscopy and electrophysiological studies, none are ideal for everyday carotid practice. Commonly used methods include awake testing (LA procedures), measurement of stump pressures and transcranial Doppler (TCD). In cerebral monitoring you want a device that is simple and cheap to use, is able to identify ipsilateral cerebral blood flow, can identify embolic events and looks at neurological function. Unfortunately, none of the methods available can satisfy all of the requirements fully. Awake testing may seem the most ideal, but it will not necessarily warn you of embolisation; once cerebral compromise is apparent, inserting the shunt may be more difficult due to patent agitation. TCD can assess reduction in cerebral blood flow (>50% reduction in middle cerebral artery flow) and provide evidence of embolic events before and during shunt insertion; however, it does not demonstrate the integrity of neurology. Stump pressure measurement is cheap and readily available; stump pressure <50 mmHg are taken to indicate the need for a shunt. Stump 'pressures' are taken as a proxy measurement of cerebral blood 'flow', and will not identify changes during the shunting period, unless repeatedly measured.

How would you manage a post-operative stroke following recent carotid endarterectomy?

The management of a post-operative stroke will be contentious and dependent on the timing and facilities available as well as when the event occurs. Whatever investigations and treatments are instituted, all patients should have their cerebral perfusion and oxygenation optimised, and this will usually require admission to an area such as HDU or ITU. Intubation and ventilation may be needed if the conscious level is impaired or the patient is confused. The intention with these patients is to identify those with carotid artery thrombosis, prevent further events (correct technical problems, antiplatelet therapy, mange hyper- and hypotension) and to identify patients with haemorrhagic strokes.

When the stroke is apparent on waking, or occurs in the recovery room, the patient is in the ideal location to return to theatre to correct carotid artery thrombosis or technical problems. Ideally, a Duplex scan should be performed immediately to see if the endarterectomised vessel is patent or if there are technical problems with the endarterectomy. If the scan is normal and the surgeon was 'happy' with the operation, the benefits of reoperation will be questionable, and perhaps the best course of action is to exclude other cause of embolisation and optimise antithrombotic therapy. These patients should have a cerebral CT scan as soon as possible to exclude a haemorrhage, particularly where enhanced antithrombotic therapy is being considered. The scan should also include angiography, this is particularly important if the aortic arch and intra-cranial vessels have not been previously imaged.

In patients where the blood pressure has been labile and there have been periods of significant hypertension, a haemorrhagic stroke should be more strongly considered. In these patients a cerebral CT should be per-formed immediately to exclude a haemorrhage. It should be remembered that cerebral haemorrhage occurs in the minority of patients, and case review has suggested that this represents about 10% of post-op strokes. Strokes that occur after the immediate post-operative period are less likely to derive the same benefit from re-exploration, and should be urgently imaged with carotid Duplex (if available), CT and CT angiography.

Buerger's disease

The basics

Buerger's disease (thromboangiitis obliterans) is an inflammatory arteri-opathy that predominantly affects small and medium sized arteries. The changes are pathologically distinct from atherosclerosis. The lower extremity is predominantly affected, although this is not exclusive. The disorder classically affects young male smokers; however, the pattern of disease is changing. Leo Buerger first described the condition in patho-logical specimens in 1908, and termed the disease thromboangiitis obliterans. In contrast to the common clinical presentation of atherosclerosis with intermittent claudication, patients with Buerger's disease tend to present with rest pain and tissue loss. Near to half of all patients diagnosed with Buerger's disease who continue to smoke end up requiring an amputation of some sort. The exact pathogenic mechanism linking Buerger's disease to tobacco is unknown.

The case

Consider the diagnosis in any young patient with symptoms or signs of critical ischaemia who smokes. Patients with Buerger's disease are young and mobile enough to attend examinations, and they have good clinical signs. In the clinical encounter, the level of vascular disease should be established and other alternative diagnosis considered. Don't make this diagnosis too glibly, but suspect it in young male smokers with significant ischaemia and preserved proximal pulses.

Questions

What are the pathological and radiological features of Buerger's diseases?

- The pathological features at a microscopic level involve an acute hypercellular thrombosis causing arterial occlusion. There is a striking perivascular inflammation that can also affect veins and can cause phlebitis. Despite the intra-vascular thrombosis, patients with Buerger's disease have not been demonstrated to be hypercoagulable.
- The radiological features are of relatively normal arteries to the knee level with abrupt occlusions of the tibial vessels with 'corkscrew' collateral feeding the distal vessels at the ankle (Fig. 6).

How is the diagnosis made?

There are several diagnostic criteria described (Tel Aviv, Oregon) for Buerger's disease. The consistent factors in these schemes are as follows:

- exclusion of other causes,
- tobacco use,

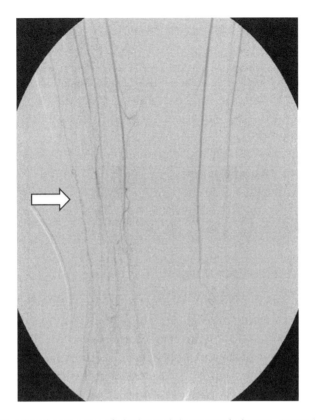

Figure 6.   Peripheral angiogram of tibial vessels in Buerger's disease. Arrow demonstrating corkscrew collaterals.

- distal extremity disease (femoral pulses nearly always preserved),
- young age of onset (<45),
- the presence of upper limb disease, phlebitis migrans or Raynaud's phenomena and radiological signs. These strengthen the diagnosis.

What other forms of vasculitis are relevant to the vascular surgeon?

- **Takayasu's arteritis** — This affects larger elastic arteries such as the aorta and its branches. The majority of patients are females and present in their second and third decade. Two phases exist, the acute pre-pulseless and chronic pulseless.
- **Giant cell (temporal arteritis)** — This is a granulomatous vasculitis affecting large and medium sized arteries, with the cranial vessels

most commonly affected. This can present with cranial ischaemia (visual loss, jaw ischaemia, headaches) or with chronic constitutional symptoms.

- **Polyarteritis nodosa** — This is a necrotising vasculitis affecting small and medium sized arteries. The disease is more common in males and usually presents in middle age. Renal and gastrointestinal involvement is common.
- **Drug induced** — Penicillins, sulphonamides, NSAIDs, cocaine, etc.
- **Connective tissue disorders** — These should be considered in patients with digital ulceration, without typical findings of atherosclerosis. Other rarer vascular disorders are also considered in the popliteal entrapment scenario.

How is Buerger's disease managed?

The absolute goal in managing Buerger's disease is establishing permanent abstinence from smoking. An antiplatelet (aspirin or clopidogrel) should be prescribed along with analgesics for pain control. Prostaglandin infusions may help with symptom control, although it is uncertain if they alter the progression of tissue loss. Distal ischaemic lesions will often auto-amputate or may require surgical amputation. Awaiting demarcation is helpful even if surgery is planned. A lumbar chemical-sympathectomy may be helpful in selected cases for chronic pain control.

Vascular malformations

The basics

Vascular anomalies fall into two main categories: haemangiomas and vascular malformations. Haemangiomas will be evident at birth, and have a distinct natural history (proliferation, plateau and involution). Most will disappear during the first decade of life. Previous terminology utilised the term 'haemangioma' for lesions appearing both around birth and those appearing later in life. More recent terminology has defined only the self-involuting tumours as haemangiomas (hence the port-wine stain is no longer considered a haemangioma). Vascular malformations grow during childhood, and may enlarge following hormonal change, trauma and sepsis. Most vascular malformations are sporadic, although some can be part of a specific syndrome, such as Klippel–Trénaunay. Vascular malformations are derived from aberrations in vasculogenesis, and generally do not undergo spontaneous involution. Although several classifications exist, they are most simply considered in two main clinically relevant categories: fast- and slow-flowing lesions.

- **Fast-flow:** Arterial malformation, arteriovenous malformations and arteriovenous fistulae
- **Slow-flow:** Venous malformations, lymphatic malformations, capillary malformations

First-line investigations include Duplex and MRI scanning. Duplex scanning demonstrates flow dynamics and morphology of the lesion. MRI scanning provides more detailed information on structure and relationship to other soft tissues. MRI is also able to differentiate slow- and fast-flow malformations. Invasive investigations such as arteriography and venography are still performed second line, and can still provide valuable additional information when planning treatment.

The case

Due to the diversity of lesions, we will run through the more common groups of malformation for this scenario.

Capillary malformations

Capillary malformations are intra-dermal vascular anomalies. The malformations appear as pink/red areas of discolouration, and can occur throughout the body. The lesions can cause hypertrophy of the surrounding soft tissues. Capillary malformations may be spontaneous or part of a syndrome such as Klippel–Trénaunay or Sturge–Weber. Imaging will often be performed to look for associated abnormalities. Pulsed dye laser is an established treatment for these lesions.

Venous malformations

Venous malformations are the most prevalent vascular malformation and tend to occur in the head and neck. Because of their slow-flow, they often take considerable time to enlarge. The lesions have previously been referred to as 'cavernous haemangiomas'. On examination, they will be deep blue in colour and easily compressible. The lesions can calcify, and local thrombosis can cause pain. Limb hypertrophy is seen with some extremity lesions. Treatment is conservative with compression where possible. Sclerosant therapy is usually the first line intervention, and repeat treatments are often needed. Surgical excision can be performed for severe symptoms, with or without pre-operative sclerotherapy. Recurrence rates are high however, due to the often diffuse nature of these lesions.

Arteriovenous malformations

Arteriovenous malformations are fast-flowing connections that bypass the capillary bed. The lesions are usually apparent at birth, and enlarge in size as their blood flow increases. The lesions are usually warm and pink/blue in colour. Arteriography is often required to establish the anatomy of their arterial supply. Small lesions can be excised (including the feeding vessel). Larger lesions often require a combination of embolisation and surgical excision. Ligation of the feeding vessel alone can cause collateralisation, making further treatment more complex. When these lesions enlarge, they can become destructive and may even lead to cardiac failure.

Lymphatic malformations

Lymphatic malformations have historically included lymphangiomas and cystic hygromas. These lesions are slow-flow and usually occur in the cervical region. The majority will be apparent within the first years of life. These lesions can be associated with both soft tissue and skeletal overgrowth.

- **Cystic hygroma:** These lesions are now known as macrocystic lymphatic malformations and are the most common type of lymphangioma. They are often found in the posterior triangle at the base of the neck, although can occur anywhere in the body. Clinically, they feel like fluid filled sacs, and can become very large. On palpation, the lesion will be smooth and transilluminate spectacularly.

- **Lymphangioma circumscriptum:** Small localised lymphatic vesicles are present that do not connect to the normal lymphatic system. They are usually found around the shoulder, axilla, groin and buttocks. If these lesions contain old blood, they may turn brown in colour.
- **Cavernous lymphangiomas:** There are generally present at birth, but may appear later in the child's life. These bulging masses occur deep under the skin, typically on the neck, tongue and lips, and vary widely in size. Although they are usually painless, the patient may feel mild pain when pressure is exerted on the area.

MRI scanning is useful in defining the anatomy of the larger lesions. The main sources of symptoms for these lesions are infection and intra-lesional bleeding. Sclerotherapy has been performed with a variety of agents with acceptable results. Surgery is reserved for severe symptoms and recurrence is high. The aim of surgery is complete excision of the lesion to minimise the risk of recurrence. Surgery can be complex and involve multiple procedures. Lymphangioma circumscriptum requires wide local excision if treatment is required.

Vascular Malformations (Specific Syndromes)

Klippel–Trénaunay syndrome

The basics

KTS was first described by the French physicians Maurice Klippel and Paul Trénaunay in 1900. Most cases are sporadic, although there have been reports that the condition has occurred in an autosomal dominant pattern. KTS is a complex and variable syndrome; hence treatment is planned on a case-by-case basis. The venous component of the disease tends to be the most problematic. The physical signs will become evident early in life and there is no gender predominance.

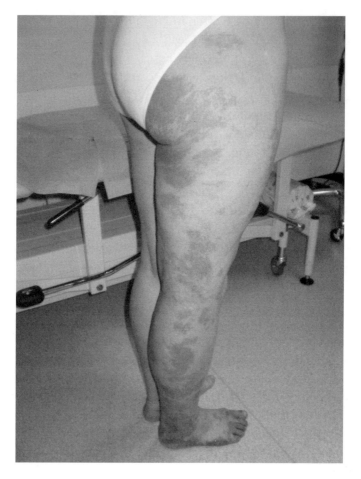

Figure 7.   'Port-wine' staining and varicose veins in KTS. There is a scar over the hip from a leg shortening procedure.

The case

KTS is an excellent vascular case with its various manifestations and physical signs (Fig. 7). The clinical findings are discussed below.

Questions

What are the pathological components of KTS?

• Venous abnormalities (varicosities)

- Bony and soft tissues hypertrophy
- Cutaneous angiomata ('port wine' stains)

Each component of the syndrome may be present to a varying degree. The limb hypertrophy can be secondary to increased bone length and/or increased soft-tissue girth. Abnormally developed lymphatics have also been associated with this syndrome.

What is the distribution of varicosities in KTS?

Unlike the typical distribution of greater or lesser saphenous varicosities, the varicosities seen in KTS tend to be located on the lateral side of the thigh and lower leg and there may be a large lateral vein (of Servelle) which may replace the deep veins. The 'port wine' stains from cutaneous angiomata tend to be located in similar lateral distribution to the varicosities. The 'port wine' stain has a distinct, linear border, and the lesion possesses neither a proliferative nor a regressing phase. There may also be GI and genitourinary vascular malformations in association.

What concerns would you have over performing superficial venous surgery in KTS?

In KTS, the deep venous system can be abnormally developed or replaced by a lateral vein. The superficial veins may provide an important role in venous function; hence, they should be left intact unless adequate venous drainage has been demonstrated. In addition, the varicosities present are frequently large and may bleed more than anticipated when surgically removed (in fact phlebectomies may require ligation of the residual vessels to stop bleeding).

What surgical options are available to treat KTS?

The surgical options for KTS have mainly included debulking procedures and venous surgery. The debulking procedures are only really considered for severe cases where conservative options have failed. Venous surgery in KTS is associated with a higher rate of recurrence than with conventional venous anatomy.

What non-surgical options are available?

Compression therapy is an important treatment modality in the management of limb swelling. Maintaining good compression therapy can reduce pain, swelling and inflammation. The potential side effects of compression therapy include displacement of fluid into other locations, and that the compression therapy itself may impede circulation through the limb. As with lymphoedema management, massage therapy can provide an improvement in symptoms. Liquid or foam sclerotherapy offer a less invasive option to treat the varicosities than conventional surgery.

Parkes-Weber syndrome

Parkes-Weber syndrome was first described by Frederick Parkes-Weber, an English dermatologist and physician to Queen Victoria. Parkes-Weber syndrome is similar in many of its features to KTS; however, in KTS the cutaneous malformations are slow-flowing, whereas in Parkes-Weber syndrome the vascular malformations are fast-flowing arteriovenous abnormalities, with associated limb hypertrophy (haemangiectatic hypertrophy). So in essence, Parkes-Weber syndrome is a fast-flow arteriovenous malformation in association with the other abnormalities found in KTS, such as cutaneous capillary malformation and skeletal or soft-tissue hypertrophy.

Proteus syndrome

Proteus syndrome is an extremely rare congenital condition and unlikely to been seen in a clinical examination. The condition is highly variable in appearance, and is named after the Greek sea-god Proteus, who could change his shape at will. The condition consists of cutaneous abnormalities (nevi), vascular abnormalities (capillary, venous or combined), plus skeletal and soft-tissue abnormalities such as hemihypertrophy. Proteus syndrome is extremely disfiguring as a result of an overgrowth of skin, bones, muscles, fatty tissues, and blood and lymphatic vessels. The changes often only occur over half of the body. The condition was publicised in the 1980s' film the 'Elephant Man', about the life of Joseph Merrick, a Proteus sufferer.

A young patient with intermittent claudication: Popliteal entrapment syndrome and other differential diagnoses

The basics

Popliteal entrapment usually presents with calf claudication in young athletic individuals. The symptoms may commence following a period of strenuous activity. Foot pulses will be normal at rest unless a complication of the disease process has occurred. Sudden onset claudication in a young person may indicate a vessel occlusion. Popliteal entrapment syndrome can be classified into its anatomical and functional varieties. Long-term complications include localised fibrosis and stenosis, aneurysmal dilatation and distal embolisation from the diseased segment of artery.

Making the diagnosis in this condition is particularly problematic for the functional group, as at least 10% of the asymptomatic population demonstrate compression of the popliteal artery with active dorsal or plantar flexion of the ankle joint. The diagnosis of popliteal entrapment is usually made in younger individuals with symptoms of claudication and evidence of vascular compromise on active ankle flexion. Primary atherosclerosis, other arterial disorders and alternative causes of leg pain must be excluded. Anatomical entrapment should be corrected by removal of the entrapment mechanism (usually release of the medial head of gastrocnemius) +/− resection of the involved segment of artery. This prevents further damage to the artery and distal vasculature.

The case

The patient should have a lower limb vascular examination. Attention should be given to assessing the quality of the ankle pulses in the plantar- and dorsiflexed positions. The patient should be inspected for venous skin changes, vasculitic lesions and examined for sources of embolisation. The candidate should also indicate to the examiner that they would perform a musculoskeletal examination of the lower limb.

Questions

What two important embryological factors are pertinent in the development of anatomical popliteal entrapment?

Two important embryological factors that can be implicated in the development of popliteal entrapment involve the differing embryonic origins of the mid portion and the distal popliteal artery, and secondly, the migration of the medial head of gastrocnemius.

- In the definitive human anatomy, the mid portion of the popliteal artery is a remnant part of the primitive axial artery and definitive distal vessel (original axial vessel lying beneath popliteus muscle) from a more superficially placed vascular plexus. This process of vascular development occurs between the 8 and 12 weeks of embryology.
- The medial head of gastrocnemius migrates from a lateral location during the embryonic development. This process occurs around a similar time to the changes in the popliteal artery.

What are the common configurations causing popliteal artery compression?

- The popliteal artery can be located medially to the medial head of the gastrocnemius. This abnormal position can occur to a varying degree depending on the final location of the gastrocnemius muscle.
- The popliteal artery may be located within the medial head of the gastrocnemius muscle.
- The popliteal artery may exist deep to the popliteus muscle.

In functional cases it is thought that muscle hypertrophy from exercise plus a 'vulnerable' location of the artery between the gastrocnemius heads predisposes to the condition. This is often more challenging to diagnose and treat than the anatomical variants.

What other structure can be involved in the compression syndrome?

Popliteal vein and the tibial nerves can also be compressed.

Do you know any classification schemes for popliteal entrapment?

A classification scheme for popliteal entrapment has been suggested by Levien and Veller. Types I to III involve misplacement of the artery in relation to all, or part of, the medial head of gastrocnemius. In type IV, the popliteal artery is anomalously developed beneath the popliteus muscle. This layout is therefore unrelated to the positioning of the gastrocnemius muscle. Type V was subsequently suggested as an addition to include cases where the popliteal vein is involved. Functional entrapment where there is compression of the vessel in stressed positions, without any apparent anatomic abnormality, is termed type VI.

What other rare vascular disorders can cause arterial claudication in the younger patient?

- **Fibromuscular dysplasia (FMD)** — FMD is the commonest cause of 'renal' hypertension in children. Most FMD affects the media of the arterial wall. The renal and carotid vessels are most commonly affected, although the external iliac artery (EIA) is the most commonly involved vessel in the lower limb vasculature. Disease of the EIA usually presents with claudication, although it can be complicated by embolisation, aneurysm or thrombosis. The classic appearance on arterial imaging is of a 'string of beads'; angioplasty has been successfully used to treat this disease.
- **Persistent sciatic artery** — The sciatic artery is the embryonic axial limb artery. In the normal individual, the majority of the vessel obliterates, apart from the segments which become the internal iliac artery, part of the popliteal artery and the peroneal artery. The condition may present with a pulsatile mass in the buttock. Aneurysmal degeneration of the anomalous artery can occur due to trauma in the sciatic foramen. The patent sciatic artery is associated with hypoplasia of the iliofemoral vessels. The blood supply through these abnormal vessels may be inadequate during exercise, and the diseased sciatic artery may acutely thrombose.

- **Cystic adventitial disease (CAD)** — CAD of popliteal artery is thought to exist due to inclusion, or extension, of mucin secreting structures between the media and adventitia of the popliteal artery. The condition usually presents with claudication in the fourth and fifth decades and is usually unilateral. On clinical examination, flexing the knee joint may cause the distal pulses to disappear. The typical appearance on angiography is of an 'hourglass' narrowing of the popliteal artery with normal distal vessels. On ultrasound or CTA, the cysts may be seen. Treatment is by open drainage of the cysts or by excision and reconstruction of the abnormal vessel portion. Simple cyst aspiration usually leads to recurrence.
- **Endofibrosis** — Arterial endofibrosis is a relatively recently described condition that can affect highly trained athletes, with cyclists predominantly at risk. Repetitive movement of the hip joint and the cycling posture are thought to lead to chronic arterial injury, resulting in progressive intimal thickening. The endofibrosis most often affects the external iliac arteries. The presence of an arterial pressure drop is a useful sign as peripheral pulses and ABPI will usually be normal at rest. The condition has been treated with resection and revascularisation using autologous vein. Prosthetic materials should be avoided due to compliance issues.
- **Premature atherosclerosis** — Lipid disorders and hyperhomocysteinemia should be considered.
- **Dissection** — Aortic dissection can be complicated by acute limb ischaemia. Claudication may be a longer-term consequence of the event. Young patients with acute dissection usually have significant hypertension or a collagen disorder such as Marfan's. Isolated spontaneous dissections have been described in the peripheral vasculature.
- **Embolisation** — As with dissection, embolisation should present with a well defined acute event. Claudication may be an ongoing consequence if the presentation is delayed or embolus is left untreated. Proximal sources of embolisation should be sought.
- **Drug induced arteriopathies** — These include cocaine, amphetamines, ergot, etc.
- **Pseudoxanthoma elasticum (PXE)** — PXE is a rare genetic disorder that produces progressive calcification and fragmentation of elastic

fibres in the skin, cardiovascular system and retina. Extensive arterio-sclerosis often occurs in the third or fourth decade of life. The disease tends to spare the aorta, but involves lower limb arteries, producing intermittent claudication. Patients with PXE often have coronary and valvular heart diseases.

- **Vasculitis**

Venous disease: Varicose veins

The basics

Varicose veins are a common clinical condition and an extremely common examination case. Although many patients may seek treatment for cosmetic reasons, a broad range of symptoms such as heaviness, itching, aching, mild swelling and cramps can be attributed to varicose veins. Symptoms tend to be worse towards the end of the day, or after prolonged episodes of standing. In females the symptoms are often worse around the time of menstruation. Varicose veins frequently present as uncomplicated entities, but can also be associated with changes of chronic venous insufficiency (CVI). The main patterns of venous incompetence involve the long (greater) and short (lesser) saphenous veins. In modern practice, all cases where intervention is being planned should have a Duplex scan; however, you should still understand the principles of clinical assessment. With the advent of Duplex scanning, a Giacomini vein is often mentioned in reports. This is a thigh extension from the short saphenous vein that usually runs medially and joins with the LSV, first described by Giacomini: when present there may not be a normal saphenopopliteal junction.

The case

Varicose veins should initially be examined in the standing position.

- **Inspection** — Comment on the extent of varicosities and their distribution in relation to the superficial venous systems. The lower abdominal wall and perineal areas should also be inspected for venous collaterals. Inspect for associated skin changes or areas of ulceration suggestive of CVI. Look for a bluish tinge to the skin in the groin suggestive of a saphena varix. Later in the examination you will want to examine the patient in the supine position to ensure that the varicosities disappear on leg elevation (venous occlusion, tricuspid disease?).

- **Palpation** — The skin should be examined for oedema, thickening, and the veins compressed to establish their patency. The saphenofemoral and saphenopopliteal junctions should be palpated for the presence of a varix. The lower limb pulses should be examined for co-existing arterial disease (+/− ABPI). Where abdominal wall venous collaterals are seen, Harvey's test can be performed to determine the direction of the flow in the veins. The test is performed by placing two fingers on a segment of vein several centimetres apart. By sliding one finger along the vein to empty it and then releasing one finger (repeated in both directions) the direction of venous filling can be determined.

- **Percussion and auscultation** — The 'Tap' test is best performed where a long segment of LSV is palpable. Normally when a column of blood is present in the LSV, transmission of a percussion wave should only occur in an antegrade direction. Where the valves in the system are incompetent, a percussion wave can also travel in a retrograde direction. Auscultation may be useful when looking for evidence of an arteriovenous shunt (machinery bruit).

- **Tourniquet test** — It is worth understanding (and being able to perform) the tourniquet test, although it is infrequently performed in modern clinical practice.

- **Hand held Doppler (HHD)** — This is an examination for junction reflux. The HHD can be used to identify reflux at the saphenofemoral junction, popliteal fossa and also in the LSV itself, whilst the patient is in the standing position. When listening for reflux, care must be taken to only apply light pressure to the area of interest, as veins can easily be compressed, hence abolishing audible venous flow. Significant reflux (bidirectional venous blood flow) is taken as >0.5 s in duration. The saphenofemoral junction is located medial to the femoral artery, 2 cm below the level of the pubic tubercle. Reflux can be augmented by compression of the calf muscle or during a Valsalva manoeuvre. The sapenopopliteal junction is much more variable in location, hence HHD examination is less reliable. Reflux in the popliteal fossa is detected by identifying the arterial signal close to the midline, and then moving the probe laterally. The calf muscle is again squeezed to augment reflux. Popliteal fossa reflux will either relate to short saphenous, gastrocnemius or popliteal venous incompetence. Examining the LSV at the knee level with HHD is useful where junction reflux is not present, but the varicosities appear distributed in the LSV territory.

Following the peripheral venous examination, you may suggest examination of the abdomen, and rectum, vagina and testes where appropriate, for evidence of malignancy or pelvic mass. Prior to intervention, or where varicosities have newly developed, a pregnancy test should be performed (pregnancy causes pelvic venous compression, and increased progesterone levels cause smooth muscle relaxation and alterations in the structure of collagen).

Venous disease: Chronic venous insufficiency (CVI) and ulceration

The basics

The prevalence of venous ulceration increases with age, with a rate of 20 per 1000 in subjects over 80 years of age. Healing of venous ulcers is a major cost burden to society with the best healing rates in specialist centres of 70% at 3 months. Venous ulcers are often recurrent and usually have a history of venous disease. The skin at the site of the ulcer is often tender, painful and inflamed prior to the development of the ulcer, and ulcer formation may be triggered by relatively minor trauma or scratching of the skin. Around half of patients with venous ulcers have superficial venous incompetence without deep incompetence or obstruction. Chronic leg ulcers are attributable to venous disease in 60–80% of cases; in around 20% of cases there is associated underlying arterial insufficiency. Venous ulcers are also often associated with diabetes. Pure venous ulcers are usually relatively painless; if pain is a significant feature, you should consider an inflammatory or arterial condition as a cause. Patients with chronic ulcers often develop limited mobility at the ankle joint, and this process further compromises function of the calf pump mechanism.

CVI is a complex condition whereby venous hypertension causes inflammation, thickening with, and fibrin deposition within, the skin and subcutaneous tissues. Clinical features of CVI include swelling, ulceration, pain and skin changes (sclerosis, pigmentation, eczema) (Fig. 8). Hypotheses for the formation of CVI skin changes include the white cell trapping, perivascular fibrin cuff formation, tissue pressure effect and macromolecule leakage theories.

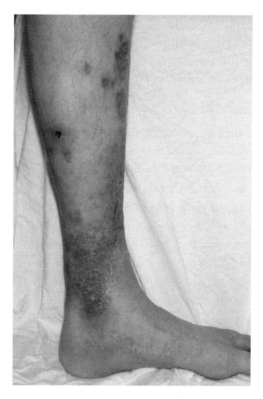

Figure 8.   Image of lower limb venous skin changes — lipodermatosclerosis and pigmentation.

The case

Venous ulceration classically occurs in the gaiter area, usually in the medial location. Ulceration occurring primarily in the foot is unlikely (but not impossible!) to have a venous cause. The venous ulcer is usually shallow and irregular, with gentle sloping edges. The surrounding skin will usually have at least some skin changes of CVI. Although the ulcer base may contain slough, once removed there should be pink or congested looking epithelium where healing is taking place. There may be areas of white fibrous tissue scarring in the ulcer from the healing process. Where there have been previous venous ulcers, there may be pale scars visible ('atrophie blanche'). The absence of visible varicosities does not exclude a venous cause to an ulcer.

Questions

What are the secondary causes of varicose veins?

- **Venous obstruction**
  Extrinsic compression — Pelvic mass (including pregnancy), increased abdominal pressure, and retroperitoneal fibrosis.
  Intrinsic obstruction — Post-DVT, May–Thurner syndrome (compression of the left common iliac vein by the overlying right common iliac artery and the subsequent fibrotic reaction).
- **Valve destruction** — Post-phlebitic limb.
- **High flow** — Arteriovenous fistula.

How does the calf muscle pump function?

The calf muscle pump is an integral part of process for recirculating blood from peripheral veins back into the centre venous system. The soleal muscles contain large valve-less venous sinusoids with a total capacity of over 100 mL in the adult. At rest the sinusoids fill, and during muscular activity blood is expelled from, these veins. Valves in the deep and perforating veins direct blood from the superficial system through the deep system in a proximal direction. In the standing subject at rest, there is standing column of blood that exerts a hydrostatic pressure down to the foot level of around 90 mmHg (equivalent to its vertical weight from the point of measurement to the right auricle of the heart). Following repeated calf muscle contraction, the hydrostatic venous pressure in the foot falls until it reaches a lower plateau level of 20–30 mmHg (ambulatory venous pressure). If the patient stands still, the pressure returns back to a resting pressure of around 90 mmHg. Where deep venous obstruction or incompetence occurs (following a DVT) the pressure produced by the calf muscle pump forces blood into the superficial system causing superficial venous hypertension.

What are physiological mechanisms of venous hypertension?

- Superficial venous reflux
- Deep venous reflux
- Perforator incompetence
- Deep venous obstruction
- Calf pump failure

(any of the above may exist in isolation or combination)

How does venous claudication differ from arterial claudication?

Exercise in the presence of venous insufficiency causes an increase in blood flow to the limb with a compromise to normal venous return. The process can cause distension and a 'bursting' type discomfort to the leg. Unlike the rapidly resolving pain in IC, relief in venous claudication takes much longer to occur, and often requires sustained elevation of the limb.

How do you manage venous ulcers?

- **Debridement** — Slough and debris should be regularly cleaned from the surface of an ulcer. Soaking the limb in a bowl of tap water often helps local dressing removal and the debridement of slough.
- **Emollients** — Surrounding areas of dry skin should be kept moist with emollients. (Topical steroids are occasionally used to treat surrounding venous eczema, if there are persistent problems with eczema, always consider an allergy to the dressings.)
- **Dressing** — Ulcers can be dressed with non-adherent, hydrocolloid and foam dressings. The benefits of each depend on the current state of the wound. An important factor in dressing performance is that is does not stick to the wound, hence remove valuable granulation tissue on dressing change.

- **Graduated compression** — The mainstay in managing venous ulcers is with graduated compression therapy. It is useful to try and minimise pre-existing swelling of the limb with rest and elevation prior to commencing therapy. Compression therapy should produce maximum pressure at the ankle, gradually reducing towards the knee level. Compression bandaging is multilayer, with a variety of layers for dressing support, padding, elastic compression and an outer cover. The layers vary between compression systems.
- **Antibiotics** — Antibiotics are only prescribed for ulcers where there is evidence of active infection (i.e., progressing cellulitis) rather than just colonisation. Topical antibiotics are generally not given to treat infections, although metronidazole gel is sometimes used for malodorous wounds.

What is the role of superficial venous surgery in managing venous ulcers?

The 'long-term results of compression therapy alone vs. compression plus surgery in chronic venous ulceration' (ESCHAR) trial addressed the question of correction of superficial venous reflux in addition to standard compression therapy. The study assessed 500 legs managed in specialist nurse led leg ulcer clinics (three centres). The investigators demonstrated that surgical correction of superficial venous reflux in addition to compression bandaging did not improve ulcer healing. However, superficial venous surgery did reduce ulcer recurrence at 4 years and also resulted in patients having a greater proportion of ulcer-free time. It should be noted that this trial was undertaken before the widespread introduction of endovenous therapies (e.g., RFA, EVLT and foam), and a large number of patients in the treatment arm did not receive an operation for their venous disease due to comorbidities.

What factors influence sub-bandage pressure?

Sub-bandage pressure is proportional to: TN/CW, where,

T is bandage tension,
C is circumference of limb,
W is width of bandage,
N is number of layers.

From analysing the formula, it is clear that a bandage applied with a constant tension will automatically produce a graduated fall in sub-bandage pressure from the narrow ankle to the wider calf. The ankle being the lowest diameter will have the highest area of pressure, providing the bandage tension remains the same throughout the dressing. Hence, there is an inverse relationship between leg circumference and pressure applied. Bandages are generally applied with a 50% overlap. Care must be taken when applying bandaging around bony prominences (malleoli and tibial crest) not to form areas of localised pressure. Ankle sub-bandage pressure of 40 mmHg are often utilised in treating venous ulcers.

How is compression hosiery classified?

Compression hosiery has commonly been prescribed by the 'Class' system. This system often leads to confusion due to the differing British standard (BS 6612:1985) and European standard (SS-ENV 12718) categories. Whereas the British system is divided into three classes, the European has four classes according to the level of ankle compression. The pressure levels in the European 'classes' are higher than those in the British system. In clinical practice, the best way to prescribe compression hosiery is by the level of compression in mmHg, hence 18–24 mmHg compression hosiery should be requested, rather than simply 'class II'.

Class	British	European
I	14–17 mmHg	18–21 mmHg
II	18–24 mmHg	25–32 mmHg
III	25–35 mmHg	36–46 mmHg
IV	NA	Over 59 mmHg

Aortic aneurysm suitability for EVAR

The basics

EVAR is now established based upon the EVAR, DREAM and OVER trials, but techniques, suitability and assessment methods are continually evolving. Assessment of suitability requires a CT angiogram with a minimum slice thickness of 3 mm (ideally 1 mm). Axial images produced by CT should be assessed to gain a general picture of the aneurysm, patency of visceral arteries and anatomy of the thoracic aorta and arch. Multi-planar reconstructions are then performed on CT workstations to allow measurements of diameters perpendicular to the axis of the aorta and length measurements. Diameters that must be measured are the neck of the aneurysm (ensuring it is disease free with parallel sides and no thrombus), the distal landing zone (usually common iliac arteries) and the aortic bifurcation. Important length measurements are length of aortic neck, distal sealing zone, distance from lowest renal artery to aortic bifurcation and distance from aortic bifurcation to intended landing zone (e.g., iliac bifurcation). 3D volume rendering modes using automated techniques to plot the centreline can give the described lengths, but these may prove inaccurate once a stiff wire and delivery system straighten the anatomy, and experience is needed to judge how aneurysms may react to EVAR.

The case

You are shown an abdominal CT scan with an AAA. These will be axial scans, but may contain reconstructed images.

Questions

What CT features of an AAA would you consider in assessing it for a conventional stent graft?

Adverse anatomical factors vary for different types of stents, but in general these can be classified as shown below. The limitations for standard EVAR are decreasing. In the EVAR trials, 50% of AAAs were suitable for stenting, whereas currently using a variety of different devices approximately 80% can be treated using EVAR. Although no single anatomical problem should prevent one from performing EVAR, several anatomical constraints may prevent sealing and fixation, thereby increasing the risk of endoleak, migration or late graft failure. Manufacturers provide indications for use (IFUs) for devices for features such as neck length, diameter and angle, but many stents are currently inserted for anatomy outside of strict IFUs. This is probably acceptable if there are reasons to favour EVAR over open repair, but overall use of EVAR outside of IFUs is associated with a higher endoleak rate and need for secondary interventions.

Graft introduction

Factors making insertion of the stent difficult include iliac artery tortuosity, especially in combination with circumferential calcification preventing straightening of the vessels. Stenotic or occlusive disease of the iliac arteries may prevent access, although minor degrees can be overcome by angioplasty, use of hydrophilic sheaths or even dilating within a sheath for more severe cases. Ultimately, a uni-iliac device may be used if one sided access is impossible with a femoro-femoral crossover graft used to perfuse the limb with the diseased iliac arteries.

Proximal sealing and fixation

A non-favourable neck may have angulation of more than 60° (although newer devices may allow greater degrees of angulation up to 90°), conical neck (more than 3 mm increase in diameter distally for 1 cm length of neck for sealing), thrombus or calcification. The length of the neck should be at least 10–15 mm (graft dependent) for an adequate proximal seal. Stent grafts come in various diameters and there will be a few AAAs that have a neck diameter that is too large (normally 32 mm diameter of neck, which requires 20% oversizing).

Distal sealing zone

Similar principles apply to the distal sealing zone as they do to the neck. Ideally, this should be close to the iliac bifurcation with sealing length of 10–15 mm. With modern devices, iliac diameters as large as 25 mm can be treated. If the landing zone involves the EIA and coverage of the internal iliac artery, there may be a risk of buttock claudication or ischaemic colitis if done bilaterally. Coverage would in addition require embolisation of the internal iliac artery to prevent a type II endoleak. The internal iliac artery may be preserved by using an iliac-branched graft, but not all cases are suitable (they need room in the CIA to open and a decent IIA to seal in), and this adds complexity.

Length from renal arteries to aortic bifurcation

The length of the aneurysm from the renal arteries has to be appropriate to allow the short stump of the contralateral limb to fully open. In practice, there are seldom cases where this is an issue with the modern portfolio of grafts available (although a short bodied design may be required). Similarly, any 'waisting' at the aortic bifurcation may not allow the two iliac limbs to pass through without compressing them, hence the importance of measuring the diameter of the aortic bifurcation. This can be overcome in some cases by relining the limbs with further stents at the bifurcation.

If the patient has no suitable neck or has a thoracoabdominal aneurysm, what endovascular options are available?

Patients with juxtarenal or thoracoabdominal aneurysms can still be treated by endovascular means, but normally require custom-made devices. Fenestrated EVAR is used to gain neck for an adequate seal in the visceral segment. The risk and complexity relates to the number of fenestrations (i.e., visceral arteries) involved. These grafts are custom made for the individual patient and take time to plan and construct, but offer a solution to patients with short or unsuitable infrarenal necks.

Branched EVAR is used to treat thoracoabdominal aneurysms where the proximal seal is often in the thoracic aorta. The extensive coverage of the aorta and associated lumbar arteries increases the risk of spinal cord ischaemia. Several strategies are advocated for spinal cord protection including blood-pressure manipulation, spinal CSF drainage, left subclavian revascularisation (if covered) and temporary perfusion branches.

Endovascular aneurysm sealing (EVAS) is an option for short or unsuitable aortic necks. Two long covered stents are deployed from below the renals to the common iliacs, and two polymer filled bags used to seal the stents in the aneurysm sac. Advantages of this system include a reported lower type II endoleak occurrence rate and a 'one solution fits all'/'off the shelf' approach to infrarenal aneurysms, including those with shorter necks. Longer-term data on efficacy is awaited.

Endoanchors (or 'staples') have been used to augment the seal in angulated or diseased necks, and may have a future in the difficult anatomy both for fixation and seal (primary and secondary). Again, more data are required before these become mainstream.

How do you classify endoleaks and how are they managed?

Endoleaks are classified into four different types. Types I, III and IV endoleak require intervention, whereas most type II leaks are benign and can be monitored conservatively unless there is continued sac expansion. The table below summarises classification, pathogenesis and management.

Type	Pathogenesis	Management
Ia (proximal)	Poor seal at neck	Balloon moulding (at first procedure) Cuff extension (if sufficient room) Palmaz stent Open banding of aortic neck Fenestrated cuff extension Endoanchors ('Staples')
Ib (distal)	Poor seal or fixation at distal landing zone	Balloon moulding (at first procedure) Upsizing distal limb with extension +/− internal iliac embolisation.
II	Feeding IMA or iliolumbar vessels	Conservative treatment If AAA not expanding. If it expands, then CT or selective catheter angiography to diagnose the cause. These may be embolised, IMA may be ligated surgically (open or laparoscopic) or translumbar injection of thrombotic material directly into AAA.
III	Modular disconnection or tears in stent graft	Intra-operatively junctional zones can be ballooned. Post-operatively, bridging stents are required.

(Continued)

IV	Porosity of stent graft or undetected endoleak	Intra-operative porosity or 'sweating' is benign. Relining with a new stent graft or explantation are options to treat this largely historical problem.

Consent for an AAA repair

The basics

The discussion about consent will depend on whether the patient is to undergo open or endovascular repair and also the ability to obtain consent. The GMC has published guidelines for good practice in obtaining consent. A key principle is of shared decision-making.

The case

There will usually be a patient who most likely is about to or has undergone the procedure. Communication is the key. You must assess how much the patient knows about the procedure and then go on to describe the procedure, its benefits and its risks. The risks as stated on the consent form should be those that are frequent or serious, and in addition should take into account the patient's personal circumstances. These can be divided into general and specific and furthermore early and late.

The benefits of surgery depend on the presentation. For asymptomatic AAAs, the reason for intervention is to prevent future rupture. In cases of distal embolisation, the aim is limb salvage and in acute cases of rupture, the aim is to save life. Rarely, large aneurysms may cause obstruction of the duodenum.

The risks of open AAA repair

- **Early complications**
1. These are related to aortic cross clamping and the systemic inflammatory response. Although cardiac complications were the main causes of early mortality, more modern series suggest that multiorgan failure (MOF) is an equal cause of deaths in elective repair,

including both primary MOF and secondary MOF to visceral ischaemia and pneumonia.

2. Isolated respiratory failure is the other prominent cause of mortality.
   With improvements in optimisation of cardiac function, patient selection, advancements in anaesthetic and post-operative critical care,
   early mortality rates have been reduced to 5%.

3. Other complications to mention include distal embolisation leading to
   limb loss, ischaemic colitis requiring a colostomy, renal failure and
   impotence. The frequency of these complications will depend on the
   complexity of the aneurysm, including suprarenal clamping, thrombus adjacent to the renal artery origins and patency of visceral and
   internal iliac arteries.

- **Late complications**
1. Poor coverage of the graft by either the sac of the aneurysm or by an
   omental flap may lead to graft-to enteric fistulae and graft infection.
2. False aneurysm, particularly with anastomosis onto the femoral
   artery.

The risks of EVAR

- **Early complications**
1. *General* complications are related to vascular surgical (groin seroma, haematoma and false aneurysm) and radiological procedures
   involving contrast agents (direct effects of contrast related to volume including renal failure and idiosyncratic reactions).
2. *Specific* complications are classified as those relating to the stent and
   those relating to the surgery. Stent related complications include
   endoleak and rupture (1% lifetime risk). Coverage of both internal
   iliac arteries in the presence of diseased visceral vessels may lead to
   ischaemic colitis. Coverage of one internal iliac artery may lead to buttock claudication. Inadvertent coverage of renal arteries may necessitate stenting the renal artery to 'open' the ostium covered by the
   stent graft. Bilateral occlusion normally necessitates open conversion
   with renal revascularisation. Balloon moulding has a small risk of

rupture in addition, which may be treated by a covered stent graft or open conversion. The 30-day mortality for EVAR is 1–2%.

- **Late complications**
1. Continued expansion and rupture can occur because of either endoleak or stent migration.
2. Limbs of the stents may occlude from kinking as a result of changes in conformation of the stent due to sac shrinkage.
3. Although the risk of graft infections is lower than open repair, procedures utilising uni-iliac stents that need a femoro-femoral crossover graft may have a higher risk.

In the UK, EVAR trials after 8 years of follow-up, open-repair had a significantly lower mortality, mainly attributable to excess secondary aneurysm sac rupture in the EVAR group and increased cancer mortality also observed in the EVAR group.

Type B aortic dissection (TBAD)

This subject has attracted significant recent attention, and whilst a patient is unlikely to be readily available for exams with an acute dissection, it is possible that a patient now in surveillance for a chronic dissection (or indeed following treatment of a type B aortic dissection (TBAD)) could be an exam case.

How do we classify aortic dissections?

There are several ways of classifying aortic dissections based on anatomy, chronology and complications.

Stanford categorised dissections into type A (dissection arising in ascending aorta) and type B (dissection arising in descending aorta). Debakey further divided dissections into type I (ascending and descending affected), type II (ascending only) and type III (descending only). DeBakey types I and II equate to Stanford A, whilst type III equates to Stanford B.

Type B aortic dissections are traditionally classified as acute (<2 weeks old) and chronic (>2 weeks old). Recent updates to this classification have included a 'subacute' category (2 weeks to 3 months). This is felt to be an important window of plasticity in the aorta, such that intervention is relatively safe, but remodelling of the aorta is possible following repair.

Complicated TBAD generally refers to dissections with evidence of either of the following:

- rupture or impending rupture (e.g., severe ongoing pain or rapid expansion),
- end-organ malperfusion (brain, bowel, kidney or limb),
- Intractable hypertension (e.g., requiring IV agents >4 days).

Uncomplicated TBAD have no evidence of these, although the name is somewhat confusing as they may develop complications later on, or indeed still rupture despite their reassuring title!

How do you manage acute uncomplicated TBAD?

Initial management should be with tight blood-pressure control with invasive monitoring on a critical care unit. This often requires multiple IV agents in the early phase, although getting the patient established on oral antihypertensives should be an early treatment goal. Endovascular intervention is an area of emerging evidence, with no one trial giving a clear picture of optimal management. There appears to be no short-term advantage to intervention over best medical therapy alone. However, there is some evidence that treatment may reduce medium- to long-term risk of rupture by promoting remodelling of the aorta whilst it is still pliable. Much of vascular surgery uses a similar risk-management strategy (compare to carotid and AAA surgery), and consideration should be given to intervention in all cases. If a simple endovascular solution exists in an otherwise fit patient, and risk factors for poor long-term outcomes are present (e.g., patient <60 years, aorta >4 cm, large false lumen, large entry tear), then intervention should be offered. More complex treatment solutions in less fit patients may be best managed conservatively in the first instance. It is best to consider each case by its own merits, rather than to have a generic rule to apply to all, at least until more robust evidence is available.

What are the risks of intervention in acute or subacute TBAD?

The risks are as follows:

- retrograde type A dissection,
- spinal cord ischaemia (from coverage of the aortic branches),
- ongoing malperfusion of viscera/limbs,
- distal stent graft induced new entry (dSINE),
- rupture,
- failure to remodel/need for reintervention.

Section 2

Final FRCS Vascular: Topics

Chapter 2

Vascular Risk Factors and Their Management

Peng Wong and Julie Brittenden

Key Points

- Peripheral arterial disease (PAD) is an under-diagnosed, under-treated condition and its prevalence is increasing.
- Patients with PAD have a cardiovascular risk profile equivalent to or worse than those with coronary or cerebrovascular disease.
- PAD patients with concomitant symptomatic cardiac or cerebrovascular disease, diabetes or a low ankle pressure index are at even higher risk of sustaining a vascular event.
- Patients with PAD should receive the same risk factor management as patients with other cardiovascular diseases.
- Patient awareness of the need for cardiovascular secondary prevention therapy in PAD is low.
- All PAD patients should be prescribed antiplatelet (clopidogrel preferably, if not on an anticoagulant) and statin, if tolerated.

The Need for Cardiovascular Risk Factor Management in Patients with Peripheral Arterial Disease (PAD)

Globally, more than 202 million people are affected by PAD. PAD is uncommon in population under the age of 50, but its prevalence rises with age, such that more than 15% of population over the age of 70 will have PAD. Its prevalence is increasing due to an ageing population, smoking, and epidemics of obesity, hypertension and diabetes. PAD is a frequently under-diagnosed condition and is often the subject of sub-optimal care. ABPI of less than 0.9 has been commonly used in both clinical and epidemiological research to diagnose PAD. ABPI of less than 0.9 has up to a 95% sensitivity and 99% specificity for diagnosing PAD. Absence of peripheral pulses is not a reliable method to diagnose PAD as up to 10% of population may have an absent dorsalis pedis pulse.

The first-line treatment for patients with PAD is cardiovascular risk factor management with the aim of improving patient survival. This is because patients with PAD have a 2–3 times increased risk of cardiovascular mortality compared to an age- and sex-matched control population. The risk of a patient with PAD dying from a myocardial infarction (MI) is believed to be equivalent to those patients who have already survived their first MI.

The global Reduction of Atherothrombosis for Continued Health (REACH) registry was established to determine atherothrombotic risk in more than 68,000 at-risk patients [1]. It has shown that those with PAD had the highest rates of cardiovascular death, MI, stroke or hospitalisation for atherothrombotic events at 1-year follow-up compared to patients with coronary heart disease (CHD) or cerebrovascular disease (CVD) (Fig. 1). It also showed that the number of events increased with the number of clinically involved vascular beds. Thus patients with PAD and symptomatic CHD or CVD have increased risk compared to those with PAD alone (Fig. 1). Subsequent 4 years follow-up data [2] showed that the risk of future ischaemic events in all patients is substantially increased by diabetes. History of ischaemic events, especially within the preceding 12 months is a strong predictor of future ischaemic events. However, in those with established atherothrombosis, polyvascular disease was again noted to be the strongest independent risk factor of future ischaemic events.

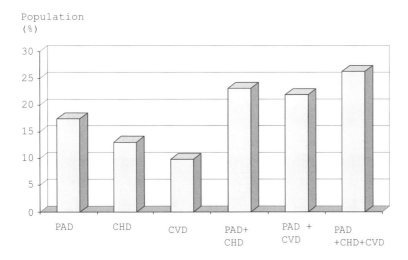

Figure 1.   One-year cardiovascular event rates in outpatients with atherothrombosis.
Source: Data for graph obtained from Ref. [1].

The risk of developing cardiovascular events in patients with PAD is also known to increase with the severity of disease, such that patients with critical limb ischaemia (CLI, defined as rest pain for more than 2 weeks unremitting to analgesia or tissue loss or ankle pressure less than 50 mmHg) have a worse prognosis than patients with intermittent claudication (Fig. 2) [3]. In one study, patients who had PAD involving the large vessels were found to have a 6.6-fold (95% confidence interval 2.9–14.9%) increased risk of death from CHD at 10-year follow-up compared to patients with no PAD. Overall, less than a quarter of patients with severe symptomatic large vessel PAD survived 10 years (Fig. 2) [3]. Patients with asymptomatic PAD have also been shown to have a reduced survival compared to a sex- and age-matched control population.

The use of ABPI has been proposed to help identify and medically optimise asymptomatic PAD patients to prevent cardiovascular events. ABPI has been shown to predict overall survival, independently of the metabolic syndrome and other conventional cardiovascular risk factors. The hazard ratio for mortality has been shown to increase consistently with decreasing ABPI for both males and females (Fig. 3) [4]. In fact, there is a U-shaped relationship between all-cause and cardiovascular

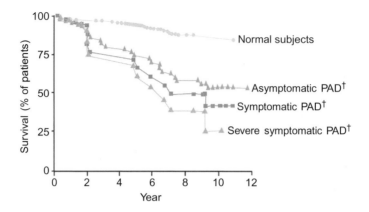

Figure 2.   Kaplan–Meier Survival curves based on mortality from all causes in patients with large vessel disease.

Note: †PAD, peripheral arterial disease.

Source: From Ref. [3]. Reproduced with permission.

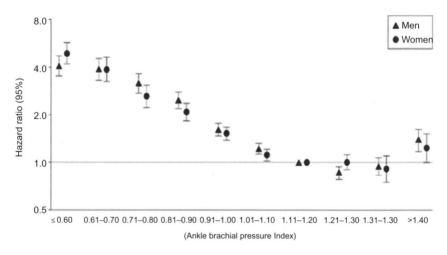

Figure 3.   Hazard ratios for total mortality in men and women by ankle brachial pressure index (ABPI) for all studies in the ABPI collaboration.

Source: From Ref. [4]. Reproduced with permission.

mortality and the ABPI. Patients with increased ABPI (more than 1.4) have also been noted to have an increase in all-cause (hazard ratio, HR: 1.77) and cardiovascular (HR 2.09) mortality (Fig. 4) compared to patients with normal ABPI [5].

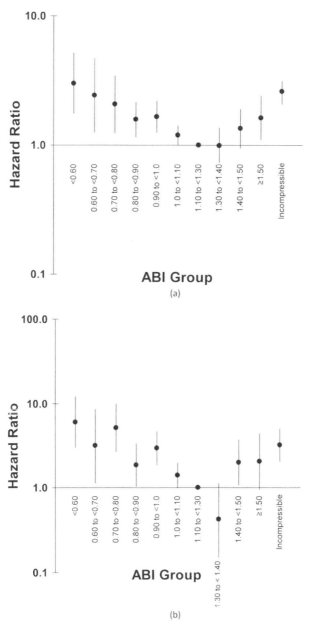

Figure 4. (a) Adjusted hazard ratios for all-cause mortality by baseline ABPI, 1988–1999. (b) Adjusted hazard ratios for CVD mortality by baseline ABPI, 1988–1999.

Source: From Ref. [5].

Why Do We As Vascular Surgeons Need to Treat Risk Factors?

Despite the increased cardiovascular risk in patients with PAD, risk factor management in these patients has been shown to be inadequate in both primary and secondary care settings. In particular, when compared to patients with CHD, patients with PAD (despite comparable risk) received less intensive treatment for lipid disorders and hypertension and were prescribed antiplatelet therapy less frequently than were patients with CHD. In addition to being under-treated, PAD is often under-diagnosed and public awareness of the condition has been shown to be poor throughout Europe and the United States.

Patients are also unaware of the need for secondary prevention therapy. Thus it is the responsibility of the vascular surgeon to initiate risk factor management if this has not already been commenced in primary care and also to educate the patient on the need for this treatment.

Risk Factors

The major risk factors for PAD are similar to CHD and can be classified into either 'modifiable' or 'non-modifiable' factors. Of all the modifiable risk factors, smoking is the most important, but others include management of dyslipidaemia, hypertension, diabetes, and the use of anti-platelet therapy. Evidence-based medicine has shown that reducing cardiovascular risk in patients with symptomatic PAD improves survival. The rationale and targets for treating these risks factors have been addressed in a number of national and international guidelines.

All vascular surgeons should check that their PAD patients have stopped smoking, that they are on an antiplatelet and a statin unless contraindicated, that their hypertension is adequately treated, exclude diabetes and give lifestyle advice. The management of these risk factors is further summarised below.

Smoking

Smoking cessation is the most important component of secondary pre-vention in patients with PAD. Cigarette smoking doubles the risk of a patient developing PAD. In fact, a meta-analysis has shown that the mag-nitude of association with smoking is even greater for PAD (pooled odds ratio of 2.71) than CHD (relative risks of 1.72 for men and 1.92 for women) [6]. Patients with PAD who continue to smoke increase the chance of disease progression by two-fold and likelihood of necessitating revascularisation or amputation. Even though cessation of smoking may not improving walking capacity in patients with PAD, it can prevent the onset of CLI and reduces the risk of bypass graft occlusion by three-fold. Smoking increases risk of aortic aneurysm development, size expansion and rupture by two-fold. Most importantly, smoking cessation is associated with a reduction in all major cardiovascular events, where it reduces overall cardiovascular risk to the level of non-smokers to within 5–7 years and 2–4 years for men and women, respectively.

The vascular surgeon has an important role in promoting smoking cessation and should 'strongly and repeatedly advise patients to stop smoking' (Fig. 5) [7], and arrange referral to a smoking cessation programme. Encouraging patients to stop smoking through smoking cessation support programmes has been shown to double the smoking cessation rate.

There are three pharmacological approaches currently proven effective in smoking cessation — nicotine replacement therapy (NRT), bupropion and varenicline. NRT increases the quit rate by approximately two-fold. Antidepressants such as bupropion have been found to be useful in achieving smoking cessation and have a synergistic effect when

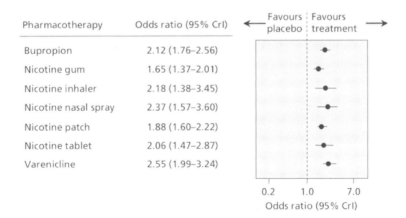

Figure 5.   Summary estimates of the effect of pharmacotherapies for smoking cessation on the odds of smoking cessation.

Source: Eisenberg MJ, Filion KB, Belisle P *et al*. Pharmacotherapies for smoking cessation: A meta-analysis of randomised controlled trials. CMAJ 2008; 179: 135–144 . Reproduced with permission.

used with NRT. Interest has focused on the role of the nicotine receptor partial agonist varenicline in smoking cessation. This may reduce dependence by mimicking the actions of nicotine on neuronal nicotinic receptors in the brain, thus maintaining some dopamine levels and reducing withdrawal symptoms that are associated with reduced dopamine release. In addition to this action, varenicline may also competitively inhibit binding of cigarette nicotine to these receptors. A randomised controlled trial has shown that varenicline results in four times greater odds of stopping smoking compared to a placebo and two times greater odds than bupropion. Although effective, these drugs may have side effects (bupropion can cause seizures, varenicline can cause depression and suicidal ideation). Pharmacotherapy treatments are usually provided within a smoking cessation programme that involves counselling and usually uses nicotine replacement as first-line treatment (Fig. 6). The combination of counselling and pharmacological approaches have been associated with a 22% cessation rate at 5 years.

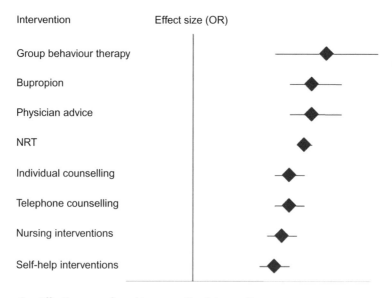

Figure 6.   Effectiveness of smoking cessation interventions.

Source: From Ref. [7]. Reproduced with permission.

Passive smoke exposure has been associated with the development of PAD. Observational studies since enforcement of smoke free legislation on the other hand have shown lower cardiovascular and cerebrovascular events. PAD patients should hence avoid exposure to environmental tobacco smoke. The effects of passive smoke on limb related events remains unknown.

Smoking: current recommendations

- Patients with PAD who smoke should be advised to quit.
- Vascular surgeons should take the opportunity to advise all patients who smoke with PAD to quit each time they attend for a consultation.
- Patients with PAD who smoke should be referred to a smoking cessation programme to develop a plan for quitting.
- Patients with PAD who are planning to stop smoking should be offered NRT or varenicline or bupropion.
- Patients with PAD should avoid exposure to environmental tobacco smoke.

Dyslipidaemia

Epidemiological, post-mortem and angiographic studies have consistently shown a strong positive correlation between plasma total cholesterol and the incidence of cardiovascular disease. In Western populations, the increased risk of future cardiovascular events is observed with serum cholesterol levels that were considered to be in the normal range and increase progressively in a linear manner with rising cholesterol concentrations. In patients with PAD, elevated levels of total cholesterol, low density lipoprotein cholesterol (LDL-C), triglycerides (TG) and lipoprotein A are independent risk factors for adverse vascular events. In contrast, increased levels of high density lipoprotein cholesterol (HDL-C) are protective.

Statins competitively inhibit the enzyme 3-hydroxyl-3-methylglutaryl coenzyme A (HMG-CoA), which catalyses the conversion of HMG-CoA to mevalonate, an early step in the biosynthesis of cholesterol. This leads to a reduction in hepatocyte cholesterol concentration and increased expression of LDL receptors, which are involved in the clearance of LDLs and LDL precursors from the circulation. Statin therapy to lower LDL-C is recommended in all patients with PAD, even in those patients whose cholesterol levels are within what is considered the normal range. The Heart Protection study showed that treatment with Simvastatin 40 mg daily resulted in a 22% (95% confidence interval 15–29%) relative risk reduction in the rates of MI, stroke and of revascularisation in patients with PAD who had a cholesterol level greater than 3.5 mmol/L [8]. There was also a significant reduction in all-cause mortality and in particular that due to cardiac causes in patients with PAD allocated to simvastatin therapy compared to placebo (Fig. 7). These benefits were observed irrespective of the baseline level of cholesterol and occurred in patients with

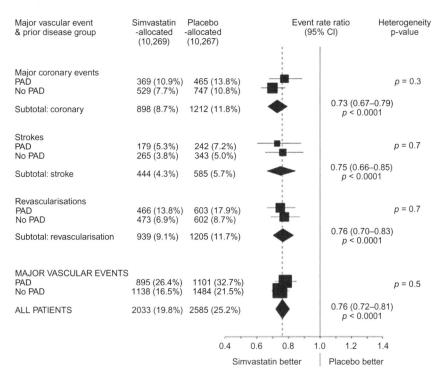

Figure 7.   Heart protection study. Randomised trial of the effects of cholesterol-lowering with simvastatin on peripheral vascular and other major vascular outcomes in 20,536 people with PAD and other high-risk conditions.

Note: PAD, peripheral arterial disease.

Source: From Ref. [8].

and without clinical disease in other arterial beds. The reduction in cardiovascular risk achieved by statin therapy has been shown to be proportional to the achieved reduction in LDL-C reduction (Fig. 8) [9]. Overall, statins reduce the 5-year incidence of major coronary events, coronary revascularisation and stroke by one fifth per mmol/L reduction in LDL-C, irrespective of the patient's baseline lipid profile. Furthermore, trials involving patients with acute coronary syndromes and stable coronary disease have shown a greater reduction in cardiac events in patients receiving high-dose compared to conventional dose statin therapy [9]. This is likely to be the case for patients with PAD and as such the Transatlantic Inter-Society Consensus (TASC) II guidelines [10] recommend more aggressive lowering of cholesterol in those patients with PAD most at risk, such as those with concurrent disease in other vascular beds. This should also be considered for those with diabetes or a low ABPI.

Current NICE guidelines on lipid modification (CG181) advocate using non-HDL-C (non-HDL cholesterol = total cholesterol − HDL cholesterol) as opposed to LDL-C level, as this will provide a better estimate of all

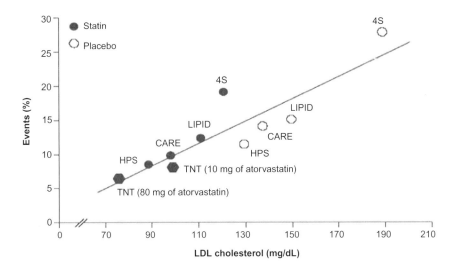

Figure 8.   Relationship between level of cholesterol reduction achieved with statin therapy and reduction in events.

Note: 100 mg dL^{-1} = 2.6 mmol.

Source: From Ref. [9]. Reproduced with permission.

atherogenic lipid particles (LDL-C: intermediate density lipoprotein cholesterol, IDL-C; very low density lipoprotein cholesterol, VLDL-C; and TG remnants). In addition, fasting samples are not required to measure non-HDL-C. Patients who have achieved the LDL-C targets can often be left with a heightened residual CVD risk due to incomplete clearance of remnant atherogenic lipid particles, which could be better ascertained by using non-HDL-C. In addition to starting patient with PAD on a statin, it is also important to monitor the reduction in non-HDL-C levels achieved. Response to treatment is monitored using percentage reduction of non-HDL-C (aiming for more than 40% reduction) rather than same target for all patients. Current NICE guideline (CG181) recommends high intensity statin dose (which reduces LDL-C by more than 40%) (Table 1) in patients with symptomatic or prior occlusive vascular disease as secondary prevention, unless there are concerns about tolerability or interactions. Atorvastatin 80 mg is the current recommended dose for secondary prevention as it is cost-effective in reducing cardiovascular events. The dose of atorvastatin should be reduced for patients with increased risk of adverse side effects, such as chronic kidney disease (estimated glomerular filtration rate < 30 mL/min/1.73 m^2), frail elderly patients with low muscle mass, untreated muscle disorder and chronic alcoholism.

Apart from cardiovascular events, statin has also been shown to reduce limb related events (worsening claudication, onset of CLI,

Table 1.   Statin dose according to intensity and percentage LDL-C reduction (based on NICE CG 181).

Intensity	Statin dose	LDL-C reduction (%)
Low intensity	Fluvastatin 20 mg, 40 mg Pravastatin 10 mg, 20 mg, 40 mg Simvastatin 10 mg	20–30
Medium intensity	Atorvastatin 10 mg Fluvastatin 80 mg Rosuvastatin 5 mg Simvastatin 20 mg, 40 mg	31–40
High intensity	Atorvastatin 20 mg, 40 mg, 80 mg Rosuvastatin 10 mg, 20 mg, 40 mg Simvastatin 80 mg	More than 40

requirement for revascularisation and amputation) compared to placebo, based on a multinational registry [11]. A multicentre randomised controlled trial (RCT) has shown that use of atorvastatin 80 mg daily improved pain-free walking time and community based walking at 12 months compared with placebo. Statin use has also been shown to improve 1-year limb salvage rates, with relative risk reduction of 18% [12]. There is some evidence to suggest that statins may reduce abdominal aortic aneurysm (AAA) growth and rupture rates.

In addition to statin therapy, dietary measures (intake of saturated fat should be reduced to less than 10% of total fat intake) are also recommended, but when used alone have been shown to result in only a 10% reduction in LDL-C, and long-term compliance is known to be low. The main limitations to using statins are their side effects, principally myopathy, elevated transaminases and rarely rhabdomyolysis. Statin treatment carries a small risk of new onset diabetes. However, there was no regular trend for the rates of adverse events and intensity of statins, but simvastatin 80 mg appears to have a consistently higher adverse events rate compared with other higher intensity statins.

Real statin intolerance is uncommon. Patients unable to tolerate statin due to side effects should be considered for a different statin with similar intensity prior to switching to a statin of lower intensity. A lower dose statin is still more beneficial than any other lipid lowering drug. Patients with primary hypercholesterolaemia should be considered for ezetimibe treatment when statin is contraindicated or not tolerated. Fibrates usage is currently limited to treatment of very severe hypertriglyceridemia. Niacin, a form of vitamin B3, has been shown to raise HDL-C by up to 25%. However, most patients cannot tolerate the dose required to achieve that level and clinical trials have not shown any significant clinical benefits.

Statins and inflammatory response

There is growing evidence that statins appear to do more than just lower cholesterol. LDL-C is oxidised by free radicals and may cause direct oxidative damage. A reduction in the levels of LDL-C by the use of statin therapy will result in reduced superoxide production. While many of the anti-inflammatory effects may be due to the reduction in LDL-C, the reduction in vascular events achieved by statin therapy is greater and occurs earlier than would be predicted from the lipid lowering effects alone. The non-lipid lowering effects of statins have been attributed to their ability to inhibit the generation of proteins called isoprenoids. Mevalonate is the precursor of these compounds and is inhibited by statins. The isoprenoids bind to a number of signalling proteins (Rho and Ras) on the cell membrane, which are involved in the inflammatory response. Through these mechanisms, statins have widespread effects on the endothelium, coagulation pathways and platelet function, all of which are implicated in the pathogenesis of acute ischaemic events and have been shown to be activated in patients with PAD.

Vascular surgery has been shown to result in endothelial activation and a pro-thrombotic state, as indeed has lower limb angioplasty. Statin therapy leads to plaque stabilisation, which translates into reduced incidence of peri-operative cardiac events, major limb adverse events and survival in patients undergoing vascular surgery.

Dyslipidaemia: current recommendations

- All patients with PAD should be commenced on Atorvastatin 80 mg if not contraindicated. PAD patients with chronic kidney disease (eGFR < 30 mL/min/1.73 m^2) should be started on Atorvastatin 20 mg.
- Measure the lipid profile (total cholesterol, HDL-C, non-HDL-C and TG) prior to starting statin. Fasting is not required.
- Repeat lipid profile at 3 and 12 months. The aim is to lower the non-HDL-C by more than 40% (rather than same target for all patients), 3 months after commencing statin. If this level is not achieved, discuss compliance, lifestyle measures and increasing dose (if started on less than atorvastatin 80 mg).
- Patients who developed side-effects with statin should be switched to a different statin of similar intensity prior to converting to statin of lower intensity. The evidence and cost-effectiveness of lower intensity statin is still better than ezetimibe or fibrates.
- Measure creatine kinase (CK) in patients with unexplained muscular pain prior to starting statin. If CK level is less than 5 times of the

upper limit of normal, start statin at a lower dose. If CK level is more than 5 times the upper limit of normal, repeat in 7 days' time. Do not start statin unless repeat CK level is less than 5 times of upper limit.

- Measure baseline liver transaminase (alanine transaminase or aspartate transaminase) level prior to starting statin. Repeat liver transaminase level at 3 and 12 months following commencement of statin, and continue if liver enzyme level is less than 3 times the upper limit of normal.

Hypertension

Hypertension is an independent risk factor for cardiovascular and cerebrovascular morbidity and mortality. The risk of cardiovascular events doubles for every 20/10 mmHg rise in blood pressure above 115/70. In the Framingham trial, the age-adjusted risk ratio for intermittent claudication in hypertensive patients compared to controls was increased two and half- to four-fold. Up to 35–55% of PAD patients at presentation have hypertension. The British Hypertension Society and NICE Guidelines on hypertension (CG 127) recommend a blood pressure target level of less than 140/90 mmHg. A meta-analysis has found poor evidence of different hypertensive classes in PAD patients and it is unknown whether significant benefits or risks accrue from their use as majority of patients are already on antiplatelet therapy and statin. Nevertheless, the current guidelines recommend lowering blood pressure in PAD in line with risk reductions for other cardiovascular patients. It can be seen from Fig. 9 that the recommended first-line drug treatment varies depending on the age and race of the patient. Angiotensin converting enzyme (ACE) inhibitor or angiotensin receptor blocker (ARB) are first-line drugs for the treatment of hypertension in patients with PAD, but should be commenced with careful monitoring due to the possibility of co-existing renal artery stenosis. The prevalence of this is difficult to ascertain, but one study, involving a selective group of patients with PAD who were undergoing angiography, found renal artery stenosis in a quarter of patients. Since the publication of the Heart Outcomes Prevention Evaluation (HOPE) and Anglo-Scandinavian Cardiac Outcomes Trial (ASCOT) studies, there has

Choosing drugs for patients newly diagnosed with hypertension

Abbreviations:

A = ACE inhibitor
(consider angiotensin-II receptor
antagonist if ACE intolerant)

C = calcium-channel blocker
D = thiazide-type diuretic

Black patients are those of African or
Caribbean descent, and not mixed-
race, Asian or Chinese patients

Younger than 55 years

55 years or older or black patients of any age

A — Step 1

C or D — Step 1

A + C or A + D — Step 2

A + C + D — Step 3

Add
- *further diuretic therapy*
or
- *alpha-blocker*
or
- *beta-blocker*

Step

Consider seeking specialist advice

BHS

NHS
National Institute for
Health and Clinical Excellence

Figure 9.   Current British Hypertensive Society and National Institute for Health and Clinical Excellence (NICE) guidelines for treatment of newly diagnosed hypertension.

been a move towards recommending the use of ACE inhibitors in patients with PAD even in the absence of hypertension. The latter trial compared regimen of calcium channel blocker +/− ACE inhibitor against beta-blocker +/− thiazide diuretic and found significant reductions in cardio-vascular events and mortality with the former regimen. ACE inhibitors have been shown to have various pleiotropic effects beyond their blood pressure lowering capacity. Whilst there appears to be a promising reduction in cardiovascular mortality, morbidity and stroke associated with ACE inhibitors, the NICE and TASC II guidelines do not recommend their use in patients with PAD other than for their blood pressure lower-ing effects. Only 30% of patients in the HOPE study were on statin ther-apy, and thus the pleiotropic effects of ACE inhibitors, in addition to standard medical therapy in patients with PAD who do not have hyper-tension, requires to be evaluated further. Some evidence suggests that the ACE inhibitor ramipril may improve pain-free and maximum walking time in patients with PAD.

Beta-adrenergic blocking agents (β-blockers), in particular those with vasoconstrictor properties, were previously not recommended in patients with PAD. However, a meta-analysis of 11 randomised controlled trials has shown that they do not worsen the symptoms of claudication and can be used safely in patients with PAD. Furthermore, β-blockers may offer additional cardio-protection to patients with symptomatic PAD and cardiovascular disease. A number of studies have shown that peri-operative use of β-blockers may reduce the post-operative cardiovascular events in PAD patients undergoing major vascular surgery. However, this is still a controversial area and the PeriOperative ISchemic Evaluation Trial (POISE) study has shown that even though β-blockers reduce peri-opera-tive MIs compared to placebo, the patients experience significantly higher rates of stroke and mortality. Current advice would be to continue β-blockers if the patient is already on them, but not to use them as first line for blood pressure control or general risk reduction.

Hypertension: current recommendations

- Patients with PAD and hypertension should be treated to reduce their blood pressure to <140/90 mmHg.
- Patients with PAD should be commenced on calcium channel blocker if they are 55 years old or older, and ACE inhibitor or ARB if they are younger than 55 years. Add in second anti-hypertensive agent if tar-get blood pressure is not achieved (Fig. 8).
- Beta-adrenergic blocking drugs are not contraindicated in patients with PAD.

Antiplatelet therapy

Patients with PAD or AAA have a higher degree of platelet aggregation, suggestive of an underlying prothrombotic state. Antiplatelet therapy is recommended in all patients with PAD and AAA. The Antithrombotic Trialists' Collaboration found that antiplatelet therapy (aspirin, ticlopi-dine or dipyridamole) was associated with a 23% reduction in non-fatal MI, non-fatal stroke and vascular death in patients with PAD [13]. A Cochrane review [14] on antiplatelet agents in patients with intermittent

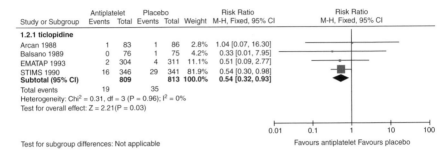

Figure 10.   Cardiovascular mortality — Antiplatelet vs. placebo in patients with intermittent claudication.

Source: From Ref. [14].

claudication reported that compared to placebo, antiplatelet therapy is associated with a 46% relative risk reduction in cardiovascular mortality (Fig. 10). In comparing different antiplatelet agents against aspirin, clopidogrel (a thienopyridine) has been shown to significantly improve cardiovascular risk. The Clopidogrel vs. Aspirin in Patients at Risk of Ischaemic Events (CAPRIE) trial showed that clopidogrel in patients at high risk of ischaemic events reduced the relative risk of major vascular events by 8.7% (95% confidence interval 0.3–16.5%) compared to aspirin. In a subgroup analysis, clopidogrel reduced the relative risk of major vascular events by 23.8% (95% confidence interval 8.9–36.2%) compared to aspirin in patients with PAD. This benefit was seen in patients with PAD with and without other vascular site involvement and represents a number needed to treat with clopidogrel vs. aspirin of 87 patients. Clopidogrel is available in generic formulations and due to the significant price drop, NICE technology appraisal committee have reported that it is cost-effective in patients with PAD. In addition, clopidogrel has been noted to have fewer severe side effects (especially gastrointestinal side effects) than aspirin or modified-release dipyridamole. A combination antiplatelet therapy of aspirin and clopidogrel has not been shown to be of benefit to patients with PAD, and is not recommended due to the increased risk of bleeding complications.

Platelet activation, despite the use of antiplatelet therapy, has been shown to be increased in patients with PAD compared to healthy controls. Studies have shown 'aspirin resistance' occurs in 11–40% of patients with PAD. Similarly, a large variation in response to clopidogrel has also been shown to occur in patients with intermittent claudication, with up to 30% of patients showing no reduction in platelet activation after a loading dose. Clopidogrel competitively and irreversibly inhibits the adenosine diphosphate $P2Y_{12}$ platelet receptor. It is currently postulated that genetic polymorphism of the $P2Y_{12}$ receptors and gene-producing enzyme (CYP2C19) to convert clopidogrel to its active metabolite form, and drug interactions (proton pump inhibitor) affecting the same enzyme may contribute to clopidogrel resistance. There are suggestions that doubling the dose of clopidogrel (150 mg) may be beneficial in patients who are resistant to clopidogrel, based on studies of patients undergoing percutaneous coronary intervention. Although several platelet function tests are available to determine *in vitro* antiplatelet resistance, none are currently being recommended for routine clinical use due to lack of evidence to prove that tailored antiplatelet activity based on platelet function tests improves clinical outcome.

Numerous studies have shown that oral anticoagulant aimed at reducing major cardiovascular ischaemic events in PAD patients do not confer any benefit, but conversely resulted in increased morbidity.

Antiplatelet therapy: current guidelines

- Patients with PAD should be prescribed antiplatelet therapy to reduce major cardiovascular risks.
- Clopidogrel 75 mg is the current recommended antiplatelet therapy and should be used as monotherapy. Patients who cannot tolerate clopidogrel, should be commenced on aspirin 75 mg.
- There is currently no evidence for the use of dual antiplatelet therapy or oral anticoagulant in reducing cardiovascular risks in PAD.

Diabetes

Diabetes and its poor control have long been recognised as a major risk factor for PAD. Incidence of type II diabetes is increasing due to global spread of diabetes. Diabetes increases the risk of PAD by two- to three-fold. Approximately 30% of patients with PAD will have diabetes, but undiagnosed diabetes is common and may occur in 12% or more of new patients referred to a vascular clinic. PAD patients with diabetes often have peripheral neuropathy with impaired sensory feedback, making presentation of claudication symptoms less common and ulcer occurrence more frequent. In contrast to the focal and proximal atherosclerotic lesions in PAD, diabetic PAD patients often have more diffuse and distal lesions. Diabetes increases risk of adverse outcomes in patients with PAD, including progression to CLI, amputation and death. The use of haemoglobin A1c (HbA1c) of more than 48 mmol/L (6.5%) has been recommended by the World Health Organisation as a diagnostic test for diabetes, and this can obviate the inconvenience of using fasting plasma glucose ($\geq$ 7 mmol/L) or oral glucose tolerance test ($\geq$ 11 mmol/L). However, HbA1c measurements can be affected by haemoglobinopathies, such as sickle cell trait, haemolytic anaemia and renal failure. HbA1c reflects plasma glucose over the previous 8 to 12 weeks and has long been utilised as a monitoring tool.

Tight diabetic control has been shown to reduce the risk of developing microvascular and macrovascular complications. The UK diabetes prospective study showed that each 1% rise in HbA1c was associated with a 28% increased incidence of PAD and a 28% increased risk of death [15]. Furthermore, each 1% reduction in HbA1c achieved by treatment was found to correlate with a 14% reduction in MI and a 43% decrease in amputation or death from PAD (Fig. 11).

The current Diabetes Association Guidelines recommend an HbA1c of less than 48 mmol/L (6.5%) to minimise risk of developing complications, such as peripheral neuropathy, retinopathy, nephropathy and CHD. Patients with an HbA1c level of greater than 48 mmol/L should be started on a medical therapy after a trial of lifestyle measures. All too often patients have been maintained on 'lifestyle measures' alone despite persistently elevated HbA1c levels. Furthermore, the presence of PAD and diabetes means that the patient falls into a high-risk category and should have aggressive cardiovascular risk factor management and appropriate foot care. In patients with type II diabetes and PAD, intensive blood pressure control has been shown to significantly reduce the risk of cardiovascular events, as has intensive treatment of dyslipidaemia.

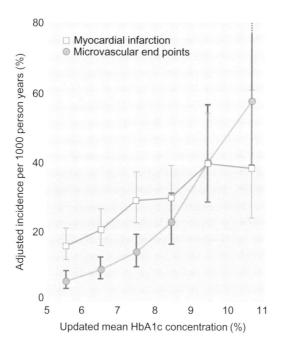

Figure 11.   Diabetes, haemoglobin A1c and macrovascular events.

Source: From Ref. [15]. Reproduced with permission.

Diabetes: current recommendations

- Patients with diabetes and PAD should have aggressive control of blood glucose, with the aim of obtaining a HbA1c level of < 48 mmol/L (6.5%).
- Patients with PAD should be screened for the presence of diabetes due to the increased risk of cardiovascular and limb ischaemic events.
- HbA1c can be used as a diagnostic test for diabetes and an HbA1c of more than 48 mmol/L (6.5%) will be diagnostic of underlying diabetes.

Lifestyle: weight reduction, diet and exercise

Obesity (body mass index, BMI, greater than 30 kg/m^2) is recognised as an independent risk factor for metabolic and cardiovascular diseases.

Thus obese patients with PAD should be offered help with weight reduction in terms of diet and exercise. Currently, patients with BMI > 40 kg/m^2 or BMI between 35 and 40 kg/m^2 with significant diseases that can be improved with weight reduction (such as diabetes and hypertension) will qualify for referral to bariatric surgical team. PAD patients with intermittent claudication who are physically active have been shown to have reduced cardiovascular risks compared to patients who are sedentary [16]. There is abundant evidence to show that exercise can improve walking distance in claudicants if it is provided as a supervised exercise programme. There is little evidence that simple advice to exercise more is effective on its own. Where they are available, patients with claudication should be referred to a local exercise programme. There are no studies looking at long-term risk reduction benefits of exercise in PAD specifically, however, they are proven to be effective in coronary disease and heart failure patients and prevent both future events and need for hospitalisation.

Weight reduction: current recommendations

- Patients with PAD who are obese (BMI > 30 kg/m^2) should be treated to reduce their weight.

Exercise: current recommendations

- Patients with PAD should be encouraged to exercise and, when available, referred to a supervised exercise programme.

Homocysteine

High plasma levels of the non-essential sulphur-containing amino acid homocysteine appear to be an independent risk factor for all types of atherosclerosis, including PAD. Vitamins B6, B12 and folate are involved in its metabolism. Hyperhomocysteinemia is common, present in up to 60% of patients with PAD, and may be treated by folic acid and vitamin B6 supplements. However, currently there is no evidence from randomised trials that treatment in patients with PAD will alter the natural history of the disease, and indeed evidence from one study in patients with cardiovascular disease suggests that treatment may have the potential of causing harm. There is still debate about whether homocysteine itself, or cofactors such as folic acid, are the causative agents.

Patients with PAD should not be given folate supplements routinely due to the lack of clinical benefits. Homocysteine should probably only be measured in patients who develop PAD at a young age in the absence of traditional risk factors.

Homocysteine: current recommendations

- Patients with PAD should not routinely have homocysteine levels measured.
- Patients with PAD should not routinely be given folate supplements.

References

1. Steg PH, Bhatt D, Wilson PWF *et al*. One-year cardiovascular event rates in outpatients with atherothrombosis. *JAMA* 2007;297:1197–1206.
2. Bhatt DL, Eagle KA, Ohman EM *et al*. Comparative determinants of 4-year cardiovascular event rates in stable outpatients at risk of or with atherothrombosis. *JAMA* 2010;304:1350–1357.
3. Criqui MH, Langer RD, Fronek A *et al*. Mortality over a period of 10 years in patients with peripheral arterial disease. *N Engl J Med* 1992;326:381–386.
4. Ankle Brachial Index Collaboration. Ankle Brachial Index combined with Framingham Risk Score to predict cardiovascular events and mortality. *JAMA* 2008;300:197–208.
5. Resnick HE, Lindsay RS, McDermott MM *et al*. Relationship of high and low ankle brachial index to all-cause and cardiovascular disease mortality: The Strong Heart Study. *Circulation* 2004;109:733–739.
6. Lu L, Mackay DF, Pell JP. Meta-analysis of the association between cigarette smoking and peripheral arterial disease. *Heart* 2014;100:414–423.
7. Lemmens V, Oenema A, Knut IK *et al*. Effectiveness of smoking cessation interventions among adults: A systemic review of reviews. *Eur J Cancer Prev* 2008;17:535–544.
8. Heart Protection Study Collaborative Group. MRC/BHF Heart Protection Study of cholesterol lowering with Simvastatin in 20, 536 high risk individuals: a randomised placebo controlled trial . *Lancet* 2002;360:7–22.

9. LaRosa JC, Grundy SM, Walters DD *et al*. Intensive lipid lowering with atorvastatin in patients with stable coronary heart disease. *N Engl J Med* 2005; 352:1425–1435.
10. Norgren L, Hiatt WR, Dormandy JA *et al*. Inter-society consensus for the management of peripheral arterial disease (TASC II). *J Vasc Surg* 2007; 45:S5–S67.
11. Kumbhani DJ, Steg PG, Cannon CP *et al*. Statin therapy and long-term adverse limb outcomes in patients with peripheral artery disease: Insights from the REACH registry. *Eur Heart J* 2014;35:2864–2872.
12. Vogel TR, Dombrovskiy VY, Galiñanes EL *et al*. Preoperative statins and limb salvage after lower extremity revascularization in the Medicare population. *Circ Cardiovasc Interv* 2013;6:694–700.
13. Antithrombotic Trialists' Collaboration. Collaborative meta-analysis of randomised trials of antiplatelet therapy for the prevention of death, myocardial infarction and stroke in high risk patients. *BMJ* 2002;324:71–86.
14. Wong PF, Chong LY, Mikhailidis *et al*. Antiplatelet agents for intermittent claudication. *Cochrane Database Syst Rev* 2011;11:CD001272.
15. Stratton IM, Adler AI, Neil HAW *et al*. Association of macrovascular and microvascular complications of type 2 diabetes (UKPDS:35): Prospective observational study. *BMJ* 2000;321:401–412.
16. Hamburg NM, Balady GJ. Exercise rehabilitation in peripheral arterial disease: Functional impact and mechanism of benefits. *Circulation* 2011;23:87–97.

Recommended Reading

Joint British Societies' 3 Board. Joint British Societies' recommendations for the prevention of cardiovascular disease (JBS3). *Heart* 2014;100:ii1–ii7.

National Institute for Health and Clinical Excellence (2010) Clopidogrel and modified-release dipyridamole for the prevention of occlusive vascular events. NICE technology appraisal guidance (TA 210).

National Institute for Health and Clinical Excellence (2011) Hypertension in adults: diagnosis and management. NICE guideline (CG 127).

National Institute for Health and Clinical Excellence (2012) Peripheral arterial disease: diagnosis and management. NICE guideline (CG 147).

National Institute for Health and Clinical Excellence (2014) Lipid modification: cardiovascular risk assessment and the modification of blood lipids for the primary and secondary prevention of cardiovascular disease. NICE guideline (CG 181).

Chapter 3

An Introduction to New Oral Anticoagulants

Saroj Das and Catherine Pye

Key Points

- New oral anticoagulants (NOACs) are growing in popularity as an alternative to warfarin.
- No monitoring of coagulation is required.
- Fixed once or twice daily dosing.
- Bridging with low molecular weight heparin (LMWH) is not required when commencing treatment with NOACs due to their quick onset of action.
- Dose adjustments are required in renal failure.
- NOACs have a favourable safety profile in comparison to warfarin, but care is required for the elderly who may be at risk of a gastrointestinal bleed.
- NOACs can be used in VTE prevention for elective orthopaedic surgery, VTE treatment and prevention of arterial thromboembolism in patients with atrial fibrillation.
- NOACs are not yet recommended for anticoagulation control in patients with prosthetic heart valve and acute coronary syndrome.

Introduction

What are new oral anticoagulants?

Warfarin is a vitamin K antagonist (VKA) and has been used for the last 60 years as the primary choice for anticoagulation. However, use of warfarin is not without problem. Hence, there has been an urgent need for cheaper new agents with an improved safety and therapeutic profile. In response to this demand, there are emerging new oral anticoagulants (NOACs) that are now in clinical use for over 5 years. In this chapter, we will discuss dabigatran etexilate, a direct thrombin inhibitor, and Factor Xa Inhibitors including rivaroxaban, apixaban and edoxaban. These NOACs unlike heparin and warfarin have specific targeted action and therefore do not affect the global clotting essay (Fig. 1).

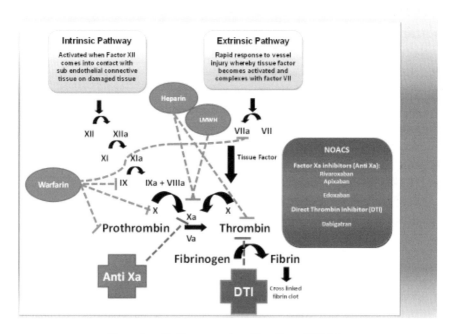

Figure 1.   Clotting cascade with action of NOACs.

Advantages of NOACs Compared to Vitamin K Antagonists (Table 1)

Efficacy

NOACs are non-inferior to VKAs in the treatment of acute DVT and PE [3–6], the prevention of recurrence [3, 7–9], and the prevention of stroke and embolism secondary to Atrial Fibrillation [10, 11]. They have also demonstrated efficacy in thromboprophylaxis for elective hip and knee replacement surgery [12–15]

Safety

NOACs have a favourable safety profile with reduced mortality, intra-cranial haemorrhage and similar or reduced major bleeding rates

Table 1.   Pharmacological properties of warfarin and the NOACs [1, 2].

	Warfarin	Dabigatran	Rivaroxaban	Apixaban	Edoxaban
Target	Epoxide reductase enzyme	Thrombin	Factor Xa	Factor Xa	Factor Xa
Bioavailability (%)	100	7	80	60	62
Dosing	OD	BID	OD	BID	OD
Time to peak action	4–5 days	1–3 h	2–4 h	1–2 h	1–2 h
Half-life (h)	40	14–17	7–11	8–14	5–11
Renal clearance	None	80%	33%	27%	50%
Monitoring	Yes	No	No	No	No
Interactions	Multiple	P-gp	3A4/P-gp	3A4/P-gp	P-gp
Pediatric, pregnancy and breastfeeding	NOACs are not recommended				
Hepatic impairment	Avoid NOACs in liver disease with coagulopathy				
Renal impairment	For NOACs — Dose reductions required if creatinine clearance <50 mL/min, avoid if creatinine clearance <30 mL/min, should not be used if creatinine clearance <15 mL/min				

Notes: 3A4 — Cytochrome P450 3A4 isoenzyme, BID — twice daily, OD — once daily, P-gp — P-glycoprotein.

compared with VKAs [16, 17]. There is some uncertainty with regard to a potential increase in GI bleeding in elderly [17, 18] and more research is required here to clarify.

Monitoring

Dabigatran, rivaroxaban, edoxaban and apixaban do not require coagulation monitoring. This has advantages for patient's quality of life and cost in comparison to Warfarin [19]. However, renal function must be checked prior to commencement.

Bridging [20]

Traditionally bridging with low molecular weight heparin (LMWH) is required when starting VKAs. This is not necessary when commencing NOACs due to the short time taken by them to reach peak serum concentration.

In patients on NOACs requiring elective surgery, the medication should be stopped 5 days before. There is no LMWH bridging required for those taking Dabigatran in high or low thromboembolic risk patients. With Apixaban, Rivaroxaban and Edoxaban, for those who have a low thromboembolic risk, no bridging is needed. In high-risk patients, 3 days of LMWH bridging is required.

Food interactions

There are no known food interactions with NOACs.

Adherence

NOACs are prescribed as fixed drug dosing. There is some evidence that the reduced need for monitoring may reduce adherence to NOACs, especially with the twice daily dosing preparations [21]. However, adherence is multifactorial and there are variable results in different studies when comparing NOAC adherence to warfarin and more research is needed in this area.

Clinical Use (Table 2)

(a) *Prophylactic anticoagulation using NOACs in orthopaedic surgery*

Elective hip and knee replacement

Venous thromboembolism prophylaxis is recommended after an elective hip replacement in patients provided there are no contraindications. NICE recommends Dabigatran, Apixaban and Rivaroxaban as thromboprophylaxis [28–30].

- Dabigatran initial dose 1–4 h after surgery [28].
- Rivaroxaban initial dose 6–10 h after surgery [29].
- Apixaban initial dose 12–24 h after surgery [30].

Thromboprophylaxis should be continued for 28–35 days postoperatively for an elective hip replacement and 10–14 days for an elective knee replacement.

Emergency orthopaedic surgery

NOACs are not currently recommended by NICE as thromboprophylaxis in emergency orthopaedic surgery [28 31].

Table 2.   Clinical use [1].

	Dabigatran	Rivaroxaban	Apixaban	Edoxaban
Treating and preventing recurrent PE and DVT	√	√	√	√
Atrial fibrillation (prevention of stroke and systemic embolus)	√	√	√	√
MI	×	√	×	×
Prosthetic heart valves, indwelling catheters and APLS	×	×	×	×
Thromboprophylaxis hip/knee surgery	√	√	√	×

(b) *Use of NOACs in the treatment of venous thromboembolism*

All the four NOACs are licensed for the treatment and prevention of recurrent venous thromboembolism. For detailed guidance about dose schedule, refer to BNF.

(c) *Use of NOACs in the prevention of thromboembolism*
     in atrial fibrillation

All the four NOACs are licensed for the prevention of stroke and systemic embolism in atrial fibrillation. For detailed guidance about dose schedule, refer to BNF.

There are currently ongoing studies in order to evaluate the long-term use of NOACs in venous and arterial diseases.

The Management of Patients on NOACs

(a) **Elective Surgery:** NOACs can be stopped ~24 h (2–3 half-lives) before a procedure that has a low bleeding risk, but 5 days before procedures with a medium or high bleeding risk, depending on which NOAC is used and on the patient's renal function [22, 23] Other expert consensus documents recommend 24- to 48-h discontinuation windows [23]. Additional studies remain ongoing [24, 25].

(b) **Emergency Surgery:** For life-threatening bleeding, the off-label therapeutic use of prothrombin concentration complex (PCC) may be considered to attempt to overcome the anti-FXa or anti-FIIa activities of NOACs by increasing the plasma concentration of these clotting factors, although clinical evidence is lacking. Specific antidotes for NOACs are now available, namely, a specific reversal agent for factor Xa inhibitors (Andexanet alfa) [26], and a potent monoclonal antibody directed against dabigatran, called idarucizumab [27].

(c) **Recommencing Anticoagulants after Surgery:** If the patient's risk of thrombosis is high and anticoagulation after peri-procedural cessation is required, NOAC administration can be resumed 12–24 h after procedures associated with rapid and complete restoration of hemostasis [24]. In general, evidence suggests that NOACs may be resumed within 24 h for a procedure with a low risk of bleeding, and within 48–72 h for a procedure with a high risk of bleeding [24].

Antidotes for NOAC

Antidotes for thrombin inhibitors and facor Xa inhibitors have been developed and are currently available for clinical use.

Idarucizumab (Praxbind) is a fully humanised monoclonal antibody fragment which has a highly specific binding affinity with dabigatran etexilate and has been developed by Boehringer Ingelheim. The compound has been approved by NICE [32], FDA and European Commission for clinical use. The recommended dose of idarucizumab is 5 g given intravenously as two consecutive infusions of 2.5 g/50 mL over 5–10 min each or as two consecutive 2.5 g bolus injections. Administration of a second 5 g dose of idarucizumab may be considered in any of the following clinical situations:

- recurrence of clinically relevant bleeding together with prolonged clotting times,
- if potential rebleeding would be life-threatening and prolonged clotting times are observed,
- patients require a second emergency surgery or urgent procedure and have prolonged clotting times.

Andexanet, a recombinant, modified factor Xa molecule is developed as a direct reversal agent for patients receiving a factor-Xa inhibitor with a major bleeding episode or requiring emergency surgery. The compound is under development and is an antidote for Apixaban, Edoxaban and Rivaroxaban.

References

1. British National Formulary, 2015. Available at: http://www.bnf.org/products/bnf-online/.
2. Electronic Medicines Compendium, 2016. Available at: http://www.medicines.org.uk/emc/medicine/30513.

3. Büller HR, Décousus H, Grosso MA, Mercuri M, Middeldorp S, Prins MH *et al*. Edoxaban versus warfarin for the treatment of symptomatic venous thromboembolism. *N Engl J Med* 2013;369(15):1406–1415.

4. Bauersachs R, Berkowitz SD, Brenner B, Buller HR, Decousus H, Gallus AS *et al*. Oral rivaroxaban for symptomatic venous thromboembolism. *N Engl J Med* 2010;363(26):2499–2510.

5. Agnelli G, Buller HR, Cohen A, Curto M, Gallus AS, Johnson M *et al*. Oral apixaban for the treatment of acute venous thromboembolism. *N Engl J Med* 2013;369(9):799–808.

6. Schulman S, Kearon C, Kakkar AK, Mismetti P, Schellong S, Eriksson H *et al*. Dabigatran versus warfarin in the treatment of acute venous thromboembolism. *N Engl J Med* 2009;361(24):2342–2352.

7. Schulman S, Kearon C, Kakkar AK, Schellong S, Eriksson H, Baanstra D *et al*. Extended use of dabigatran, warfarin, or placebo in venous thromboembolism. *N Engl J Med* 2013;368(8):709–718.

8. Agnelli G, Buller HR, Cohen A, Curto M, Gallus AS, Johnson M *et al*. Apixaban for extended treatment of venous thromboembolism. *N Engl J Med* 2013;368(8):699–708.

9. Büller HR, Prins MH, Lensin AW, Decousus H, Jacobson BF, Minar E *et al*. Oral rivaroxaban for the treatment of symptomatic pulmonary embolism. *N Engl J Med* 2012;366(14):1287–1297.

10. Miller CS, Grandi SM, Shimony A, Filion KB, Eisenberg MJ. Meta-analysis of efficacy and safety of new oral anticoagulants (dabigatran, rivaroxaban, apixaban) versus warfarin in patients with atrial fibrillation. *Am J Cardiol* 2012;110(3):453–460.

11. Giugliano RP, Ruff CT, Braunwald E, Murphy SA, Wiviott SD, Halperin JL *et al*. Edoxaban versus warfarin in patients with atrial fibrillation. *N Engl J Med* 2013;369(22):2093–2104.

12. Eriksson BI, Dahl OE, Rosencher N, Kurth AA, van Dijk CN, Frostick SP *et al*. Dabigatran etexilate versus enoxaparin for prevention of venous thromboembolism after total hip replacement: A randomised, double-blind, non-inferiority trial. *Lancet* 2007;370(9591):949–956.

13. Eriksson BI, Dahl OE, Rosencher N, Kurth AA, van Dijk CN, Frostick SP *et al*. Oral dabigatran etexilate vs. subcutaneous enoxaparin for the prevention of venous thromboembolism after total knee replacement: The RE-MODEL randomized trial. *J Thromb Haemost* 2007;5(11):2178–2185.

14. Gómez-Outes A, Terleira-Fernández AI, Suárez-Gea ML, Vargas-Castrillón E. Dabigatran, rivaroxaban, or apixaban versus enoxaparin for thromboprophylaxis after total hip or knee replacement: Systematic review, meta-analysis, and indirect treatment comparisons. *Brit Med J* 2012;344:e3675.

15. Turpie AG, Lassen MR, Davidson BL, Bauer KA, Gent M, Kwong LM *et al.* Rivaroxaban versus enoxaparin for thromboprophylaxis after total knee arthroplasty (RECORD4): A randomised trial. *Lancet* 2009;373(9676): 1673–1680.

16. Schulman S, Kakkar AK, Goldhaber SZ, Schellong S, Eriksson H, Mismetti P *et al.* Treatment of acute venous thromboembolism with dabigatran or warfarin and pooled analysis. *Circulation* 2014;129(7):764–772.

17. Ruff CT, Giugliano RP, Braunwald E, Hoffman EB, Deenadayalu N, Ezekowitz MD *et al.* Comparison of the efficacy and safety of new oral anticoagulants with warfarin in patients with atrial fibrillation: A meta-analysis of randomised trials. *Lancet* 2014;383(9921):955–962.

18. Vaughan Sarrazin MS, Rose A. Safety of new oral anticoagulants. *Brit Med J* 2015;350:h1679.

19. Zheng Y, Sorensen SV, Gonschior AK, Noack H, Heinrich-Nols J, Sunderland T *et al.* Comparison of the cost-effectiveness of new oral anticoagulants for the prevention of stroke and systemic embolism in atrial fibrillation in a UK setting. *Clin Ther* 2014;36(12):2015–2028.e2.

20. Kozek-Langenecker SA, Afshari A, Albaladejo P, Santullano CA, De Robertis E, Filipescu DC *et al.* Management of severe perioperative bleeding: Guidelines from the European Society of Anaesthesiology. *Eur J Anaesthesiol* 2013;30(6):270–382.

21. Rodriguez RA, Carrier M, Wells PS. Non-adherence to new oral anticoagulants: A reason for concern during long-term anticoagulation? *J Thromb Haemost* 2013;11(2):390–394.

22. Gogarten W, Vandermeulen E, Van Aken H, Kozek S, Llau JV, Samama CM. Regional anaesthesia and antithrombotic agents: Recommendations of the European Society of Anaesthesiology. *Eur J Anaesthesiol* 2010;27: 999–1015.

23. Sié P, Samama CM, Godier A. *et al.* Surgery and invasive procedures in patients on long-term treatment with direct oral anticoagulants: Thrombin or factor-xa inhibitors. Recommendations of the working group on perioperative haemostasis and the French study group on thrombosis and haemostasis. *Arch Cardiovasc Dis* 2011;104:669–676.

24. Spyropoulos AC, Douketis JD. How I treat anticoagulated patients undergoing an elective procedure or surgery. *Blood* 2012;120:2954–2962.

25. van Veen JJ, Makris M. Management of peri-operative anti-thrombotic therapy. *Anaesthesia* 2015;70:58–e23.

26. Deborah M, Siegal John T, Curnutte Stuart J, Connolly, Genmin Lu, Pamela B Conley, Brian L Wiens, Vandana S Mathur, Janice Castillo, Michele D Bronson, Janet M Leeds, Florie A Mar, Alex Gold, and Mark A Crowther,

Andexanet alfa for the reversal of factor Xa inhibitor activity. *N Engl J Med* 2015;373:2413–2424. DOI: 10.1056/NEJMoa1510991.

27. Tiffany Y Hu, Vaibhav R Vaidya, Samuel J Asirvatham. Reversing anticoagulant effects of novel oral anticoagulants: Role of ciraparantag, andexanet alfa, and idarucizumab. *Vascular Health Risk Manag* 2016;(12):35–44.

28. National Institute for Health and Care Excellence. Dabigatran Etexilate for the prevention of venous thromboembolism in adults. NICE technology appraisal guidance [TA157] [Internet]. 2008. Available at: https://www.nice.org.uk/guidance/ta157/chapter/1-guidance.

29. National Institute for Health and Care Excellence. Rivaroxaban for the prevention of venous thromboembolism after a total hip or total knee replacement in adults. NICE technology appraisal guidance [TA170] [Internet]. 2009 17/3/2016. Available at: https://www.nice.org.uk/guidance/ta170.

30. National Institute for Health and Care Excellence. Apixaban for the prevention of venous thromboembolism after total hip or knee replacement in adults. NICE technology appraisal guidance [TA245] [Internet]. 2012 17/3/16. Available at: https://www.nice.org.uk/guidance/TA245/chapter/2-The-technology.

31. National Institute for Health and Care Excellence. Venous thromboembolism: Reducing the risk for patients in hospital. NICE guidelines [CG92] [Internet]. 2010 17/3/16. Available at: https://www.nice.org.uk/guidance/cg92/chapter/1-Recommendations.

32. Reversal of the anticoagulant effect of dabigatran: idarucizumab — NICE. Available at: https://www.nice.org.uk/advice/esnm73/chapter/key-points-from-the-evidence.

Chapter 4

Management of Acute Limb Ischaemia

Arun Prakash Balakrishnan and Ragai Makar

Key Points

- Acute limb ischaemia (ALI) is associated with significant mortality and morbidity.
- Clinical assessment is paramount for planning management.
- All cases of ALI should be assessed by a vascular specialist.
- All cases should be started on intravenous heparin as soon as possible to prevent extension of thrombus.
- Surgery is preferred with severe ALI as time is of essence.
- Thrombolysis is associated with a lower mortality rate but higher failure rates.
- Surgery is more durable but is associated with a higher mortality rate.
- If compartment syndrome is likely or suspected, a fasciotomy is required.

Definition

Acute limb ischaemia (ALI) can be defined as a sudden compromise of the blood supply to a limb, threatening its viability. Symptoms are usually of less than 2 weeks in duration. The lower limbs are more commonly affected than the upper limbs.

Background

Patients with ALI present depending on the severity of their symptoms. In patients with acute arterial occlusions and no collateral symptoms, the onset is immediate and severe. This scenario is seen in patients with embolic occlusions, trauma, thrombosed aneurysms and occluded grafts. If the acute event occurs on a background of an artery or a graft narrowing/occluding over a period of time then usually there are developed

Table 1.   Causes for arterial occlusion.

Embolic

Mural thrombus following myocardial infarction

Atrium in patients with atrial fibrillation [2]

Atrium in patients with rheumatic heart disease

Atrial myxoma

Aneurysms and atherosclerotic lesions proximal to the ischaemic limb

Paradoxical emboli from the venous system in patients with atrial septal defects

Thrombotic

Thrombosis of an artery due to atheroma

Thrombosed aneurysm with peripheral embolisation

Thrombosis of a reconstructed artery or bypass graft

Arterial dissection

External compression

Popliteal entrapment

Cystic adventitial disease

Blunt trauma resulting in disruption of the intima

Penetrating trauma resulting in division of the artery

Compartment syndrome

Low-flow states in the limb

Hypotension

Low cardiac output

Vasoconstrictor drugs

Severe venous thrombosis

collaterals. In these patients, the symptoms are not severe and they present later.

After 3–6 h of severe ischaemia, the muscle and nerve undergo irreversible changes. Ischaemia of the limb for greater than 6 h usually results in functional impairment or limb loss. Time is therefore of essence — the less the time interval between the event and treatment, the better the outcome. ALI is a genuine surgical emergency with a high incidence of mortality and morbidity. These patients are best managed by a dedicated vascular service [1].

Aetiology

ALI can be caused by occlusion of a native vessel or a graft. Arteries are mainly occluded by thrombus and emboli (Table 1).

Emboli tend to lodge in the bifurcation of an artery. The usual sites are at the bifurcation of the common femoral artery, iliac artery, popliteal artery, aorta and brachial artery. Almost all emboli are part of thrombus although foreign body or tumour emboli can occur. Emboli lodging at the aortic bifurcation is termed saddle emboli.

Assessment of the Acutely Ischaemic Limb

The limb is cool, pale with decreased sensation and muscle weakness. The clinical features of an acutely ischaemic limb are often described as the '6P's':

Pain	Sudden onset, constant and severe
Pallor	The limb is pale
Pulselessness	Unilateral loss of pulses
Paralysis	Inability to move limb
Paraesthesia	Altered sensation
Perishingly cold leg	Cool or cold skin

However, this is a rather simplistic approach best suited to medical students rather than a vascular specialist. Patients rarely complain of any of these specifically, except pain. Most commonly, they describe sudden onset of pain, inability to stand or walk on the leg and then the onset of numbness in the foot.

An acutely ischaemic limb must be carefully assessed to determine the severity of ischaemia. The main questions to answer are the following:

- Is the ischaemia reversible?
- Is the leg viable?
- Is the limb immediately threatened?

The severity of ischaemia influences its management and decision-making. A viable limb has minor or no sensory or motor impairment. The presence of rest pain, decreased sensation and muscle weakness indicates a threatened limb. Limbs with severe pain in the presence of fixed mottling and tender muscles are irreversibly ischaemia. A viable limb allows time for investigation to decide on appropriate intervention (Table 2). When the cause for limb ischaemia is thrombosis *in situ*, the symptoms/signs may be less pronounced. This is because occlusion

Table 2.   Classification of ALI.

Category	Description	Capillary return	Muscle paralysis	Sensory loss	Doppler signals	
					Arterial	Venous
I viable	Not immediately threatened	Intact	None	None	Audible	Audible
IIa threatened	Salvageable if promptly treated	Intact/ slow	None	Partial	Inaudible	Audible
IIb threatened	Salvageable if immediately treated	Slow/ absent	Partial	Partial/ complete	Audible	Audible
III irreversible	Primary amputation	Absent staining	Complete Tense compartment	Complete	Inaudible	Inaudible

Source: Reprinted with permission from Rutherford RB. Suggested standards for reports dealing with lower extremity ischaemia. *J Vasc Surg* 1986;4:80–94.

occurs in an artery/graft that has narrowed over a period of time, permitting collaterals to develop.

Management

The severity of ischaemia influences its management, urgency and decision-making (Fig. 1).

When a diagnosis of severe ALI is made, the patient should be adequately resuscitated. The following measures, in particular, should be instituted:

1. Oxygen should be administered.
2. Intravenous (IV) access and fluids should be administered to achieve adequate hydration.
3. Heparin therapy: a bolus of 5000 units is intravenously followed by the infusion of heparin at the rate of 1000 units per hour. The APTR is monitored and heparin infusion adjusted accordingly to maintain adequate anticoagulation.
4. Adequate analgesia should be administered.
5. Urine output should be monitored — usually a catheter is inserted.

Heparin is used to prevent propagation and extension of thrombus. It also reduces the incidence of cardiovascular events and improves

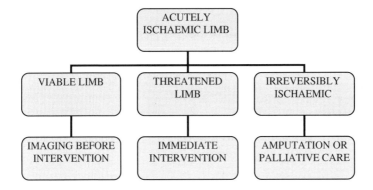

Figure 1.   Flow chart showing initial decision-making pathway.

prognosis [3]. Heparin is an anticoagulant that works by inhibiting the action of prothrombin 3.

Investigation

All patients should have the following base line tests, although treatment should not be delayed for the results:

1. Full blood count
2. Urea and electrolytes
3. Blood glucose
4. Clotting if already on anticoagulant therapy
5. Electrocardiogram (ECG)
6. CXR if suspected cardiac condition
7. Blood group and save serum

Vascular imaging is only indicated to guide treatment if the limb is viable. If the limb is threatened, then imaging will not change the planned procedure and will delay revascularisation. Imaging will define arterial anatomy and help decide if surgery or endovascular therapy is appropriate. If required on table, angiography may be preferred to avoid delays. If the limb is not immediately threatened then standard imaging modalities including Duplex and computed tomography angiography (CTA) or magnetic resonance angiography (MRA) may be appropriate.

Treatment Strategies for Acute Limb Ischaemia

The various available treatment options are:

1. Surgical revascularisation
2. Surgery in the form of an amputation
3. Endovascular including thrombolysis
4. Palliative care

If the limb is immediately threatened, then immediate intervention is indicated.

Surgical revascularisation

Femoral embolectomy is performed under a local or general anaesthetic depending upon the fitness of the patient. If performed under a local anaesthetic, then an anaesthetist should be present in theatre and the patient adequately monitored. The patient is appropriately prepared and draped. In the absence of a femoral pulse, both groins are exposed. The limbs should be visible throughout the procedure and the feet should be placed in transparent bags. The femoral vessels on the affected side should be accessed through a vertical incision centred on the mid-inguinal point. The common femoral, superficial femoral and profunda femoris arteries should be dissected free and controlled with sloops. A transverse arteriotomy should be fashioned proximal to the bifurcation of the common femoral artery into the superficial femoral and profunda femoris artery in order to permit selective catheterisation of both arteries. The embolus usually lodges in the femoral bifurcation, iliac bifurcation or the aortic bifurcation. If there is an embolus at the femoral bifurcation, this is removed by using a forceps or suction. This manoeuvre will establish good flow of blood down the common femoral artery if there are no other proximal lesions. A Fogarty catheter is passed down the superficial femoral and profunda arteries in attempt to remove any thrombus that may have dropped down these arteries. An intra-operative angiogram can be performed to check if the arteries have been adequately cleared. The arteriotomy is closed with prolene.

If the embolus is proximal to the femoral artery then a Fogarty catheter will need to be passed cranially. The balloon is inflated and the catheter withdrawn. Embolic material may be retrieved and good flow may be established. Subsequently, the superficial femoral and profunda arteries should also be cleared of possible embolic material. An angiogram may be necessary and the arteriotomy is closed in a similar fashion as above. If flow cannot be established down one side, then the patient should have a femoral to femoral artery bypass if there is a normal pulse on the other side. If this is not the case, then the patient should have an ipsilateral axillary to femoral artery bypass.

Some patients with an ischaemic limb have a good femoral pulse with an embolus at the popliteal bifurcation. If this diagnosis is suspected then the below knee popliteal artery should be exposed through an incision behind the medial border of the tibia. The below knee popliteal, anterior tibial, peroneal and the posterior tibial arteries should be dissected free and controlled with sloops. An incision should be made proximal to the bifurcation of the popliteal artery. Each of the above arteries can now be cleared by selectively catheterising them with a Fogarty balloon catheter. An angiogram can be performed to check clearance of the vessels. The arteriotomy is usually closed with a vein patch to avoid narrowing of the vessel.

If a saddle embolus is suspected at the aortic bifurcation, then the femoral arteries are dissected free and controlled in both groins. A Fogarty catheter is passed in a cranial direction on both sides and the clot removed.

In the case of upper limb ischaemia, the brachial artery and its bifurcation into the radial and ulnar arteries should be accessed through a lazy S shaped incision in the ante cubital fossa. The arteries are dissected free and controlled with sloops. A transverse arteriotomy is made just proximal to the brachial bifurcation. Clot at the bifurcation can be removed with a pair of forceps or by suction. A Fogarty catheter is then passed cranially into the distal branches to clear any possible embolic material. When good flow has been established, the arteriotomy is closed with prolene.

If an angiogram reveals the presence of residual clot in the vessels then intra-operative thrombolysis can be used to dissolve the clot. 100,000 units of Streptokinase or t-Pa 15 mg in 100 mLs of normal saline can be used as an infusion into the distal vessels over 30 mins [4]. An angiogram is repeated to check adequacy of clearance.

Thrombosed arteries, thrombosed aneurysms and grafts can also present with threatened limbs. In these scenarios, the surgical approach is different. If there is an absent femoral pulse and inflow cannot be established by embolectomy because of iliac atherosclerosis, the patient should have a femoral to femoral or axillary to femoral artery bypass.

The superficial femoral artery cannot be cleared sometimes due to atherosclerotic disease. The patient should have an on-table angiogram.

Attempts should be made to clear residual thrombus with intra-arterial thrombolysis. If there is endovascularly treatable disease, this should be treated by an angioplasty. Lesions not amenable to angioplasty may require distal bypass.

Bypass grafts may occlude in the immediate post-operative period or further down the line. Grafts that thrombose in the immediate post-operative period should be explored as this is usually due to technical reasons. Late graft occlusions are usually due to lesions proximal to, in the graft or distal to the graft due to vein valve site stenosis, neo intimal hyperplasia or progression of disease. These are better first approached by thrombolysis. These patients are sometimes primarily operated on due to the severity of their ischaemia. Late graft occlusions are unlikely to be resurrected. They should have an on-table angiogram. If a distal vessel is identified, then they should have a bypass procedure as long as good inflow is established.

Thrombosed popliteal artery aneurysms require urgent intervention. An on-table angiogram will identify patent vessels if any distal to the aneurysm. Embolic material in the runoff should be cleared by thrombolysis. A bypass procedure should be performed and the aneurysm excluded by ligation.

In the immediate post-operative period, all patients should be anticoagulated with heparin. They should be then anticoagulated with warfarin for a period of 3–6 months.

Surgery in the form of amputation

A proportion of patients will present with irreversible ischaemia. They tend to have severe rest pain, fixed staining and mottling, paralysis and profound sensory loss. No attempts should be made to revascularise these limbs as the reperfusion injury is likely to prove fatal to the patient. If the patient should have any intervention it should be an amputation. This usually is an above knee amputation. About 10% of patients present with an already non-viable limb and the 30-day amputation rate following ALI is 25–30% [5].

Endovascular treatments

Thrombolysis

Thrombolytic agents can be used intra-arterially to try and dissolve thrombus to treat ALI. Catheter directed thrombolysis is indicated in limbs that fall into categories I and IIa [5]. As the limb is not severely ischaemic, time is available to pursue thrombolysis. Agents that are available to use are streptokinase, urokinase and tissue plasminogen activator. Plasminogen in fibrin in a clot is activated to plasmin which degrades fibrin facilitating thrombolysis. Thrombolysis should be used intra-arterially and not systemically.

The advantages of thrombolysis are decreased risk of trauma to the endothelium, dissolution of clot in vessels that cannot be accessed by means of an embolectomy catheter and low pressure reperfusion of the limb. They may reveal stenotic lesions that are amenable to angioplasty. This will improve long-term patency rates if these lesions are angioplastied.

Complications associated with thrombolysis include the following:

1. Myocardial infarction
2. Cerebrovascular accidents
3. Bleeding from puncture site
4. Embolisation

If persistent bleeding is an issue then the effect of the lytic agent can be reversed by administering aprotinin. Fresh frozen plasma may be required and other clotting products may need to be replaced.

The use of thrombolysis will depend upon availability, patient's clinical condition and local expertise. There is evidence from randomised clinical trials that at similar time intervals the limb salvage rates with thrombolysis are comparable to surgery but with a lower mortality rate [6–8]. A recent Cochrane review has found no significant difference between initial thrombolysis and surgery in limb salvage or mortality at 30 days, 5 months and 12 months. However, there is a higher incidence of stroke (1.3%) and major bleeding with thrombolysis [9] (see Table 3).

Table 3.   Contraindications to thrombolysis.

Active bleeding

Cerebrovascular accident within 2 months

Recent GI bleeding

Pregnancy

Neurosurgical procedure within 2 months

Vascular surgical procedure within 2 weeks

Abdominal surgery within 2 weeks

Bleeding disorder

Extensive trauma

Other endovascular treatment options are *percutaneous aspiration thrombectomy,* percutaneous *mechanical thrombectomy and ultrasound accelerated thrombolysis* [10].

Aspiration thrombectomy involves the use of a large bore end hole catheter to aspirate thrombus.

Mechanical thrombectomy involves the use of devices that agitate, disperse and aspirate thrombus.

Ultrasound accelerated thrombolysis uses USS energy to loosen and thin strands of fibrin in the clot exposing plasminogen receptor sites. This improves permeability and penetration of the thrombolytic agent resulting in quicker dissolution of the clot.

The above procedures can be used along with thrombolysis to optimise results.

Palliative care

A proportion of patients will present with ALI whilst being very unwell. The likely outcome for these patients is death. Attempts should not be made to intervene as this will not change the outcome of their illness.

The aim of the treatment should be to alleviate their symptoms. The local palliative care team should be involved and the care of the dying pathway should be instituted.

Complications of Acute Limb Ischaemia

Compartment syndrome

This is due to reperfusion. Typically, immediately after surgery, the treated limb is noted to be perfused but the patient complains of pain in the calf and inability to dorsiflex the foot.

Reperfusion of an ischaemic muscle results in oedema of the muscle. Swelling is due to the failure of cellular membrane function and leaking of capillaries. As muscles are enclosed in a bony fascial compartment, this increases the volume and ultimately pressure within the compartment. As the pressure within the compartment increases, muscle perfusion decreases resulting in further ischaemic injury. This in turn increases muscle oedema. Thus, a vicious circle is established resulting in obstruction of veins, arteries, capillaries, nerve dysfunction and infarction of the muscle. The anterior compartment is the most vulnerable.

If clinically suspected or with compartment pressures of more than 20 mmHg, fasciotomy is indicated. A four-compartment fasciotomy should be performed.

Rhabdomyolysis

Muscle breakdown as a result of ischaemic injury can release myoglobin into the blood stream. This can cause acute tubular necrosis leading to renal failure.

Patients have dark urine, elevated levels of serum creatine kinase and myoglobin in the urine.

Treatment includes hydration, alkanising the urine and removing the source of myoglobin. Patients may require haemofiltration or dialysis.

References

1. Clason AE, Stonebridge PA, Duncan AJ *et al*. Acute ischemia of the lower limb: The effect of centralising vascular surgical services on morbidity and mortality. *Br J Surg* 1989;76:592–593.
2. Earnshaw JJ. Demography and aetiology of acute leg ischemia. *Semin Vasc Surg* 2001;14:86–92.

3. Blasidell FW, Steele M, Allen RE. Management of lower extremity arterial ischemia due to embolism and thrombosis. *Surgery* 1978;84:822–834.

4. Earnshaw JJ, Gaines PA, Beard JD. Management of acute lower limb ischemia. In: Beard JD, Gaines PA (eds.), *Vascular and Endovascular Surgery*. Elsevier, 2006, p. 169.

5. Norgren L, Hiatt WR *et al.* Acute limb ischemia. In TASC II inter-society consensus on peripheral arterial disease. *Eur J Vasc Endovasc Surg* 2007; 33(1):S5–S67.

6. Results of a prospective randomized trial evaluating surgery versus thrombolysis for ischemia of the lower extremity. The STILE trial. *Ann Surg* 1994;220:251–266.

7. Ouriel K, Shortell C, Deweese J, Green R, Francis C, Azodo M *et al.* A comparison of thrombolytic therapy with operative revascularisation in the initial treatment of acute peripheral arterial ischemia. *J Vasc Surg* 1994;19:1021–1030.

8. Ouriel K, Veith F, Sasahara A. A comparison of recombinant urokinase with vascular surgery as initial treatment for acute arterial occlusion of the legs. Thrombolysis or Peripheral Arterial Surgery (TOPAS) Investigators. *N Eng J Med* 1998;338:1105–1111.

9. Berridge DC, Kessel DO, Robertson I. Surgery versus thrombolysis for initial management of acute limb ischemia. *Cochrane Database Syst Rev* 2013;6(6):CD002784. DOI:10.1002/14651858.CD002784.pub2.

10. Marjolein Schrijver A, Van Leersum M, Fioole B *et al.* Dutch randomized trial comparing standard catheter-directed thrombolysis and ultrasound-accelerated thrombolysis for arterial thromboembolic infrainguinal disease (DUET). *J Endovas Therapy* 2015;22(1):87–95.

Chapter 5

Chronic Lower Limb Ischaemia, Critical Ischaemia and the Diabetic Foot

Abigail H. M. Morbi and Cliff Shearman

Key Points

- Peripheral arterial disease (PAD) affects approximately 30% of the adult population.
- PAD is a powerful marker of cardiovascular risk and the risk is related to the severity of PAD.
- Risk factor management has been proven to reduce cardiovascular risk, but many patients do not receive adequate treatment.
- The optimum treatment to improve walking in patients with intermittent claudication is best medical treatment (BMT) and supervised exercise, with angioplasty for those who do not improve with exercise therapy.
- Angioplasty and surgery appear to be equivalent in treating critical limb ischaemia (CLI), but there is insufficient evidence comparing long-term outcomes. Angioplasty is cheaper due to reduced length of hospital stay, but surgery is better for patients who survive over 2 years. There is some evidence that patients have worse outcomes if they undergo surgery after having endovascular intervention.

- Diabetic foot complications are a common cause of hospital admission and often precede amputation. The majority of amputations in the UK are carried out in patients with diabetes, and many of these are avoidable.
- Patients with diabetes should be screened annually for neuropathy and PAD and those at increased risk of foot ulceration seen regularly in a specialised foot clinic.
- Multi-professional team approach to the management of diabetic foot complications and timely recognition and treatment of the acute diabetic foot can reduce amputation rates.

Epidemiology

Atherosclerotic arterial disease affecting the legs, peripheral arterial disease (PAD), is very common. In many patients it is asymptomatic, but commonly the first manifestation of PAD is pain in the leg on walking, intermittent claudication. Claudication distance is reproducible and the pain resolves at rest. In some patients the blood supply to the leg becomes further reduced to a level where pain is experienced at rest and ulceration and gangrene occur (critical limb ischaemia, CLI). In the Edinburgh Artery study [1] it was found that 4.5% of men and women over 55 years of age had intermittent claudication, but a further 25% had asymptomatic disease. In one third of the asymptomatic group, evidence of a major vessel occlusion was found. At 5-year follow up, those that had subsequently developed claudication were found to have come from the asymptomatic group [1], suggesting there may be a window of opportunity to prevent disease progression. Further evidence of this high prevalence comes from the PARTNERS study [2], which screened 6979 subjects over 70 years of age or over 50–69 with a risk factor for vascular disease in 320 primary care practices in the USA. The study found 5.5% had symptomatic PAD and in total 29% of subjects had PAD [2]. Further, it is estimated that the prevalence of limb-threatening ischaemia or CLI is 220 per million of the population [3].

A number of studies have identified that the majority of patients with PAD do not significantly deteriorate from the point of view of their legs. In the Edinburgh Artery study, the annual risk of limb loss was less than 1–2%. However, 5–10% of subjects suffered a cardiovascular event per year, commonly a myocardial infarction or stroke [1]. This is an extraordinarily high cardiovascular risk and patients with PAD are 6 times more likely to die from cardiovascular disease over 10 years than non-PAD subjects.

The severity of PAD is a prognostic indicator of cardiovascular risk, those with the most severe symptoms faring worse. In patients with CLI, the cardiovascular death rate is even worse and one in five will be dead within 1 year of diagnosis. Although less marked, even the asymptomatic group have an increased cardiovascular risk. Over the past decade, this observation has often led to the main focus of treatment shifting to address cardiovascular risk in patients with PAD by attempting to modify their risk factors. However, it is important to remember that many patients with intermittent claudication are extremely handicapped by their symptoms and these may need addressing in their own right. Although it might seem appealing to screen the adult population for PAD, there is currently no strong evidence that this approach would reduce cardiovascular risk or be cost effective.

Intermittent Claudication

History

Tight, cramp like pain in the muscles of the calf, thigh or buttock is characteristic. Calf claudication is the most common symptom, simply because the most common site of PAD is in the superficial femoral or popliteal arteries. More proximal disease more commonly causes buttock or thigh claudication. Occasionally, buttock claudication can occur from isolated internal iliac artery blocks, usually bilateral. This is rare although it is increasingly seen after endovascular treatment of aortic aneurysms if one or both internal iliac arteries are covered.

Typically, the pain of claudication comes on only after walking for a certain distance, which is reproducible (the pain-free walking distance) and is usually worse on hills. It may stop the patient from walking and is relieved by resting in the standing position. Most other causes of hip or leg pain, such as arthritis, may be exacerbated by walking, but will also cause some pain at rest or in certain positions or postures. If the pain only subsides when the patient sits down, this suggests the symptoms may be related to their back rather than arterial disease. Spinal canal claudication typically produces numbness, weakness or heaviness in the leg rather than pain localised to a specific muscle group. Spinal canal claudication, due to a narrow spinal canal, may actually be easier going uphill as leaning forwards opens the spinal canal up and is usually only relieved when the patient sits down.

It is usual, when taking a history of claudication, to ask the patient to quantify their walking distance, but this is notoriously inaccurate as it will vary with speed and terrain. Additionally, patients are often extremely poor at estimating distances. For research purposes walking distances are usually assessed by walking on a treadmill at a set speed and degree of slope. Usually the 'initial claudication distance', which is the distance at which the pain first starts, and the 'absolute claudication distance', which is the distance at which the patient stops, are recorded.

It is important to take a full history of cardiovascular risk factors, in a patient with intermittent, claudication to allow appropriate risk factor management, as these patients have significant cardiovascular morbidity and mortality.

Examination

A full cardiovascular examination is important to detect other manifestations of cardiovascular disease. Upper limb peripheral pulses should be palpated and the cardiac rhythm checked. Measurement of blood pressure, cardiac auscultation and abdominal examination for the presence of an abdominal aortic aneurysm should be performed. An abdominal aortic aneurysm cannot be fully excluded by clinical examination and any suspicion should prompt an ultrasound scan.

Examination of the peripheral circulation should include inspection for clinical signs such as ulceration and gangrene. Other, less definitive signs of ischaemia such as cracked skin, hair loss and nail damage should be recorded, but are not very useful in their own right. Capillary return is notoriously unreliable unless particularly prolonged, but it should probably also be assessed. In a patient with diabetes, it is important to look for signs of abnormal foot shape and callus formation. Skin colour and temperature should also be recorded.

The most important aspect of the peripheral examination is peripheral pulse palpation. The femoral, popliteal, posterior tibial and anterior tibial/dorsalis pedis pulses should be identified. In a small number of normal subjects (10–15%) the dorsalis pedis may be absent and in some individuals it is possible to palpate the anterior communicating branch of the peroneal artery on the lateral side of the ankle.

Usually, it is sufficient to judge whether a pulse is present or absent. Lower limb pulses can be difficult to feel and trying to judge whether a pulse is strong or weak is rarely of great use. In some patients a hard calcified vessel may be palpated, which is important to identify as it may have implications for treatment. A rough rule is that in patients with calf claudication, the disease will be predominantly in the superficial femoral artery and so the popliteal pulse will be absent. For thigh and buttock claudication, the disease is predominantly in the aortoiliac segment and the femoral pulse will be weak or absent. Although this is not infallible, it is a useful concept to bear in mind when examining the peripheral circulation.

Thigh and buttock claudication may be associated with male impotence (Leriche syndrome). It may therefore also be appropriate to enquire about the ability for a male to attain an erection. A small number of patients will have isolated disease of their internal iliac arteries causing their claudication and so will have palpable femoral pulses. This may also be seen in patients who have had therapeutic occlusion of their internal iliac arteries to allow endovascular repair of an aortoiliac aneurysm.

Auscultation over the femoral artery may detect the presence of a bruit. We believe this is of limited significance as it simply implies turbulent flow proximally. However, in patients with a good history of claudication but palpable pulses a bruit may signify proximal disease, which is only haemodynamically significant during exercise.

Ankle brachial pressure index (ABPI) measurement

Measurement of the ABPI is the third part of the diagnostic triad. The ankle pressure is expressed as a ratio compared to the brachial pressure. An ABPI of 0.9 or less is usually taken to be abnormal. In some patients, especially those with diabetes, the peripheral arteries may be stiff or calcified, which can give an artificially high ankle pressure. This is usually obvious, but if doubt remains further investigation may be required. In symptomatic patients with an ABPI of <0.9, there is a 95% sensitivity of diagnosing PAD. To measure the ABPI, you need a hand held Doppler with an 8 MHz probe, 15 cm sphygmomanometer and cuff. Make sure the patient is lying flat, ideally for 10 min before starting. The test is invalid if the patient's legs are not at the same level as the heart. Secure the cuff around the arm as if taking a blood pressure reading in the normal manner. Apply gel over the brachial pulse and apply the Doppler probe over the brachial artery, at an angle of 60° to the skin. Repeat on the other arm and use the higher of the two systolic readings to calculate the ABPI. When measuring pressures in the dorsalis pedis and posterior tibial arteries, make sure the cuff is placed on the lower calf about two fingerbreadths above the malleoli. The ABPI is calculated for each leg, by dividing the highest ankle pressure by the brachial pressure [4].

Toe pressures/pole test

Patients with diabetes, renal failure and other conditions causing vascular calcification can develop incompressible tibial arteries, causing falsely high systolic pressures when measuring the ABPI. Measurement of toe pressures provides an accurate alternative measurement. The toe pressure is normally about 30 mmHg less than the ankle pressure and an abnormal toe brachial index (TBI) is defined as <0.70. Usually, this is not done using a hand-held Doppler but by using a system of automatically inflating cuffs on the great toes (sometimes other toes as well) and by recording the pulse using a plethysmographic technique or laser Doppler.

To measure ABPI using the pole test, the leg is slowly elevated from the horizontal position until the Doppler signal disappears. The height above the left ventricle is measured using a calibrated pole (i.e., a ruler) to record the hydrostatic pressure in equivalents to mmHg. For example 70 cm is equivalent to 50 mmHg.

Differential diagnosis

In the majority of patients the diagnosis of intermittent claudication due to PAD can be confidently confirmed by the simple measures outlined above. Other conditions that should be considered in the differential diagnosis are nerve root irritation due to degenerative lumbar spine disease in which the pain often takes longer to wear off and may only be relieved by sitting. True spinal canal stenosis is relatively uncommon, and again, the pain is characteristically relieved by sitting or flexing the lumbar spine. Other musculoskeletal conditions such as osteoarthritis are usually possible to identify due to their associated symptoms of nocturnal pain, early morning stiffness and pain that persists for hours after ceasing walking. Venous claudication is rare and usually the patients will have a history of previous venous problems or signs of chronic venous insufficiency.

There is a small group of patients who have a non-atherosclerotic cause of their vascular intermittent claudication They are often younger, have no other manifestations of cardiovascular disease and their symptoms may only occur after walking some distance. These patients should however be investigated further to exclude other rare causes of exercise induced ischaemia, which may need specific treatment. These include cystic adventitial disease, popliteal entrapment syndrome, congenital abnormalities such as persistent sciatic arteries and fibromuscular dysplasia.

Investigations

In some patients, the diagnosis of intermittent claudication may remain uncertain. They may have other comorbidities that make it difficult to determine the dominant cause of the symptoms or they may have non-compressible vessels. In these patients treadmill exercise testing by an experienced technician may be of value. Observation of the patient walking and determination of the distance walked on a treadmill may be helpful in determining the origin of the pain. However, relatively few patients will need this level of investigation. Treadmill walking (the distance to the onset of pain, the claudication distance, and the maximum distance they can walk, absolute walking distance) is most commonly used when new therapies are being evaluated.

If there still remains doubt as to the presence of PAD, such as in a patient with diabetes or if intervention is being considered, then colour-flow duplex (CFD) ultrasound scanning should be undertaken. CFD utilises the B mode ultrasound component to identify the vessel and then interrogates them with Doppler ultrasound to determine the velocity of blood flow through them. Direction of flow is colour-coded on the display, which makes it easier and quicker to identify areas of disease due to turbulence or cessation of flow. This will display the extent of the PAD and also, using the Doppler component, give an objective evaluation of the haemodynamic severity of the disease based on the velocity shift across the diseased segment. Duplex is ideal for the infra-inguinal vessels, but can be more difficult in the aortoiliac segments. Usually an experienced ultrasonographer can get enough information to determine the extent and severity of the disease. Bubble contrast enhancing agents have been used, but currently have not been found to be of great value in the investigation of PAD. Duplex ultrasound will confirm the diagnosis of PAD, but will also usually give a strong indication of what interventions are likely to be applicable to an individual, e.g., angioplasty or bypass surgery. In many patients with clear Duplex scans, no further imaging is required although some clinicians prefer more detailed imaging prior to intervention.

Depending on the pattern of disease and nature of the planned intervention, more detailed information may be required. Digital subtraction angiography (DSA) is now rarely used for diagnostic imaging. It is invasive and requires a significant volume of contrast medium, which is nephrotoxic. Multi-slice computed tomography angiography (CTA) is the preferred mode of imaging in many units (see Fig. 1).

It is relatively non-invasive with very rapid acquisition times under 30 s. However, an intravenous contrast medium is required and contrast induced nephropathy can occur, particularly in patients with impaired renal function. The radiation dose is also significant, being 80–200 chest X-ray equivalent and, although for single studies this is not an issue, in patients having repeated scans, this must be borne in mind. Image

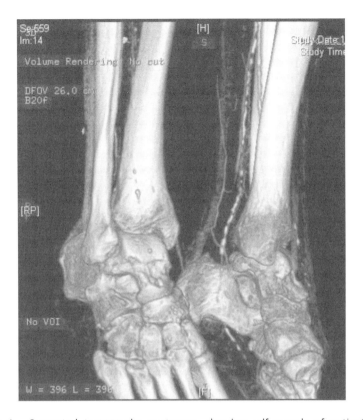

Figure 1. Computed tomography angiogram showing calf vessels of patient with diabetes. Calcification is clearly seen.

interpretation can pose problems, particularly with calcification in the vessel wall.

Magnetic resonance angiography (MRA) is also widely used (see Fig. 2) and is recommended by NICE as the optimum method to visualise the peripheral vessels.

Calcification does not cause the same problems for CTA, but acquisition times are longer. Recognition of nephrogenic systemic fibrosis, which may be induced by the contrast agent gadolinium in patients with impaired renal function, has limited its role in these patients. Both of these techniques are ideal to use as outpatient investigations.

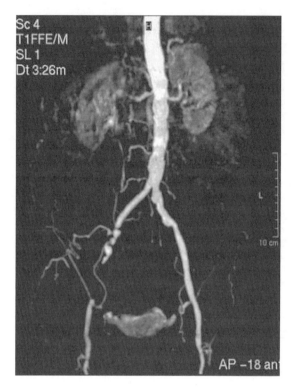

Figure 2.   Magnetic resonance angiogram of patient with right iliac artery occlusion.

Management

The two aims of treatment are to reduce the cardiovascular risk and improve the walking ability of the patient with intermittent claudication. It should be remembered that intervention for these patients is for symptomatic relief, compared to patients with CLI who require intervention for limb salvage.

Reducing cardiovascular risk

Despite evidence of increased cardiovascular risk in patients with PAD, and a clear need to address and modify cardiovascular risk factors in this cohort, evidence suggests many patients do not receive the correct treatment and advice. There needs to be a focus on modification of risk factors, to reduce the burden of cardiovascular morbidity and mortality in patients with PAD.

Smoking is the most important risk factor for the development of PAD and even passive smoking increases cardiovascular risk. Smokers are more than 4 times more likely to develop PAD than non-smokers. Not only is disease progression and amputation more likely in smokers, but smoking increases the risk of hypertension and raised cholesterol. Excess cardiovascular risk is halved within 1 year of cessation and is the same as non-smokers within 5 years in those patients who successfully give up smoking. There is no strong evidence for the benefits of smoking cessation to the limb, but some observational studies have suggested an improvement in walking distance and a reduction in amputation rates. Smoking affects graft patency and wound healing, affecting those patients who undergo bypass or amputation. Smoking cessation advice, when combined with nicotine replacement therapy, improves quit rates to around 30%. Success rates are highest with programmes that combine counselling, group therapy and pharmacotherapy. There is limited evidence for the use of electronic cigarettes and a Cochrane review recommended further research is needed in this area.

The prevalence of diabetes is increasing, affecting more than 382 million people worldwide. Patients with type 2 diabetes have 3–5 times more chance of developing PAD compared to the non-diabetic population. The UK Prospective Diabetes Study suggested that each 1% increase in HbA1C was associated with a 28% increase in PAD. Diabetes is associated with 1–16 times increased risk of amputation and this has 80% mortality at 5 years. Also, the effects of other risk factors such as hypertension and hypercholesterolaemia are amplified in patients with diabetes. Studies looking at tight diabetic control in type 1 diabetes show a reduction in all cardiovascular events [5] and studies in type 2 diabetes have shown a reduction in cardiovascular events but no evidence for reduction in mortality [6].

For patients with diabetes and PAD, every attempt should be made to identify and reduce any other risk factors, and diabetic control should be optimised for the individual patient. Patients with diabetes should also have regular checks of their feet for signs of neuropathy or PAD. For patients with PAD who require intervention, it must be considered that poorly controlled diabetes affects surgical outcomes, and NICE guidelines recommend monitoring HbA1c pre-operatively and delaying surgery in patients with poor diabetic control.

There is a strong association between serum cholesterol, atherosclerosis and cardiovascular mortality. The Framingham Heart Study showed fasting cholesterol >7 mmol/L doubled the risk of intermittent claudication [7]. In the Heart Protection Study, patients with PAD and a total cholesterol over 3.5 mmol L^{-1} who took simvastatin (a HMG-CoA reductase inhibitor) had a 17.6% reduction in cardiovascular events compared to those on placebo [8]. There was also a reduction in the subsequent need for both cardiac and non-cardiac revascularisation procedures. Based on these results, nearly all patients with PAD should be prescribed statin therapy. There is also emerging evidence that statins have a direct effect on atherosclerotic plaque, stabilising it and possibly causing plaque regression in high doses. In the Asteroid Study, high dose rosuvastatin resulted in reduced plaque volume over 24 months. NICE recommends for all patients with PAD, starting with 20 mg atorvastatin for primary prevention and 80 mg atorvastatin for secondary prevention. There is still debate as to whether primary prevention reduces cardiovascular events in low-risk patients, and current guidance from NICE is that evidence does not support the use of statins in patients with <20% 10-year cardiovascular risk.

Up to 24% of the adult population are hypertensive, and hypertension is associated with a three-fold increased risk of PAD as well as being strongly associated with stroke and myo cardial infarction. Up to 55% of the PAD cohort have hypertension. Treatment of hypertension will reduce stroke rates by 38% and cardiovascular deaths by 14%. Angiotensin converting enzyme (ACE) inhibitors and calcium channel blockers are the main first-line antihypertensive agents used in PAD. In patients over 55 years of age or of Afro-Caribbean descent, NICE guidelines recommend that calcium channel blockers should be used as initial treatment with ACE-inhibitors or angiotensin II receptor blocker used as first-line therapy in those under 55 years of age. The Heart Outcomes Prevention Evaluation (HOPE) Study of the angiotensin converting enzyme inhibitor, ramipril, demonstrated an advantage in reducing cardiovascular events, even in those patients whose blood pressure was not elevated [9].

However, there are potential problems with the widespread use of ramipril in patients with PAD, as many will have renal artery disease. At present, in those with PAD and hypertension ramipril should be considered as the first-line treatment, but there is not enough evidence to suggest widespread use in non-hypertensive patients. The UK Prospective Diabetes Study demonstrated a reduction of systolic blood pressure by 10 mmHg, resulting in a 16% decrease in limb amputation or death from PAD.

The Antithrombotic Trialists' Collaboration meta-analysis found that antiplatelet agents (predominantly aspirin, a cyclo-oxygenase inhibitor) reduced the risk of cardiovascular events by 23% in patients with PAD [10]. A dose of 75 mg was as effective as higher doses. Approximately 20% of patients are unable to take aspirin largely due to gastrointestinal disturbance, and it is emerging that a similar proportion of patients have aspirin resistance. Clopidogrel is a thienopyridine derivative that blocks ADP induced platelet activity. In the Clopidogrel vs. Aspirin in Patients at Risk of Ischaemic Events (CAPRIE) study, clopidogrel showed a relative decrease in cardiovascular events compared to aspirin (particularly in the PAD group), with a relative risk reduction of 8.7% compared to aspirin and was associated with less gastrointestinal side effects [11]. In the subgroup of patients with PAD, clopidogrel showed a 23.8% relative risk reduction compared to aspirin at 2 years of follow up [11]. At the time of the CAPRIE study, clopidogrel was more expensive and was therefore reserved for use in patients resistant to aspirin or unable to tolerate the gastrointestinal side effects. However, now that clopidogrel is out of patent, NICE recommends it as first-line antiplatelet therapy in patients with PAD.

The CHARISMA trial investigated the effect of dual therapy, with aspirin and clopidogrel in patients with PAD. There was no overall advantage for dual therapy, but there was some benefit in patients at high risk of cardiovascular events although significant bleeding complications increased. The CASPAR trial found no improvement in limb salvage or survival after below-knee bypass grafting, in patients on dual therapy compared to aspirin.

A number of other lifestyle changes should be advocated. Weight reduction and regular exercise have proven cardiovascular benefit. They also have a positive effect on other risk factors. Omega 3 fatty acids (fish oils) appear to have some beneficial effects, but their clinical role in PAD has not been established. Likewise, antioxidants and other dietary additives have not demonstrated to be of clinical benefit.

Despite the overwhelming evidence for the benefit of risk factor management, recent epidemiological studies have found that only around 30–50% of patients get adequate treatment for these.

Improving walking distance

In many patients, confirmation of the diagnosis of intermittent claudication, reassurance of the natural history of the condition as regards the leg and risk factor management will be all that is required. The decision to directly attempt to improve walking distance is something that should be decided by the patient balanced by the impact of their symptoms on their day-to-day life compared to the chance of success vs. the risks of treatment. Patients who have claudication are a heterogeneous group. Many will only be mildly troubled by their symptoms or have other significant comorbidity that reduces their mobility. Others, however, may be severely restricted by their claudication, which can significantly alter their lifestyle. It is the role of the clinician to help the patient decide on the best therapeutic option for them based on the impact of their symptoms on their quality of life.

A number of vasoactive drugs have been promoted to increase walking distance. In the UK, two drugs are currently used, naftidrofuryl oxalate (Praxilene) and cilostazol (Pletal). In a meta-analysis of eight studies, cilostazol has been demonstrated to improve walking by 50% with some improvement in quality of life. Studies have shown no conclusive evidence of an advantage of one agent over the other and as naftidrofuryl costs less than cilostazol, it was recommended that if vasoactive drugs were indicated, naftidrofuryl should be used. However, if symptoms do not improve after 3 months, the drug should be discontinued. NICE guidelines do not recommend cilostazol, pentoxifylline and inositol nicotinate for the treatment of intermittent claudication [4].

The benefits of exercise have been realised for over a decade, with exercise therapy improving walking distance in patients with intermittent claudication and hence improving functional ability and quality of life. A meta-analysis of 21 studies suggested an improvement in walking distance of 124% with exercise therapy. Supervised exercise programmes requiring three sessions of 30 min per week for 6 months seemed to provide the most benefit. A Cochrane review of 30 studies showed exercise to improve walking ability by 50–200% in patients with intermittent claudication, and NICE recommends exercise therapy as first-line treatment for this group of patients [4]. Supervised exercise therapy has been shown to improve treadmill walking time and improve maximal and pain-free walking distance compared to non-supervised exercise. The main problem with this approach is making it appealing to patients and generally less than 30% of them will either want to try exercise or continue on a programme. Not all patients have access to supervised exercise programmes, and when left to their own devices, compliance is poor, resulting in a lack of benefit from unsupervised exercise therapy.

Two small randomised trials of angioplasty vs. exercise showed the benefit of exercise in terms of walking distance. The Mimic Trial compared best medical treatment (BMT) and exercise to BMT, exercise and angioplasty [12]. In this study of 144 patients with stable claudication, they found a significant advantage for angioplasty above exercise and BMT alone, especially for patients with aortoiliac disease. These results strongly suggest a broad approach to the treatment of patients with claudication and combining exercise with angioplasty, if indicated, to gain the maximum benefit. However, in a direct comparison of supervised exercise, supervised exercise and angioplasty or angioplasty alone for superficial femoral artery disease, there was no difference in outcome, all treatment regimens giving the same benefit [13].

Generally, percutaneous angioplasty should be appealing for patients with intermittent claudication. It is relatively non-invasive, often can be done as a day case and significant complications occur in less than 3% and limb loss in around 0.3%. However, restenosis rates, particularly in more distal disease, are significant and can be as high as 40% for distal superficial femoral artery disease. If patients with short stenoses or occlusion in the proximal vessels only are treated, then about 50–60% of patients will be suitable. Stent placement after angioplasty may improve the initial technical success rates, but has not been demonstrated to improve clinical outcome.

Surgical reconstruction (bypass or common femoral endarterectomy) has been demonstrated to improve quality of life in patients with claudication. However, the risks of morbidity and mortality are significant. There are still a few patients with simple lesions who may be offered surgery. Usually, for some reason they will not be suitable for endovascular treatment or will have had multiple restenoses after angioplasty. However, the expectation of a good result should be high and the patient should be fully aware of the potential risks. It should be considered that surgery in this cohort of patients is for symptomatic improvement (walking distance) not for limb salvage, and so the risks of limb-threatening morbidity and mortality with surgery may outweigh the benefits.

Critical limb ischaemia (CLI)

A large number of patients who present with limb-threatening ischaemia have not had a previous history of claudication. They are often less mobile, so may not have precipitated any symptoms, but often other factors, such as infection, cause a sudden deterioration. For this reason it has proved difficult to accurately define CLI. The Inter-Society Consensus for the Management of Peripheral Arterial Disease (TASC II) suggests that a patient with persistent pain, ulcers or gangrene, considered to be due to proven arterial disease, should be considered to have CLI [3]. This definition is based on previous attempts to define the condition in the Trans-Atlantic Inter-Society Consensus (TASC) of 2000. The diagnosis is usually confirmed by a low ankle blood pressure (under 50 mmHg), but this is not always the case in some patient groups, e.g., for diabetes. The need to intervene in patients with CLI is obviously much greater as a significant proportion will deteriorate and face limb loss without revascularisation.

Patients with CLI face an enormous cardiovascular risk and 50% will be dead within 1 year of diagnosis. It is important to recognise, and when possible correct, any associated risk factors, as described above for patients with claudication. These patients with CLI also tend to be older and have significant comorbidities that need to be optimised.

Options for revascularisation include angioplasty or surgery. Conventional transluminal angioplasty has limited results for more distal disease, but the development of low profile catheters and stents for coronary artery work has improved outcomes. Subintimal angioplasty seems to have greater initial success, but the medium-term patency rates tend to be variable. However, in many patients even if the original angioplasty site reoccludes, ulcers have often healed and it seems the angioplasty worked long enough to achieve wound healing.

Surgical bypass

Surgical bypass can either be inflow procedures to the femoral artery, anatomical bypasses such as aortobifemoral bypass or extra-anatomical bypasses such as cross femoral bypass or axillo-femoral bypass. Distal bypass is technically demanding, but if carried out in experienced units can achieve excellent results. A meta-analysis of infrageniculate bypass in high-risk patients found limb salvage rates of over 78% at 5 years. The optimum bypass graft is autologous vein and if long saphenous vein is not available, excellent results can be obtained using arm vein, short saphenous vein or the deep veins. Although moderate results can be obtained, there is little role now for the use of prosthetic grafts below the knee due to the high risk of infection.

In patients selected for surgery, great care needs to be taken to identify the optimum run-off vessel and it is also important to carry out Duplex ultrasound scanning of the veins to ascertain if they will be suitable and to minimise the dissection required to harvest them. There is no clear advantage of *in situ* vs. reversed vein techniques and it is really dependant on the experience of the surgeon.

Up to 30% of vein bypass grafts will develop stenoses and if left, many will go onto occlude. It is not possible to detect these stenoses clinically and many patients are asymptomatic. Many units therefore carry out regular Duplex ultrasound surveillance of the grafts and correct any significant stenosis (greater than 50% or 3 times velocity shift across the narrowed segment). However, a randomised controlled study has brought this practice into question. Although the study found it was possible to detect stenoses, it found no difference in outcome between patients in surveillance and those simply followed up. As Duplex surveillance is time consuming and costly it was found not to be cost effective. Many units, however, continue to monitor these patients, arguing that there are other benefits, such as checking on risk factor , management and long-term outcomes.

There are a number of options available to revascularise a critically ischaemic limb. The TASC II document has classified lesion in the aortoiliac and femoropopliteal segment and reviewed the evidence for treatment options [3]. However, a randomised controlled study, the Bypass vs. Angioplasty in Severe Ischaemia of the Leg (BASIL) study compared surgery vs. angioplasty for the treatment of CLI and severe limb ischaemia [14]. This study found no difference in amputation free survival, which was 55% during the study period, between either treatment. There was also no difference in mortality, 3% and 5%, respectively, for angioplasty and surgery. However, although there was an initial 20% failure rate from angioplasty, length of stay in hospital was much shorter, making angioplasty more economical [14]. There are a number of important points that arise from this study. First, only 30% admitted to the units involved in the study were randomised, suggesting a large proportion were not revascularised. Also, 37% died during the study period, largely from cardiovascular disease, emphasising the high cardiovascular event rate in these patients. Few patients were made worse by angioplasty, suggesting that in most of these patients who are elderly and frail it is worth trying angioplasty initially as even if it does not succeed it will not prevent a surgical approach. That said, there is some suggestion that patients who undergo endovascular intervention initially, have worse outcomes if they then go on to require surgical bypass.

The purpose of the multi-disciplinary team is to decide upon the best treatment option for a particular patient, and often there will be a clear preferred option for endovascular or bypass surgery, based on the patient's history, comorbidities and imaging. These patients were not included in BASIL, as patients had to be equally suitable for endovascular and surgical intervention. BASIL 2 is currently underway, which will help to elicit what happens to those patients who are not deemed fit for randomisation to angioplasty or surgery and to investigate more long-term outcomes after intervention, aiming to definitively answer the question about whether endovascular or surgical intervention is the better treatment strategy in this cohort.

One group of patients in whom surgery is usually the optimum treatment are those with disease in the common femoral artery. Angioplasty here may put the profunda artery origin at risk and often these patients are treated by common femoral endarterectomy. There still remains some doubt over which is the optimum technique to revascularise the distal tissues in patients with diabetes, and further studies are needed to determine this. The role of surgical profundaplasty (usually an endarterectomy of the common femoral artery into the profunda artery with patch closure) remains contentious. If no other options are available, or a distal procedure is not appealing due to poor quality distal vessels, it is worth attempting.

Amputation

Amputation is the only option possible in some patients who have no options for revascularisation. Extensive infection may require urgent intervention. If the patient is very sick, then guillotine amputation of the infected tissue with subsequent conversion to formal amputation may be the best option. It will achieve control of sepsis and avoid infection of a definitive amputation stump. The patient can be returned to theatre when they are stable for conversion of the guillotine stump to the optimal formal amputation.

Primary amputation may also be required in patients in whom there is extensive tissue loss and no obvious method of revascularisation of the limb. Secondary amputation is required when a revascularisation attempt has failed to achieve tissue healing or relief of pain. Below-knee amputation has the advantage of greater mobility with a prosthesis due to preservation of the knee joint. However, the primary healing rate of below-knee amputations is approximately 80% compared to 90% with above-knee amputation.

Selection of amputation level can be difficult. The presence of a good femoral pulse together with a well developed profunda femoris artery is encouraging for a below-knee amputation. The quality of the tissues in the leg, previous wounds and the presence of sepsis and the general condition of the patient also make a major contribution to the decision at what level to amputate. The multi-disciplinary team should be involved pre-operatively, with input from the therapy team regarding the patient's mobility and options for prostheses aiding the decision about the level of amputation. The use of measurements such as $TcPO_2$ at the level of amputation has been found to be helpful by some units, but the general application of these techniques has not been widespread. Often the decision has to be made based on the clinical factors outlined above and the appearances of the tissues at the time of surgery.

Diabetic Vascular Disease

Diabetes affects more than 382 million people worldwide [15]. In recent epidemiological studies, it has been found that over 40% of patients presenting with PAD have diabetes and 20% of all hospital admissions for complications of diabetes are due to foot problems. An estimated 15% of patients with diabetes develop a foot ulcer every year, and 25% of people with diabetes will develop a foot ulcer during their lifetime [16].

The ultimate consequence of foot disease without adequate management is amputation and the relative risk of amputation, associated with all types of diabetes, is 13 times compared to that of a non-diabetic [17] with 1/5 of patients with a diabetic foot requiring amputation [18], which has a severe impact on quality of life and up to 80% mortality at 5 years. The diabetic foot places a huge burden not only on patients but also on healthcare systems, accounting for £639–£662 million of NHS expenditure [19]. It has been estimated that 85% of amputations could have been avoided with adequate care.

There are two main reasons why patients with diabetes are so prone to foot complications: neuropathy and ischaemia. Screening patients with diabetes is essential to detect early signs of neuropathy and PAD (Table 1). This can be simply done by the use of a 10-g monofilament test, peripheral pulse palpation and ankle blood pressure measurement. Patients who have any evidence of neuropathy or PAD should be given help and advice to detect problems early and seek help. There is encouraging evidence that a multi-disciplinary approach to diabetic foot complications can reduce major amputation rates and is highly cost effective.

Table 1.   Eight clinical features to look
for in the diabetic foot.

- Neuropathy
- Ischaemia
- Deformity
- Callus
- Swelling
- Skin breakdown/ulceration
- Infection/redness
- Necrosis

Neuropathy

1. Sensory neuropathy reduces the patient's ability to appreciate damage to the foot, such as rubbing of ill-fitting footwear. Thus small lesions, such as from ill-fitting shoes, are not appreciated at an early stage by the patient. Also, lack of proprioception means that when the patient is standing, subtle movements in posture that would normally offload pressure do not happen.

2. Motor neuropathy results in reduced power of the short flexor muscles of the foot. The resulting imbalance between these and the long extensors results in an 'intrinsic minus' foot with clawing of the toes and prominence of the metatarsal heads. Abnormal weight bearing on the metatarsal heads (combined with reduced sensory proprioception) causes tissue damage and ulceration (Fig. 3, Table 1).

3. Finally, autonomic neuropathy causes reduction in sweating and dry skin, which is more prone to cracking and damage. The failure of the autonomic system also has effects on the vasomotor tone in the skin circulation with abnormal arteriovenous shunting. All of these factors make the foot prone to damage and ulceration.

Ischaemia

Patients with diabetes have a four-fold increased risk of developing PAD and the resulting ischaemia is another factor predisposing the foot to injury and poor healing. Patients with diabetes and PAD have the greatest

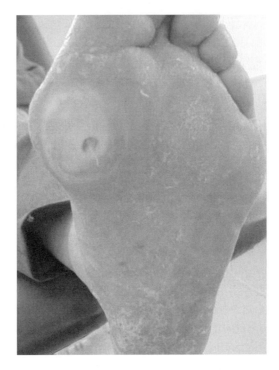

Figure 3.   Typical neuropathic foot ulcer. The ulcer is surrounded by a ring of keratinised skin.

risk of suffering an amputation. There are also abnormalities of the microcirculation such as thickening of the basement membrane, increased capillary permeability and increased platelet adherence, which reduce tissue perfusion.

It has been estimated that of patients with foot complications, approximately 10% will be due to ischaemia, 45–60% will be due to neuropathy and 25–45% will be a combination of the two (= neuro-ischaemia). However, the final common presenting factor is often infection. The immunosuppressive effect of hyperglycaemia predisposes the patient with damaged ischaemic tissue to infection, which can be extensive.

Management of the diabetic foot

The first-line treatment of a patient with a diabetic foot complication is to ensure that their diabetes is controlled, and this may require a sliding scale or correction of a keto acidosis. Ensuring good blood sugar control is of key importance in the peri-operative period and will aid wound healing.

Treatment of infection involves cultures and local wound swabs followed by intravenous antibiotics. Units should have agreed regimens with their microbiology team, which will cover the common causative agents such as staphylococcus aureus, streptococcus, pseudomonas and anaerobic bacteria. Superficial wound swabs may fail to identify the causative organism and aspiration of tissue fluid using a 10 mL syringe and a green needle is advocated by some groups to obtain more accurate deep tissue cultures. The extent of the infection is determined by careful inspection of the foot and palpation of the tissues. Tenderness or crepitus suggests extensive infection. Often infection of a digit will spread to the associated web space and infect the tissue between the metatarsals. This may only be apparent by a slight redness and tenderness over the dorsum of the foot. Plain X-rays should be undertaken. They may reveal osteomyelitis or gas in the tissues. Surgical drainage of any collection and removal of dead infected tissue should be undertaken within 24 h of admission, and further tissue sent for microbiological culture. Where infection is localised to one digit and the patient is systemically well, antibiotics may be sufficient in the emergency setting. If the patient is severely unwell with extensive infection, not responding to antibiotics, amputation may be required. Where amputation is required, and more than one digit is affected, there is limited evidence as to whether it is better to remove the affected digits or proceed to trans-metatarsal amputation.

Once the situation has been stabilised by the above, full assessment of the neurological and vascular status of the limb can be undertaken. The absence of pedal pulses together with a low ankle blood pressure indicate a high-risk foot. Further investigation, starting with a Duplex scan and probably including a CTA, should be obtained. Unless the foot shows signs of healing, revascularisation either by angioplasty or surgery should be performed.

Wounds on the foot should not be sutured but generally left to heal by secondary intention Attempting to suture the skin may reduce skin edge blood flow and trap infected material leading to abscess formation. Care should be taken to avoid oedema of the limb, and the patients should rest with their leg elevated for the first few days. The use of negative pressure wound therapy has transformed management of these patients. Although the precise way in which it works is not clearly understood, negative pressure therapy will remove excess tissue fluid, increase microcirculatory blood flow beneath the wound and reduce the wound size.

Response to negative pressure therapy is variable, and robust evidence for its clinical benefit and mechanism of action is lacking. NICE currently recommends its use only in the trial setting or as an attempt at limb salvage, and suggests further research is needed to evaluate its clinical effectiveness.

Patients can be mobilised early using total contact casts. A cast is placed on the lower limb with a window to allow inspection of any wound. These need to be expertly fitted as if there are abnormal areas of pressure the cast itself will cause damage.

Conclusion

PAD is a common problem and is strongly associated with cardiovascular risk factors and cardiovascular morbidity and mortality. Despite overwhelming evidence for the benefit of the treatment of cardiovascular risk factors, many patients remain undiagnosed and under-treated. Recent evidence has suggested that combining BMT, exercise and intervention has the best results for symptomatic disease. Endovascular treatments seem to have the same result as surgical treatments in term of limb salvage, but evidence for long-term outcomes is lacking. BASIL 2 trial is currently underway and may help to answer questions regarding the best intervention for those with CLI. The commonest cause of amputation is diabetes, the prevalence of which is increasing. Evidence shows that early detection of foot problems in diabetes and a multi-disciplinary approach to the problem can reduce amputation rates.

References

1. Leng GC, Lee AJ, Fowkes GR, Whiteman M, Dunbar J, Housley E, Ruckley VC. Incidence, natural history and cardiovascular events in symptomatic and asymptomatic peripheral arterial disease in the general population. *Int J Epidemiol* 1996;25:1172–1181.

2. Hirsch AT, Criqui MH, Treat-Jacobson D, Regensteiner JG, Crteager MA, Olin JW, Krook SH, Hunningake DB, Comerota AJ, Walsh ME, McDermott MM, Hiatt WR. Peripheral arterial disease detection, awareness and treatment in primary care. *JAMA* 2001;286:1317–1324.
3. Norgren L, Hiatt WR, Dormandy JA, Nehler MR, Harris KA, Fowkes FG. TASC II Working Group. Inter-Society Consensus for the Management of Peripheral Arterial Disease (TASC II). *J Vasc Surg* 2007;45(S):S5–67.
4. National Institute for Health and Clinical Excellence (NICE) Guideline, Lower-Limb Peripheral Arterial disease 2014. Available at: http://pathways.nice.org.uk/pathways/lower-limb-peripheral-arterial-disease #content=view-node%3Anodes-assessment-and-diagnosis&path=view%3A/pathways/lower-limb-peripheral-arterial-disease/lower-limb-peripheral-arterial-disease-overview.xml.
5. Nathan DM, Cleary PA, Backlund JY, Genuth SM, Lachin JM, Orchard TJ, Raskin P, Zinman B. Diabetes Control and Complications Trial/Epidemiology of Diabetes Interventions and Complications (DCCT/EDIC) Study Research Group. Intensive diabetes treatment and cardiovascular disease in patients with type diabetes. The diabetes control and complications trial, epidemiology of diabetes interventions and complications. *N Eng J Med* 2005; 353(25):2643–2653.
6. Kelly TN, Bazzano LA, Fonseca VA, Thethi TK, Reynolds K, He J. Systematic review: Glucose control and cardiovascular disease in Type 2 diabetes. *Ann Int Med* 2009;151(6):394–403.
7. Kannel WB. Skinner JJ Jr, Schwartz MJ, Shurtleff D. Intermittent claudication. Incidence in the Framingham Study. *Circulation* 1970;41(5):875–883.
8. Heart Protection Study Group Collaborative Group. MRC/BHF heart protection study of cholesterol lowering with simvastatin in 20,536 high-risk individuals: Randomised placebo controlled trial. *Lancet* 2002; 360(9326):7–22.
9. Yusuf S, Sleight P, Pogue J, Bosch J, Davies R, Dagenais G. The heart outcomes prevention evaluation study investigators. Effects of angiotensin-converting enzyme inhibitor, ramipril, on cardiovascular events in high-risk patients. *N Engl J Med* 2000;342(3):145–153.
10. Antithrombotic Trialists' Collaboration. Collaborative meta-analysis of randomised trials of antiplatelet therapy for the prevention of death, myocardial infarction, and stroke in high risk patients. *BMJ* 2002;324(7329): 71–86.
11. CAPRIE Steering Committee. A randomised, blinded, trial of clopidogrel versus aspirin in patients at risk of ischaemic events (CAPRIE). *Lancet* 1996;348(9038):1329–1339.

12. Greenhalgh RM Belch JJ Brown LC Gaines PA, Gao L, Reise JA, Thompson SG. Mimic Trial Participants. The adjuvant benefit of angioplasty in patients with mild to moderate intermittent claudication (MIMIC) managed by supervised exercise, smoking cessation advice and best medical therapy: Results from two randomised trials for stenotic emoro-popliteal and aortoiliac arterial disease. *Eur J Vasc Endovasc Surg* 2008;36(6):680–688.

13. Mazari FAK, Khan JA Carradice D, Samuel N, Abdul Rahman MNA, Gulati S, Lee HLD, Mehta TA, McCollum PT, Chetter IC. Randomized clinical trial of percutaneous transluminal angioplasty, supervised exercise and combined treatment for intermittent claudication due to femoropopliteal arterial disease. *Br J Surg* 2012;99:39–48.

14. Adam DJ, Beard JD, Cleveland T, Bell J, Bradbury AW, Forbes JF, Fowkes FG, Gillepsie I, Ruckley CV, Raab G, Storkey H; BASIL trial participants. Bypass Versus Angioplasty in Severe Ischaemia of the leg (BASIL): Multicentre, randomised controlled trial *Lancet* 2005;366(9501):1925–1934.

15. International Diabetes Federation. IDF diabetes atlas. 6th edition. Brussels (Belgium): International Diabetes Federation; 2013. Available at: http://www.idf.org/diabetesatlas.

16. Singh N, Armstrong DG, Lipsky BA. Preventing foot ulcers in patients with diabetes. *JAMA* 2005;293(2):217–228.

17. International Diabetes Federation Position Statement — The Diabetic Foot. Available at: http://www. idf.org/Position_statementsdiabetic_foot.

18. Lavery LA, Armstrong DG, Wunderlich RP, Mohler MJ, Wendel CS, Lipsky BA. Risk factors for foot infections in individuals with diabetes. *Diabetes Care* 2006;29(6):1288–1293.

19. Kerr M. Foot Care for People with Diabetes: The Economic Case for Change. NHS Diabetes, 2012. Available at: http://www.diabetes.org.uk/Documents/nhs-diabetes/footcare/footcare-for-people-with-diabetes.pdf.

Chapter 6

Basic Endovascular Skills

Craig Nesbitt, Sebastian Mafeld and Colin Nice

Key Points

- Endovascular practice involves three key elements:
  - **Safe Access:** How to get into a blood vessel safely. Ultrasound-guided Seldinger technique allows a safe approach to the arterial system. The common femoral is the most frequently used access site, but alternative access approaches like the brachial, popliteal, radial and tibiopedal also have benefits.
  - **Safe Navigation:** An understanding of the tools which can be used inside blood vessels. Guidewires have a central core and outer covering which determine their behaviour. Catheters are sized in French (Fr) which refers to their outer diameter. They come in a range of lengths and sizes and allow injection of contrast and a way to steer and support the guidewire.
  - **Safe Closure:** How to safely close the vessel at the end of a procedure. Manual compression of a vessel is a safe way to close a vessel but closure devices can produce quicker haemostasis and earlier ambulation. Vascular access up to 24Fr can also be closed percutaneously with pre-deployed suture mediated devices.

Safe Arterial Access and Closure

Safe arterial access is the critical starting point to any endovascular procedure. It requires three key components:

1. Seldinger needle — typically 18GA hollow needle, 7 cm in length.
2. J-Tip 0.035" guidewire — typically a steel wire coated with polytetrafluoroethylene (PTFE).
3. Sheath/dilator — to be passed over the guidewire.

A variety of sites can be used for vascular access, but the most common approach in day-to-day practice is via the common femoral artery (CFA). Regardless of access location, the approach (modified Seldinger technique) is the same. The technique involves the following key steps:

1. Identify a safe location for vessel puncture.
2. Angle the access needle 45° to the skin and advance the needle through the skin into the vessel.
3. Pulsatile flow through the needle should be identified to confirm the needle is safely inside the vessel lumen.
4. Advance the guidewire through the access needle.
5. Remove the needle and advance the sheath/dilator over the wire and into the vessel.

Common Femoral Artery

The CFA is a frequently used access site. It lies relatively superficially in the groin making it accessible and it may also be compressed against the underlying bone to achieve haemostasis at the end of the procedure. Access to the CFA can be in a retrograde (against direction of blood flow) or antegrade (with direction of blood flow) approach. A retrograde approach is used for iliac, aortic and visceral intervention while an antegrade approach is useful when the target lesion is in the SFA, popliteal or tibial vessels.

There are three main approaches to CFA access:

- *Ultrasound Guided Access* — Being able to directly visualise the CFA and its bifurcation and guide a Seldinger needle means the optimum site for access can be identified and hazards such as heavily calcified atherosclerotic plaques can be avoided. For ultrasound-guided access, the following approach is used:

- o Scan the access site to ensure it is patent and plan patient positioning.
- o Confirm probe is orientated correctly (gently tap on edge).
- o Transverse scan (normal veins will compress with light pressure).
- o Optimise US settings (depth, gain, focal zone).
- o Longitudinal scan and identify bifurcation and vessel plaque or calcification.
- o Plan optimal vessel entry (and closure) site.

- *Manual Palpation* — Identify the mid-inguinal point and then palpate to find the point of maximum pulsation (most superficial part) of the CFA. The Seldinger needle is advanced at 45° to the skin until it reaches the artery. At this point the arterial pulsation should be transmitted through the needle and the needle is advanced into the vessel until pulsatile flow is obtained.

  The mid-inguinal point has been shown to have a degree of reliability as a landmark for the CFA [1]. Note, however, the inguinal skin crease is an unreliable marker for the CFA.

- *Fluoroscopic Guidance* — A Seldinger needle (radiopaque) can be aimed using fluoroscopic guidance at the medial aspect of the mid femoral head where the CFA should be encountered. In patients with calcified vessels, the radiopaque vessel calcification can act as a target for the needle (although calcification may mean that this is not the best site for puncture!).

Troubleshooting

Why is it important to have pulsatile flow through the Seldinger needle prior to inserting a guidewire?

The needle has a bevelled edge and when advancing into the vessel will initially be partially luminal and partially within the vessel wall. If at this point the wire is advanced, it could enter into the vessel wall and cause a dissection.

After puncturing the CFA, the needle moved and is now no longer within the vessel. Can I repuncture directly?

No, typically 2–3 min of manual compression should be applied following failed access of the CFA with a Seldinger needle. This is to ensure adequate haemostasis.

What if my Seldinger needle is too short to reach the vessel?

This can be a problem in patients with high BMIs, instead of the standard 7 cm length Seldinger needle, a longer (9 cm) needle can be used.

Can I use a hydrophilic "slippy" guidewire through a Seldinger needle?

No, the hydrophilic coating from a slippy guidewire can get stripped off at the needle edge and embolise.

In patients with a high BMI or very scarred groins sometimes the sheath doesn't pass easily over a wire and can kink in the skin, is there anything I can do to avoid this?

Insert the J-tipped guidewire into the vessel, then instead of advancing a sheath, a 4Fr dilator may advance easier into the vessel. Then the wire can be withdrawn and exchanged for a stiff wire, e.g., Amplatz super stiff guidewire. Then the dilator can be withdrawn and the sheath will frequently pass easier over the extra support from the stiffer guidewire. Manual compression of the soft tissues and maintaining good guidewire tension will minimise the chances of the dilator or sheath looping subcutaneously.

On antegrade CFA access, what if the wire enters the profunda femoris artery, how can I redirect this into the SFA?

Provided that the puncture is above the femoral bifurcation, then an angled catheter can be inserted and contrast injected to identify the SFA origin (an ipsilateral oblique view and roadmapping are helpful). The J guidewire is exchanged for a hydrophilic guidewire which may then be redirected down the SFA instead.

Safe closure of the CFA

Once an endovascular procedure has been completed, safe closure of the vessel is critical for haemostasis. The skin incision does not reflect the entry point into a vessel, therefore when removing a sheath, compression over the skin incision may not provide adequate haemostasis. When removing the sheath, a finger should be placed above and below the sheath and compression applied. Typically for access with sizes up to 6Fr, a 10–15 min manual compression is enough to achieve haemostasis. Manual compression can be effectively applied to even larger access sites but may require longer compression times.

If manual compression has been used as a method of haemostasis, the following post-procedure observations are recommended:

Bed rest — 4 h of which the first 2 h lying flat.
Pulse, blood pressure and checking of the groin every 15 min for the first 2 h then every 30 min thereafter for a total of 6 h.
Patient advice should be given that if during the period of observation they perform any activity that may increase intra-abdominal pressure e.g., coughing/sneezing then they should apply gentle pressure to the puncture site and contact staff immediately if any bleeding or swelling is identified.

Closure devices

Closure devices have the added benefit of earlier ambulation time for patients. This must be balanced against the added cost of the device and expertise required for successful deployment. Three of the most common vascular closure devices licensed for CFA closure are summarised below. These are licensed for closure of up to 6Fr (Starclose) and (8Fr for Angio-seal).

Manufacturer	Device name	Method of closure
Abbott Vascular (Illinois, USA)	StarClose SE	Extravascular nitinol clip
Cordis (California, USA)	ExoSeal	Extravascular bio-absorbable Polyglycolic acid (PGA) plug
Terumo Medical (Tokyo, Japan)	Angio-Seal	Anchored extravascular collagen plug

Complications of common femoral artery access

With correct CFA access, the chances of complications are reduced. Minor bleeding or haematoma may occur in as many as 6–10% of cases [2] and can normally be managed conservatively.

Retroperitoneal Haematoma: This can be life threatening. If bleeding occurs into the retroperitoneal space it may not be readily identified by clinical examination so imaging with computed tomography or angiography is essential. It is important to note that ultrasound cannot be used to exclude retroperitoneal haemorrhage.

Pseudoaneurysm Formation: A pseudoaneurysm is a hole in the vessel wall secondary to a defect in the intima/media and may only be contained by the adventitia. Sometimes, all three walls of the vessel may be disrupted and only contained by the surrounding soft tissues.

A pseudoaneurysm is at the risk of rupture and therefore may require treatment. Small pseudoaneurysms (<1 cm) often resolve spontaneously but larger pseudoaneurysms should be treated. Historically, ultrasound-guided compression was used but this is uncomfortable for both the patient and operator, and now first line management is the ultrasound-guided injection of thrombin. This has a high technical success rate but if thrombin injection fails, then surgical repair should be considered.

Damage to Adjacent Vessels: The deep circumflex iliac and the inferior epigastric arteries arise from the very distal external iliac artery and their close proximity to the CFA leaves them vulnerable to damage.

Other Complications: Arteriovenous fistula formation occurs in <1% of cases but is rarely symptomatic and can be treated by surgical or endovascular means [3]. Arterial dissection and occlusion also occur very infrequently <1% [2,3].

Large Arterial Access and Closure

Large arterial access up to 24Fr can be required for treatment of the thoracic and abdominal aorta. While traditionally this has been done using a femoral cut down, more recently, percutaneous pEVAR and pTEVAR have gained popularity. This involves the pre-deployment of sutures into the vessel which are tightened at the end of the procedure. Data support a high technical success rate for pEVAR using pre-deployment of suitable closure devices [4]. The two devices most commonly used for percutaneous large vessel access are as follows:

ProStar XL — Percutaneous Vascular Surgical System (Abbott Vascular):

This device deploys two braided polyester sutures into the vessel which can be tightened at the end of a procedure. It is able to close holes between 8.5Fr and 24Fr, but its licensing varies between countries.

Perclose ProGlide Suture-Mediated Closure System (Abbott Vascular):

This device deploys a single monofilament polypropylene suture. It is licensed to close 5–21Fr holes, but any hole greater that 8Fr requires two sutures to be deployed according to the manufacturer's guidance.

Brachial Artery Access

Access to the brachial artery offers a more favourable approach to caudally orientated visceral vessels. It also offers an alternative access site in cases of severe aortoiliac disease where femoral access is not achievable. As the brachial artery is an end artery, damage to this vessel can result in limb threatening ischaemia.

Traditional teaching for Brachial access suggested a high brachial artery approach, however, this is no longer recommended for the same reason that axillary access has largely been abandoned; haematoma from a high brachial or axillary puncture can spread within a tough fibrous space called the medial brachial fascial compartment and result in compression of the median and ulnar nerves [5,6]. Therefore, the current accepted technique for brachial artery access is with a "low" approach in the antecubital fossa.

The modified Seldinger technique also applies to the brachial artery. Some operators suggest using a micropuncture set (21GA needle and 0.018" guidewire) to initially access the brachial artery. The brachial artery can frequently be palpated as it passes superficially in the antecubital fossa therefore access with manual palpation and with ultrasound have both been described.

Access to the left brachial artery is usually preferred as the operator's catheters/guidewires are only cross one arch vessel (left subclavian artery).

Vessel thrombosis, brachial pseudoaneurysm formation, dissection and haematoma formation along with median nerve injury are potential major complications.

Manual compression (10–20 min) is normally enough to achieve adequate haemostasis of a low brachial artery puncture.

Radial Artery Access

Radial artery access has been popularised by cardiologists for percutaneous coronary intervention (PCI) and is associated with less bleeding and transfusion risk than femoral arterial access [7]. More recently, interventional radiologists have used radial arterial access for non-coronary interventions with a high degree of success [8].

The hand's dual blood supply via the radial and ulnar arteries means that the damage to the radial artery should not risk the hand provided there is a patent ulnopalmar arch. Therefore, performing a modified Allen's test (Barbeau test) prior to accessing the radial artery is useful to ensure ulnopalmar patency [9].

Pre-procedural topical nitroglycerin and lidocaine followed by intra-arterial injection of nitrates, calcium channel blockers and heparin has been suggested as an approach to maximise vessel diameter and reduce chance of spasm [9]. Vessel access can be performed with manual palpation or ultrasound guidance using a 21GA Seldinger needle followed by insertion of an 0.018" wire. Sheath sizes up to 5Fr and 6Fr sheaths are most commonly used. For peripheral intervention from a radial approach, it is important to ensure adequate device length prior to commencing a procedure.

Radial artery haemostasis should be performed using non-occlusive pressure. This is based on the finding from a study which showed that non-occlusive pressure (patent haemostasis) reduced that chance of radial artery occlusion compared with occlusive radial artery compression [10]. Therefore, rather than manually compressing the radial artery, a wristband compression device with a manually adjustable inflatable component across the radial artery is frequently used. This can be inflated to a pressure enough to provide haemostasis but allowing for the radial pulse to be palpable distally [9].

Retrograde Popliteal and TibioPedal Access

This is a frequently talked about access approach, but less commonly used in day-to-day practice. In critical limb ischaemia with disease involving the femoro-politeal or below the knee vessels, an antegrade CFA approach is most commonly chosen. When this fails, a retrograde approach via the popliteal or tibiopedal vessels can be utilised to successfully cross a lesion.

Popliteal access

The popliteal artery can be accessed from a retrograde approach to treat ilio-femoropopliteal lesions or an antegrade approach to treat occlusions below the knee. The popliteal vein is often overlying the artery when approaching from the popliteal fossa, therefore oblique angulation of the access needle is sometimes required. The use of a micropuncture set can be useful for popliteal access to minimise the risk of damage to surrounding structures. Both ultrasound and fluoroscopic guided access have been described. When performing retrograde popliteal access, once the wire has crossed the lesion, it can be retrieved with a snare from the ipsilateral groin and then intervention continued from an ipsilateral antegrade CFA approach.

For adequate haemostasis following a popliteal puncture, manual compression (7–10 min) followed by compression bandaging has been suggested [11]. Off label use of a nitinol extravascular clip closure device has also been described [12].

One of the larger series of popliteal access (174 patients) demonstrated a high technical success rate and puncture related complication rate of 4.3% [13]. Similar to risks at other access site, complications of the popliteal artery access can include; haematomas, AV-fistula formation, arterial occlusion and distal embolisation [14].

Retrograde TibioPedal Access

The anterior tibial, posterior tibial and peroneal arteries are all potential targets for retrograde access. These vessels are often small and heavily diseased therefore the use of a micropuncture access kit is essential. Depending on the desired target vessel, proper foot positioning can be used to facilitate access [15]:

- plantar flexion for the dorsalis pedis and anterior tibial artery;
- foot inversion when accessing the distal peroneal artery in the leg;
- foot eversion or dorsiflexion for access to the posterior tibial artery.

Because the tibiopedal vessels are often heavily diseased and calcified, this calcification may be readily visible on fluoroscopy allows for fluoroscopically guided access. Alternatively, ultrasound-guided access can be performed.

Due to the small calibre of the tibiopedal vessels, typical sheath sizes needed for lower limb intervention (5Fr, 6Fr) cannot be advanced safely. Therefore, the main purpose of tibiopedal access is to cross the lesion retrogradely and then retrieve the wire through the ipsilateral groin and then continue the intervention from an antegrade approach. The tibiopedal access is then removed and light manual compression applied for approximately 5 min to achieve haemostasis [16].

Safe Navigation

Safe navigation of the arterial and venous system requires the same basic equipment, guidewires and catheters.

- ### Guidewires

Guidewires are used for gaining access to target vessels, crossing lesions and supporting balloon and stent delivery. The three basic components of guidewire design are its central core, outer covering and tip.

1. **Central Core:**
   1.1. *Material*: This affects the wire's flexibility, torque and trackability. Modern stainless steel wires provide good support and

torque but are susceptible to bending. Nitinol is a flexible and kink-resistant alternative but provides less tensile strength. Hybrid wires with stainless steel shafts and nitinol tips are a useful combination.

1.2. *Taper*: This describes how a wire's core tapers towards the tip. Gradual/longer tapers allow the wire to track around tortuous vessels more easily but provide less support in short distances compared to short tapers [17].

2. **Outer Covering:** The material covering the central core influences the guidewire's performance. A coiled covering as seen in the standard J-wire provides maximum tactile feedback. Polymer or plastic coverings create less friction resulting in enhanced tracking and lesion crossing capabilities. Some wires utilise a hybrid design with a polymer covered shaft and coiled tip. Hydrophobic coverings such as silicone and teflon repel water reduce wire friction and provide good tactile feedback, useful for parking and anchoring across lesions as they are less likely to slip out of the vessel. Hydrophilic coatings require activation with water to create a gel-like surface allowing the wires to glide through tortuous vessels. Their enhanced trackability comes at the expense of reduced tactile feedback and thus they are more prone to perforation and dissection.

3. **Tip:**

   3.1. *Tip-load*: A 1-piece core-to-tip wire provides a greater tip-load resulting in enhanced transmission of force, steerability and improves tactile feedback. A 2-piece (shaping ribbon) core does not reach the tip providing a floppy atraumatic end to the wire.

   3.2. *Tip morphology*: Straight and small angled tips enhance penetration. A double bend improves steerability and J tips are relatively atraumatic and thus ideal for subintimal lesion crossing.

4. **Diameter:** Wires are sized according to their functional diameter *in* inches: 0.014, 0.018, 0.035 are the most common. Smaller wires are more flexible and can be used for navigating a tortuous vessel, a larger diameter wire has more torque and support and can straighten a vessel helping sheaths and catheters to track over.

Table 1.   *Angio-speak*: Guidewire phraseology.

Term	Explanation
Steerability	Ability of a guide wire tip to be delivered to the desired position in a vessel
Support/trackability	Ability to advance balloon catheters/other devices on guidewire
Torque	Ability to transmit rotational forces from the operators hand to the tip
Tactile feedback	"Feel" of the wire tip's behaviour, as perceived by the operator
Tip load	Force needed to bend a wire when exerted on a straight guide wire tip, at 1 cm from the tip

Table 2.   Commonly used guidewires.

Wire	Characteristics	Common uses
Standard J-shape	Low support wire with atraumatic J-tip	Seldinger access, navigating the aorta
Glidewire AKA "slippy wire"	Hydrophilic coating	Crossing lesions, navigating tortuous vessels
Bentson	Outer coil around a stainless steel core. Floppy distal tip	Arterial access, basic arterial navigation
Amplatz	Supportive but with a flexible tip (1 cm or 7 cm versions)	EVAR with little tortuosity
Lunderquist	Very high support	Useful in EVAR where maximum support is required

5. **Length:** In general, wires come in standard (145 cm) and exchange lengths (260 cm or longer). A longer wire permits more distal access and catheter exchange without losing distal position. It is important to consider wire length before crossing a difficult lesion (see Tables 1 and 2).

Guidewire length required = Length inside patient to cross lesion
+ length of delivery system
+ a small margin.

Catheters

Endovascular catheters are sized according to their overall length (cm) and diameter, which is measured in *French* (*Fr*) (equal to 0.33 mm). Catheter French size refers to the *outer* diameter of the catheter.

Catheters come in a range of sizes, lengths and shapes. A catheter allows the delivery or radiopaque contrast and has an angle designed to select a target vessel (see Fig. 1).

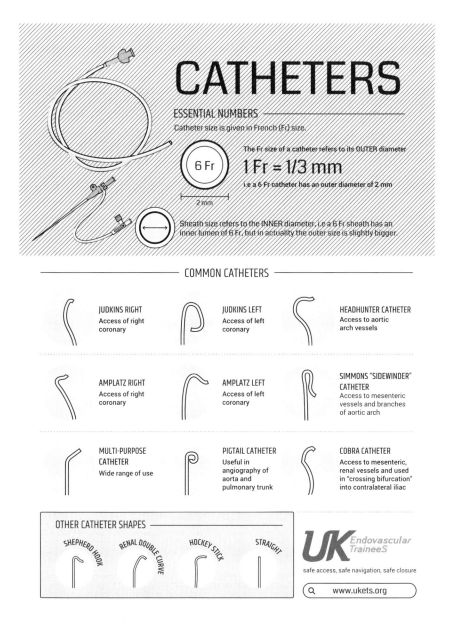

Figure 1.   Catheters (reproduced with permission from the UK Endovascular Trainees).

Catheter length is also important, shorter lengths (50 cm) are optimal for retrograde iliac work, medium lengths (65 cm) for abdominal visceral work and longer lengths (100–125 cm) for the thoracic aorta and its branches.

Catheter design

1. **Surface:** Coatings have a range of properties including friction reducing, antimicrobial, antithrombogenic.
2. **Outer layer:** This affects the catheters softness/pliability. Polyurethane tracks the wire more easily whereas nylon is stiffer and can tolerate higher pressures making them ideal for diagnostic angiography.
3. **Reinforcement:** Some catheters have a wire-braided layer in their wall which enhances the catheter torque.
4. **Tip:** Tip design varies from simple straight to complex curve.

Basic endovascular catheter practical tips for safe practice

1. Although rounded tips are less traumatic, catheters should not be advanced unless over a wire to prevent trauma including dissection and dislodging micro-emboli.
2. Always flush catheters with heparinised saline to prevent thrombus formation.
3. Before contrast injection, always aspirate on the catheter to remove any air bubbles and also to reconfirm intra-luminal position.
4. A small volume of hand-injected contrast is useful for again reconfirming position prior to larger volumes and higher flow rates of contrast.
5. Always remove catheters over a suitable guidewire to again prevent catheters traumatising the vessel wall or knotting.

Balloons

The principle of the angioplasty balloon catheter is to exert a radial force on the luminal surface of a vessel to treat occlusive disease. As the balloon is inflated, occlusive plaque is ruptured, the plaque is compressed

Table 3. *Angio-speak:* Angioplasty phraseology.

Term	Explanation
Nominal pressure	Pressure (in ATM) required for balloon to reach its labelled diameter
Rated burst pressure	Pressure at which 99.9% of balloons will survive (with 95% confidence)
A 5 × 4 balloon	A 5 mm diameter, 4 cm long angioplasty balloon.

and the artery is overstretched leading inevitably to a degree of dissection which is often visible on completion angiographic images. In a sense, angioplasty is controlled vessel injury. These dissections will almost always heal without further treatment (see Table 3).

Sizing

Balloons are available in a range of diameters and lengths. They pass over a guidewire and through an access sheath. On the outer packaging, the balloon's diameter when fully inflated (mm) is displayed alongside the balloons length (cm) which is the distance between the radiopaque markers.

The balloons are packaged fully deflated and once inflated will never quite deflate to their original profile and can be difficult to remove through the sheath or indeed readvance into a lesion.

Clinical note — Minimise the length of the balloon to minimise the damage to healthy "normal" vessel which can incite neointimal hyperplasia.

Compliance

1. Compliance is the ability of the balloon to increase in size/stretch as the pressure is increased. Two therapeutic balloon types exist:
   (i) *Semi-compliant*: These are the balloon catheters used for most therapeutic interventions. Made from polyolefin copolymer (POC), which is a softer material enabling good trackability, these balloons expand as the pressure is increased and it is often possible

to see wasting of the balloon around a stenotic lesion during inflation. They give the operator more control over dilatation of stenotic lesions compared to non-compliant balloons but can cause more dissection as the rate of inflation is quicker and in resistant lesions they will often over dilate into areas of less resistance (termed dog-boning).

(ii) *Non-compliant*: Constructed of polyethylene terephthalate (PET), a non-compliant balloon will have no appreciable change in diameter once nominal pressure is achieved even with further increases in pressure. This ensures greater force is exerted against a lesion. The walls of the balloon are generally thicker making them less trackable through a lesion but they are suitable for hard calcified or resistant lesions.

Delivery Systems

Balloon catheters have two separate lumens (analogous to a urethral catheter), one lumen accommodates the guidewire and the other dilates the balloon.

They come in two basic delivery systems with the fundamental difference being the amount of guidewire that is incorporated inside the catheter.

1. *Over the wire*: Continuous guidewire support providing enhanced control and pushability — is this the most commonly used system.
2. *Rapid exchange (monorail)*: Allow quick balloon exchanges that can be exchanged without the need for an assistant. They are more practical for simple cases where wire support is not needed.

Drug eluting balloons (DEB)

Drug eluting balloons are coated with the antiproliferative agent paclitaxel which inhibits neointimal growth and migration of vascular smooth muscle cells thus reducing rates of restenosis. Paclitaxel is bound to the balloon's outer surface with a combination with different hydrophilic excipients which facilitate the rapid transfer of the drug from the balloon to the arterial wall [5].

Evidence has shown the superiority of DEB vs. standard balloons for target lesion revascularisation and lesion restenosis rates in infra-inguinal and infra-popliteal lesions. Yet, to date, there is no strong evidence that DEB affects clinical endpoints such as amputation rates, wound healing or mortality.

Stents

Stents are supportive frameworks which apply radial force to diseased arteries and promote vessel remodelling. Most are made of stainless steel or nitinol, a nickel-titanium alloy with the ability to regain its manufactured shape once deployed.

Stent deployment is by two basic mechanisms:

1. *Balloon expandable stents* are securely mounted on a balloon angioplasty catheter by the manufacturer and deployed by pressure regulated balloon inflation. Advantages include their greater radial force and reliable accurate placement. Care must be taken when introducing balloon mounted stents through arterial sheaths and tight stenoses to prevent stent dislodgement.
2. *Self-expanding stents* are constrained by a low profile sheath and are deployed when the covering sheath is withdrawn. They apply less radial force than balloon expandable stents and may require post-dilation. Some earlier versions shortened significantly upon deployment which hindered precise placement. Current devices are much less prone to this.

Stent grafts

Stent grafts, also referred to as covered stents, consist of a fabric covering (Dacron or PTFE) applied to a stent. This increases the profile of the device and stent grafts require larger calibre arterial access than uncovered stents of the same diameter. Stent grafts allow endovascular treatment of arterial haemorrhage and exclusion of aneurysms whilst maintaining perfusion of the distal vascular bed.

Several case series describing stent graft treatment of long SFA lesions (mainly occlusions) suggest similar patency rates to prosthetic

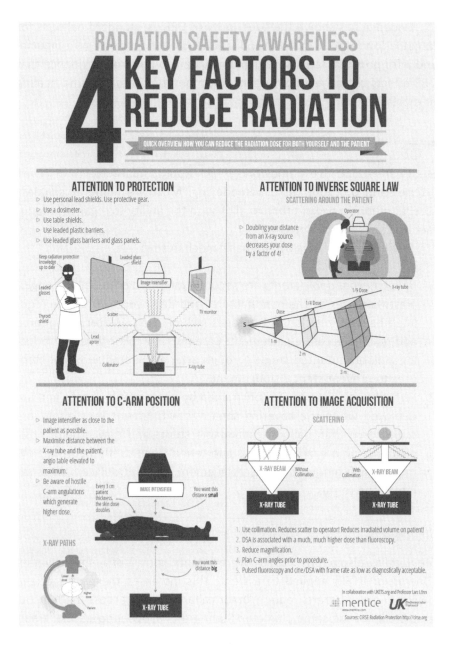

Figure 2.   Radiation Safety Awareness (reproduced with permission from the UK Endovascular Trainees) UKETS.org.

femoropopliteal bypass procedures. Great care must be taken to avoid covering the origin of profunda with the stent graft proximally. The distal extent of any stenting procedure must also be very carefully considered so that future surgical options are not compromised (i.e., conversion of an above knee femoropopliteal bypass into a below knee femoropopliteal or femorotibial bypass).

Radiation Safety

It is important to note that endovascular procedures take place under X-ray guidance thereby exposing the operator and patient to radiation. Whilst not exhaustive, we provide four key tips to enhance radiation safety (Fig. 2).

References

1. Hunt JA, Harris JP. Is the mid-inguinal point an accurate landmark for the common femoral artery in vascular patients? *Aust N Z J Surg* 1996;66(1): 43–45.
2. Rajebi H, Rajebi MR. Optimizing common femoral artery access. *Tech Vasc Interv Radiol* 2015;18(2):76–81.
3. Stone PA, Campbell JE. Complications related to femoral artery access for transcatheter procedures. *Vasc Endovas Surg* 2012;46(8):617–623.
4. Pratesi G, Barbante M, Pulli R, Fargion A, Dorigo W, Bisceglie R *et al.* Italian percutaneous EVAR (IPER) registry: Outcomes of 2381 percutaneous femoral access sites' closure for aortic stent-graft. *J Cardiovasc Surg (Torino)* 2015;56(6):889–898.
5. Tsao BE, Wilbourn AJ. The medial brachial fascial compartment syndrome following axillary arteriography. *Neurology* 2003;61(8):1037–1041.
6. Steve Lee K, Sos TA. Brachial artery access. *Tech Vasc Interv Radiol* 2015;18(2):87–92.
7. Bertrand OF, Bélisle P, Joyal D, Costerousse O, Rao SV, Jolly SS *et al.* Comparison of transradial and femoral approaches for percutaneous coronary interventions: A systematic review and hierarchical Bayesian meta-analysis. *Am Heart J* 2012;163(4):632–648.
8. Posham R, Biederman DM, Patel RS, Kim E, Tabori NE, Nowakowski FS *et al.* Transradial approach for noncoronary interventions: A single-center review

of safety and feasibility in the first 1,500 cases. *J Vasc Interv Radiol JVIR* 2016;27(2):159–166.

9. Fischman AM, Swinburne NC, Patel RS. A Technical guide describing the use of transradial access technique for endovascular interventions. *Tech Vasc Interv Radiol* 2015;18(2):58–65.

10. Pancholy S, Coppola J, Patel T, Roke-Thomas M. Prevention of radial artery occlusion — Patent hemostasis evaluation trial (PROPHET study): A randomized comparison of traditional versus patency documented hemostasis after transradial catheterization. *Catheter Cardiovasc Interv* 2008;72(3):335–340.

11. Brountzos EN, Moulakakis KG, Avgerinos ED, Dalainas I, Giannakopoulos TG, Kakisis J *et al.* Retrograde transpopliteal approach of iliofemoral lesions. *Vasc Endovas Surg* 2011;45(7):646–650.

12. Noory E, Rastan A, Sixt S, Schwarzwälder U, Leppännen O, Schwarz T *et al.* Arterial puncture closure using a clip device after transpopliteal retrograde approach for recanalization of the superficial femoral artery. *J Endovasc Ther Off J Int Soc Endovasc Spec* 2008;15(3):310–314.

13. Yilmaz S, Sindel T, Lüleci E. Ultrasound-guided retrograde popliteal artery catheterization: experience in 174 consecutive patients. *J Endovasc Ther Off J Int Soc Endovasc Spec* 2005;12(6):714–722.

14. Ye M, Zhang H, Huang X, Shi Y, Yao Q, Zhang L *et al.* Retrograde popliteal approach for challenging occlusions of the femoral-popliteal arteries. *J Vasc Surg* 2013;58(1):84–89.

15. El-Sayed HF. Retrograde pedal/tibial artery access for treatment of infragenicular arterial occlusive disease. *Methodist DeBakey Cardiovasc J* 2013; 9(2):73–78.

16. Sabri SS, Hendricks N, Stone J, Tracci MC, Matsumoto AH, Angle JF. Retrograde pedal access technique for revascularization of infrainguinal arterial occlusive disease. *J Vasc Interv Radiol* 2015;26(1):29–38.

17. Walker C. Endovascular Today — Guidewire Selection for Peripheral Vascular Interventions [Internet]. Endovascular Today. [cited 2017 May 20]. Available at: http://evtoday.com/2013/05/guidewire-selection-for-peripheral-vascular-interventions/.

Chapter 7

Endovascular and Surgical Options for Peripheral Revascularisation

Colin Nice

Key Points

- Risk factor optimisation and best medical therapy are the standard of care for all patients.
- Severe acute ischaemia is best managed with surgery, there is a role for thrombolysis in less severe cases.
- Thrombolysis requires intensive monitoring to identify and manage complications.
- Surgical or endovascular revascularisation is appropriate for patients with limiting claudication or critical limb ischaemia.
- Non-invasive imaging should be used for procedural planning.
- Bypass grafts with autologous vein produce the best long-term patency rates.
- Endovascular procedures have lower mortality and morbidity rates than the equivalent surgery.
- Stents and stent grafts improve endovascular results and are important for managing complications.

- Patient fitness, comorbidity and preference are as important as lesion characteristics in informing revascularisation decisions.
- Multi-disciplinary teams are best placed to manage individual patients in this rapidly evolving field.

Background

Many patients with peripheral arterial disease (PAD) do not require any revascularisation procedure. Identification and management of modifiable risk factors is effective in reducing the excess risk of cardiovascular mortality and preventing acute limb ischaemia (ALI) due to disease progression. Supervised exercise programmes benefit those with intermittent claudication, a Cochrane review of randomised trials in patients with stable intermittent claudication suggested an improvement in walking distance of 150% with a regime of three sessions per week of walking to near maximum pain [1].

Surgical and endovascular revascularisation procedures produce substantial additional benefits when proficiently performed upon carefully selected and prepared patients.

Treatment strategies addressing the differing aetiologies of chronic PAD and ALI determine the urgency, nature and effectiveness of attempted revascularisation.

Acute Limb Ischaemia

ALI may be due to arterial occlusion arising from *in situ* thrombosis of established atheromatous plaques or embolisation from remote sites. The majority of emboli are cardiogenic, resulting from atrial fibrillation or mural thrombus, complicating myocardial infarction. Aortic and popliteal aneurysms are other important causes and these should be sought with clinical examination and imaging.

Treatment decisions are often based on clinical assessment, complemented by hand-held Doppler ultrasound examination, due to clinical urgency or limited availability of other imaging modalities.

Basic measures

Immediately following the diagnosis of ALI, anticoagulation with intravenous heparin should be commenced to prevent thrombus propagation. Daily assessment of APTT ratio is required with a target ratio of 2 (range 1.5–2.5) considered optimal. This should be monitored at least daily and dose adjustments made according to local protocols. Intravenous fluid rehydration may be needed prior to and following endovascular revascularisation to minimise the risk of contrast induced nephropathy (CIN).

Analgesia

ALI causes severe pain. Lying flat may exacerbate symptoms and many patients are only able to tolerate a dependent limb position. Effective analgesia is needed to relieve this and also to permit the patient to lie still enough to allow surgical or endovascular procedures performed under local anaesthetic. Regional blocks of the femoral and sciatic nerve are a promising technique which alleviate ischaemic pain without the need for epidural or general anaesthetic [2].

Embolectomy

Surgical exposure and control of the common femoral artery can often be performed under local anaesthetic. Removal of emboli with balloon catheters may effectively restore limb perfusion.

Chances of technical success are greatest with larger calibre arteries and cardiogenic emboli where the likelihood of an associated stenosis or occlusion is lower. Embolectomy is effective for supra-inguinal occlusive emboli as absence of a femoral pulse hinders vascular access for catheter delivered thrombolysis. Selective catheterisation and embolectomy of below knee vessels may prove impossible without fluoroscopic imaging and guidewire compatible embolectomy catheters.

Completion angiographic appearances indicate technical success, identify associated underlying lesions and determine the need for adjunctive procedures such as thrombolysis or angioplasty.

Following successful embolectomy, anticoagulation decreases the risk of recurrent embolisation, particularly in those with atrial fibrillation. A target INR of 2.5 (range 2–3) is optimal.

If femoral embolectomy is unsuccessful, then either on-table thrombolysis or surgical exploration of the distal popliteal artery or of the anterior tibial artery and tibio-peroneal trunk may be required.

Thrombolysis

Pharmacological thrombus dissolution is used to treat embolic occlusions or resolve *in situ* thrombosis and reveal the underlying stenotic lesions. In ALI, thrombolysis delivered by an intra-arterial catheter within the thrombus is more effective and carries a lower risk of complications than systemic thrombolysis. Three main agents have been employed, they exhibit no major differences in efficacy.

Recombinant tissue plasminogen activator (rTPA) is most widely used in the UK. This acts by converting plasminogen into plasmin and promoting fibrin degradation.

Streptokinase induces antibody production, preventing repeat administration. It is ineffective in patients with prior streptococcal infections and is no longer widely used.

Urokinase has similar efficacy to rTPA and has been favoured in the US. Concurrent administration of low dose heparin through the arterial sheath is used to prevent pericatheter thrombus formation.

Newer classes of thrombolytic agents acting independently of the plasminogen system (Alfimeprase and Plasmin) offer the potential for more rapid lysis coupled with a lower risk of serious bleeding and an improved safety profile. Platelet GP2b/3a receptor antagonists such as abciximab produce a synergistic effect with thrombolytics, resulting in more rapid lysis, but this may be at the expense of increased haemorrhagic complications. The role of these agents in peripheral arterial disease is still to be defined.

The efficacy of all thrombolytic agents diminishes rapidly and most units restrict usage to within 4–6 weeks of the presumed thrombus formation (usually a major symptomatic deterioration). Beyond this therapeutic window, the low chance of successful lysis is outweighed by the relatively high complication rate.

In the acutely threatened ischaemic limb emergency, embolectomy is preferred to thrombolysis which can take up to 24 h to substantially improve limb perfusion.

Contraindications to thrombolysis

The risks and benefits of thrombolysis must be carefully considered for each patient. Situations where thrombolysis is contraindicated include the following:

- active bleeding
- previous cerebral haemorrhage
- surgery, major trauma or cardiopulmonary resuscitation within the preceding 2 weeks
- proliferative diabetic retinopathy
- recent ocular surgery or trauma
- bleeding diathesis
- pregnancy

Thrombolysis regimes

Prerequisites for successful thrombolysis are an informed, cooperative patient in whom the risk of inadvertent arterial sheath or catheter removal is low (the resulting haemorrhage may be very difficult to control) and careful supervision and monitoring, usually within a high dependency environment.

Effective analgesia during this period may require intravenous opiates or specialist pain team input.

Several different thrombolysis regimes are described.

Low dose regimes administer a continuous infusion typically for 24 h or longer. High dose regimes involve an initial bolus followed by a high dose infusion with the aim of achieving faster thrombolysis during core working hours. Both strategies are effective and confer similar limb salvage and complication rates.

Persistent thrombotic occlusion resistant to embolectomy is often managed with intra-operative rTPA thrombolysis. A typical dosage regime is 15 mg diluted to 100 mL and delivered by infusion or repeated small bolus injections over 30 min.

Complications

Thrombolysis carries substantial risks. Thirty-day mortality in a large UK based audit was 12.4% [3], with the majority of deaths attributable to myocardial infarction or stroke. Stroke occurs in approximately 3% of patients and may be haemorrhagic or thrombotic. Major arterial haemorrhage requiring cessation of thrombolysis affects about 10% of patients. This is mostly from groin puncture sites, but there is a significant risk of concealed retroperitoneal and intra-abdominal haemorrhage. Haemodynamic monitoring, frequent assessment of the puncture site, limb perfusion and neurological status are required to promptly detect serious bleeding and minimise the duration of thrombolysis. Titration of thrombolytic dose to the results of coagulation studies is necessary to avoid excessive depletion of fibrinogen.

There should be a high index of suspicion for concealed arterial bleeding and a low threshold for performing CT examination to assess for cerebral or abdominal haemorrhage.

Minor bleeding from the puncture site is common (20–40%) and can be managed by local compression and need not require thrombolytic cessation.

Distal embolisation may produce deterioration in limb perfusion or be evident on check angiography. This usually resolves with continued thrombolysis or thrombus aspiration.

Surgery vs. thrombolysis

Randomised controlled trials demonstrate no clear superiority for surgery or thrombolysis on 30-day limb salvage rates or mortality [4]. Registry data show that surgery is performed 3–5 times more frequently, suggesting that timely access to thrombolysis is limited.

Mechanical thrombectomy

A variety of adjunctive endovascular techniques involving mechanical thrombus aspiration or thrombectomy aim to promote faster thrombus resolution. They are often combined with thrombolysis. These add to the cost and complexity of treatment and are not currently widely used.

Unsalvageable limbs

Even with current techniques, a significant proportion of ischaemic limbs cannot be saved. In these patients, efforts must be directed towards pain management and resuscitation with prompt amputation and rehabilitation. Futile attempts at revascularisation pose a major risk from rhabdomyolysis and hyperkalemia.

Chronic Limb Ischaemia

In chronic arterial disease, non-invasive imaging techniques including duplex ultrasound, magnetic resonance angiography (MRA) and computed tomography angiography (CTA) have largely replaced catheter angiography for the majority of patients and allow accurate assessment of disease distribution. The haemodynamic significance of stenoses demonstrated by these techniques can be further evaluated with targeted duplex ultrasound or translesional pressure gradients obtained with catheter angiography. Typical thresholds for treatment are a peak systolic velocity ratio (PSVR) of 2.5 for ultrasound and a 5–10 mmHg pressure gradient without vasodilatation or 10–15 mmHg with vasodilator administration measured at angiography.

Lesion prioritisation

When confronted with multiple lesions in a patient with chronic limb ischaemia, treatment of significant proximal lesions is undertaken first. Symptomatic improvement following angioplasty or stenting of aorto-iliac lesions frequently exceeds that of femoro-popliteal lesions and if a good response is achieved, subsequent infra-inguinal revascularisation may be unnecessary. Even when further surgical or endovascular procedures are required, then optimisation of arterial inflow increases the likelihood of technical success. It may be unnecessary or undesirable, due to severe potential complications, to treat all identified lesions, and a staged approach with clinical review will optimise the risk/benefit balance for individual patients.

Surgical Revascularisation

Endarterectomy

Areas of bulky heavily calcified plaque respond poorly to angioplasty which may fail to fracture the plaque. Stenting is similarly ineffective as stents lack sufficient radial force to overcome these lesions. For lesions in readily accessible surgical sites, such as the common femoral artery, endarterectomy is an effective treatment.

Surgical bypass

Graft materials

Infra-inguinal bypasses may be constructed from autologous vein or prosthetic graft such as woven Dacron or polytetrafluoroethylene, PTFE) There is a major advantage to using vein grafts with 5-year patency rates of 74–76% vs. 39–52% for PTFE [5, 6]. Most commonly, the long saphenous vein (LSV) is used either as a reversed vein graft or an *in situ* vein graft, following valvotomy. Narrow calibre and varicose veins are unsuitable and many patients may have already undergone LSV harvesting for prior lower limb or coronary revascularisation. In these circumstances, short saphenous vein, cephalic vein or superficial femoral vein are alternatives. Pre-operative duplex ultrasound assessment reliably demonstrates suitable veins and avoids the unnecessary morbidity resulting from exploration of poor quality veins.

Anastomotic techniques

Venous cuffs or patches performed at anastomoses between prosthetic grafts and small (distal) arteries improve the patency of femoro-popliteal

PTFE grafts performed below the knee, but do not produce any benefit in above knee grafts [7].

Aortoiliac bypass

Surgical bypass with a prosthetic graft from the distal aorta to either the iliac or common femoral arteries is usually the preferred option for occlusive or diffuse stenotic disease. A variety of trans-peritoneal or extra-peritoneal approaches may be employed. The patency of aorto-bifemoral grafts is high (greater than 80% at 5 years).

Femoral–femoral crossover graft

Femoral-femoral crossover operations utilising prosthetic grafts are an alternative to aorto-iliac or aorto-femoral bypass for unilateral iliac occlusive disease. They are also employed following aorto-uni-iliac stent graft treatment of abdominal aortic aneurysms. As an intra-abdominal incision is avoided, this is a less invasive option better suited to higher risk patients, although the majority will require either regional or general anaesthesia.

Extra-anatomic bypass

Axillo-bifemoral prosthetic grafts (Fig. 1) are used as a less invasive alternative to aorto-iliac bypass procedures for occlusive disease or to treat aorto-iliac graft infection. Long-term graft patency rates for extra-anatomic bypasses are lower than those for aorto-bifemoral grafts, and they are usually reserved for patients with critical limb ischaemia.

Femoropopliteal bypass

Non-invasive imaging will confirm the adequacy of arterial inflow and determine whether there is sufficient outflow to promote graft patency. The proximal anastomosis is usually sited anteriorly on the common femoral artery. The distal anastomosis is into the popliteal artery and may be above or below the knee. Autologous vein grafts are preferred as they have the best long-term patency rates, but prosthetic grafts may be

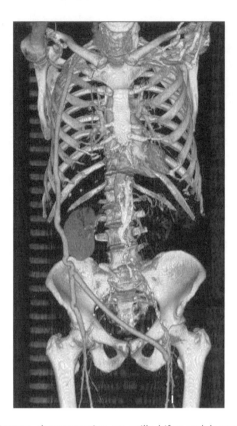

Figure 1.   CT angiogram demonstrating an axillo-bifemoral bypass graft (performed 9 years previously).

necessary for patients with insufficient suitable vein. Five-year patency rates for above knee and below knee femoropopliteal vein grafts are similar (62% and 68%, respectively). Prosthetic grafts perform much worse below the knee with 5-year patency falling from 43% above knee to 27% below. Many units restrict below knee prosthetic grafts to patients with critical limb ischaemia.

Femoro-distal bypass

The quality of the outflow artery correlates with long-term graft patency rates. The choice of distal arterial anastomotic site (tibial or peroneal artery) does not appear to affect outcome and therefore the best quality artery with uninterrupted run off to the foot should be selected. Five-year assisted patency rates for vein grafts are approximately 60% and less than 35% for prosthetic grafts.

Endovascular Techniques

Angioplasty

Angioplasty techniques use pressure-controlled balloon inflation to fracture arterial plaque and remodel the artery. As the plaque is not removed, this is most effective for short focal stenoses without heavy calcification. Excessively calcified lesions are resistant to angioplasty.

A randomised controlled trial [8] demonstrated additional benefit of angioplasty over supervised exercise programme and best medical therapy. At 24 months post angioplasty, absolute walking distance was improved by 78% for aorto-iliac lesions and 38% for femoro-popliteal lesions.

Drug eluting balloon angioplasty

In addition to the mechanical effects of plaque fracture and vessel dilatation, drug eluting balloons (DEBs) deliver an antiproliferative drug (Paclitaxel) directly to the vessel wall with the intention of reducing restenosis and the need for further reinterventions.

Comparison with simple angioplasty [9] appears favourable with randomised trials now showing markedly better primary patency and reduction in reintervention rates following DEB angioplasty in the SFA.

Procedural outline

Patient symptoms, examination and pre-procedural imaging are reviewed.
Arterial access site is planned (ultrasound guidance is a useful adjunct).

- Local anaesthetic infiltration
- Arterial puncture and guidewire passage (Seldinger technique)

- Arterial sheath placed
- Angiographic evaluation of lesion
- Heparin anticoagulation
- Guidewire passage across lesion (frequently requires a hydrophilic guidewire)
- Exchange for supportive guidewire
- Angioplasty balloon placement and inflation[a]
- Angiography to assess response
- Repeat inflation or stenting if needed
- Arterial puncture site compression/closure device

Subintimal angioplasty

This technique can be effective in recanalising iliac, SFA and long below knee occlusions. It involves intentional guidewire passage into the subintimal plane to create a channel that extends for the length of the occlusion. The guidewire is then redirected back into the vessel lumen and the entire section angioplastied to create a new flow channel between the intima and media.

Care must be taken to avoid major collateral vessels as occlusion of these can precipitate acute limb ischaemia. Heavily calcified vessels may prevent guidewire and catheter passage and it may be impossible to reenter the vessel lumen.

Although procedures performed on crural arteries in patients with critical limb ischaemia achieve lower technical success rates, compared with those performed above the knee, this remains a valuable technique as many of these patient groups are unfit for surgical revascularisation. Long-term patency rates are a less important measure for this group as patient life expectancy is short, and even a temporary increase in limb perfusion may be sufficient to achieve relief of rest pain, ulcer healing and limb salvage.

---

[a] Medicines and Healthcare products Regulatory Agency (MHRA) alert notice from May 2002 mandates use of a calibrated inflation device to minimise the risk of balloon rupture and embolisation.

Complications

Arterial puncture site haemorrhage

The risk of puncture site haemorrhage increases with the following:

- vessel wall calcification (loss of elastic recoil),
- hypertension,
- number of arterial puncture attempts,
- size of arterial sheath,
- anticoagulation.

These can mostly be controlled with manual compression, although this may need to be prolonged.

Concealed retroperitoneal haemorrhage is a life-threatening emergency occurring within a few hours of the procedure.

Pain, pallor, tachycardia, hypotension, flank tenderness or visible haemorrhage are all useful indicators of serious bleeding. Early detection prior to the onset of haemorrhagic shock is the aim and vigilant post-procedural monitoring in an appropriate environment is mandatory. Any clinical suspicion of serious bleeding must prompt emergency CT examination and surgical exploration and repair if active bleeding is confirmed.

Arterial rupture

Iliac artery rupture is a rare but potentially fatal procedural complication. Female patients requiring angioplasty of heavily diseased, narrow calibre, external iliac arteries are most at risk. Severe pain unrelieved by angioplasty balloon deflation indicates likely rupture. Immediate angiography is required to confirm the site of rupture and then balloon inflation to tamponade the site is performed.

Urgent cross-matching of blood is undertaken and experienced vascular surgical and anaesthetic assistance urgently obtained. Once this team is assembled, then the tamponade balloon may be deflated. Minor ruptures may resolve with balloon tamponade alone, but continued extravasation requires immediate placement of a covered stent placed across the rupture site. This usually resolves the problem, but if not, then emergency surgery will be required.

Rupture of infra-inguinal arteries seldom causes any major clinical problems.

Dissection

Arterial dissection is a frequent event during angioplasty. Usually, this is minor and non-flow-limiting, and no treatment is indicated. Flow-restricting dissections may resolve with prolonged (5–15 min) balloon inflation or placement of an uncovered stent.

Distal embolisation

Embolisation may be caused by plaque fracture and detachment or by thrombus. Completion angiography of the distal vascular territory will detect this complication. If limb perfusion is maintained, then further intervention is unnecessary. In cases where the limb is compromised, then thrombus aspiration or thrombolysis are often effective, but some patients will still need surgery. Symptomatic plaque embolisation is more likely to require surgery.

Contrast induced nephropathy (CIN)

Following iodinated contrast administration, there is frequently a transient deterioration in renal function which is maximal at 48 h and has generally resolved by 5 days. Patients with normal pre-procedural renal function are unlikely to suffer clinical problems, but for those with pre-existing renal impairment, there may be an irreversible worsening of renal function. Adequate hydration in the peri-procedural period is essential to minimise this risk. Pre-treatment with N-Acetylcysteine (NAC) may be beneficial. A meta-analysis showed a moderate reduction in CIN in patients pre-treated with NAC. The use of iso-osmolar contrast media lessens the degree of renal impairment in high risk patients with diabetes. The minimum possible contrast volumes consistent with high quality imaging should be used.

Carbon dioxide (CO_2) may be used as an alternative contrast agent to guide angioplasty in high-risk patients. Infra-inguinal angioplasty performed solely with ultrasound guidance is a viable alternative for centres lacking the necessary equipment or experience in CO_2 angiography.

Aortic angioplasty

Infrarenal aortic atheroma and minor stenoses are common and often clinically insignificant. The small minority of lesions which produce significant haemodynamic effects may be treated with either aortic angioplasty or uncovered stent placement. Both methods result in excellent long-term patency rates.

Iliac stenting

Iliac artery angioplasty has high technical success rates and produces 5-year patency rates of approximately 70%. Stent placement (Figs. 2 and 3) either as a primary procedure or performed selectively following suboptimal response to angioplasty significantly reduces the failure rate of endovascular treatment. Although endovascular treatment for aortoiliac occlusive disease carries lower risks than surgical revascularisation, a recent large UK registry recorded a 2% in hospital mortality rate, with deaths mainly occurring in patients with critical limb ischaemia. Mortality for those with claudication was 0.2%.

SFA stenting

Previous attempts to stent SFA stenoses and occlusions failed. There was a very high incidence of early stent fractures and the majority of these subsequently occluded.

Fundamental stent redesign has produced a generation of devices better suited to the complex series of forces affecting the SFA.

Recent trials suggest a much reduced early stent fracture rate with substantially improved vessel patency.

Two-year follow-up data comparing primary SFA stenting with a strategy of SFA angioplasty and selective stent placement for residual stenosis

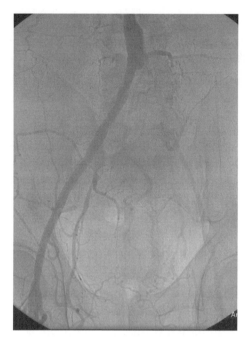

Figure 2.   Angiogram showing a left common iliac artery occlusion.

or dissection showed clinical improvement and lower reintervention rates with primary stenting. The current role of SFA stenting is as a 'bail out' procedure for significant residual stenosis or flow-limiting dissection at the time of angioplasty. Longer-term data are needed before the substantial additional costs generated by a primary stenting policy can be justified.

Below knee stenting

Treatment of short focal lesions of the tibial arteries with either coronary artery stents or dedicated below-knee stents is described. The majority of critically ischaemic limbs contain diffuse stenoses and long occlusions involving more than one run off vessel and are therefore anatomically unsuitable. There is currently little evidence to support below knee stent placement.

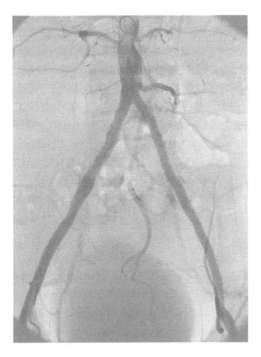

Figure 3.   Left common iliac artery occlusion treated with balloon expandable stent placement. A right-sided stent was also placed to preserve the right common iliac origin (same patient as Fig. 2).

Hybrid Procedures

Hybrid procedures typically consist of a surgical bypass combined with either angioplasty or stenting to optimise graft inflow or outflow. The order of these procedures requires careful consideration and the endovascular component is usually performed first to avoid compromising the inflow or outflow to a newly constructed graft by balloon inflation or haemostatic manoeuvres. A dedicated endovascular theatre is the optimal environment, but satisfactory results can be obtained with a fluoroscopy compatible theatre table and portable image intensifier with vascular processing software including digital subtraction.

Radiation Protection

Radiation protection legislation requires that all medical diagnostic and therapeutic procedures are justified and that exposures are as low as reasonably achievable (the ALARA principle). Endovascular operators must be adequately trained in both the principles and practicalities of radiation protection. There is an individual legal responsibility to comply with local radiation protection policies and dosimetry monitoring arrangements.

Restenosis

Angioplasty or stent-induced plaque fracture and vessel wall trauma induce a complex series of responses frequently leading to intimal hyperplasia and vessel restenosis. The incidence of restenosis varies between anatomical sites and small calibre vessels, long stenotic segments or occlusions are particularly prone.

The use of stent grafts may prevent tissue ingrowth and reduce restenosis rates. A variety of response-modifying techniques aim to reduce or prevent restenosis. In established in-stent restenosis, simple balloon angioplasty may effectively treat short focal lesions, however there is a very high recurrence rate for total in-stent occlusions. The use of drug coated balloon angioplasty provides better short-term results, however this benefit may diminish with time particularly for longer and more complex lesions.

A combination of lesion debulking with laser atherectomy and drug coated balloon angioplasty may give a more durable improvement [10].

Graft/Stent Surveillance

Occlusion of surgical bypass grafts and arterial stents is frequently preceded by progressive stenosis within or immediately adjacent to the graft or stent.

Retreatment at this stage is difficult and many units undertake graft and stent surveillance programmes in which significant stenoses identified with duplex ultrasound are treated with the aim of avoiding graft or stent occlusion.

These programmes are resource-intensive. Compliance rates with long-term follow-up are low, and patients still present requiring treatment for lesions occurring outside the surveillance zone (i.e., opposite limb).

The majority of reinterventions are required within the first year and it may be more cost effective to limit surveillance to 1 year or to stratify follow-up according to early surveillance findings.

BASIL Trial

The BASIL trial (bypass vs. angioplasty in severe ischaemia of the leg) compared the outcomes of 452 patients presenting to UK centres with severe limb ischaemia [11]. Patients were randomised to either a surgery first (*n* = 228) or an angioplasty first (*n* = 224) strategy.

Only 60% of participants received antihypertensive treatment, 54% received antiplatelet drugs and 34% were taking cholesterol-lowering agents.

The primary endpoint was survival free from amputation for the trial limb.

Trial duration was 5.5 years, with follow-up ending when the endpoints of death or above ankle amputation of the trial leg were reached. At follow-up completion,

- 248 patients (55%) were alive without amputation of the trial leg,
- 38 (8%) were alive following amputation,
- 130 patients (29%) were dead without amputation.

A surgery first strategy was associated with a higher rate of early morbidity (57% vs. 41%).

Six month amputation free survival was not significantly different between the treatment groups and health-related quality of life (HRQL) was similar.

At 2 years, surgery was associated with a reduced risk of future amputation or death.

A strategy of surgery first increased the hospital costs by about one-third.

These results indicate that there is scope to substantially improve the medical treatment of risk factors. For patients with a short life expectancy, an angioplasty first strategy reduces early morbidity and treatment costs but for relatively fit patients, expected to live beyond 2 years, a surgery first strategy is more durable and carries a reduced reintervention rate, possibly outweighing the initial costs and increased short-term morbidity.

Upper Limb Revascularisation

Although less frequently affected than the lower limbs, revascularisation may be needed for either acute or chronic ischaemia involving the arms.

Surgical embolectomy or catheter delivered thrombolysis are the main options for embolic occlusions, with severity of ischaemia and local availability and expertise again being the determining factors.

Chronic ischaemia associated with limiting symptoms may be treated by surgical bypass (carotid-subclavian or carotid-axillary) or by endovascular methods. Reduced upper limb pulses or asymmetric blood pressure measurements in the absence of limiting symptoms do not constitute an indication for revascularisation.

Trauma from cervical or rudimentary first ribs in thoracic outlet syndrome (TOS) may cause subclavian arterial stenoses or aneurysm formation and distal embolisation. Revascularisation with autologous or prosthetic graft is combined with rib resection. Adjunctive embolectomy or thrombolysis may be needed for embolic presentations.

Additional considerations for upper limb endovascular procedures include the following:

- The need for alternative arterial access sites (usually brachial artery), with associated risk of serious neurovascular complications (including median nerve compression) and higher incidence of arterial spasm.
- Manipulations around the aortic arch carry a risk of stroke. This must be explained to patients. Meticulous technique, avoidance of air

bubbles in contrast media and measures to avoid peri-catheter thrombus formation are mandatory.
- Awareness of the vertebral artery anatomy and careful planning to avoid inadvertent embolisation or occlusion.

Evidence-based Approach

The recently updated Transatlantic Inter-Society Consensus (TASC II) Guidelines on the management of peripheral vascular disease [12] are a collaboration involving international medical, vascular surgical, interventional radiology and cardiology societies. Their recommendations are graded based upon the level of supporting evidence.

Lesions are stratified according to the results of surgical and endovascular revascularisation.

- Type A lesions give very good results with endovascular treatment and this is preferred.
- Type B lesions give good results with endovascular treatment and this is recommended unless there are adjacent lesions requiring surgical treatment.
- Type C lesions with surgical revascularisation produces superior long-term results and is preferred for good risk patients.
- Type D lesions respond poorly to current endovascular methods and surgical revascularisation is preferred for fit patients.

These guidelines emphasise that 'patient's comorbidities, fully informed patient preference and the local operators long-term success rates must be considered when making treatment recommendations for type B and type C lesions'.

Decision-making

The evidence base for these interventions continues to evolve and individual management decisions are best considered by a multi-disciplinary team experienced in best medical management, anaesthesia and able to offer the full range of surgical and endovascular techniques.

References

1. Watson L, Ellis B, Leng GC. Exercise for intermittent claudication. *Cochrane Database of Syst Rev* 2008;4:CD000990. DOI: 10.1002/14651858.CD000990.
2. Marcus AJ, Lotzof K, Kamath BSK, Shanthakumar RE, Munir N, Loh A, Bird R, Howard A. A new approach: Regional nerve blockade for angioplasty of the lower limb. *Cardiovasc Intervent Radiol* 2006;29:235–240.
3. Earnshaw JJ, Whitma B, Foy C. On behalf of the Thombolysis Study Group. National audit of thrombolysis for acute limb ischaemia (NATALI) clinical factors associated with early outcome. *J Vasc Surg* 2004;39:1018–1025.
4. Berridge DC, Kessel DO, Robertson I. Surgery versus thrombolysis for initial management of acute limb ischaemia. *Cochrane Database of Syst Rev* 2002;1:CD002784.
5. AbuRahma AF *et al*. Prospective controlled study of polytetrafluoroethylene versus saphenous vein in claudicant patients with bilateral above knee femoropopliteal bypasses. *Surgery* 1999;126(4):594–602.
6. Green RM *et al*. Prosthetic above-knee femoropopliteal bypass grafting: Five year results of a randomized trial. *J Vasc Surg* 2000;31(3):417–425.
7. Stonebridge PA, Prescott RJ, Ruckley CV. Randomized trial comparing infrainguinal polytetrafluoroethylene bypass grafting with and without vein interposition cuff at the distal anastamosis. The Joint Vascular Research Group. *J Vasc Surg* 1997;26:543–550.
8. Greenhalgh RM, Belch JJ, Brown LC, Gaines PA, Gao L, Reise JA, Thompson SG; Mimic Trial Participants (December 2008). The adjuvant benefit of angioplasty in patients with mild to moderate intermittent claudication (MIMIC) managed by supervised exercise, smoking cessation advice and best medical therapy: results from two randomised trials for stenotic femoropopliteal and aortoiliac arterial disease. *Eur J Vasc Endovasc Surg* 2008;36:680–688.
9. Tepe G, Laird J, Schneider P, Brodmann M, Krishnan P, Micari A, Metzger C, Scheinert D, Zeller T, Cohen D, Snead D, Alexander B, Landiniand M, Jaff M. Drug-Coated Balloon versus Standard Percutaneous Transluminal Angioplasty for the Treatment of Superficial Femoral and/or Popliteal Peripheral Artery Disease: 12-Month Results from the IN.PACT SFA Randomized Trial. Circulation. 2014; CIRCULATIONAHA. 114.011004, published online before print December 3, 2014.
10. Dippel EL, Makam P, Kovach R *et al*. Randomized controlled trial of excimer laser atherectomy for treatment of femoropopliteal in-stent restenosis initial results from the EXCITE ISR trial. *JACC Cardiovasc Interv* 2015;8: 92–101.

11. Adam DJ, Beard JD, Cleveland T. BASIL Trial Participants: Bypass versus angioplasty in severe ischaemia of the leg (BASIL): Multicentre, randomised, controlled trial. *Lancet* 2005;366:1925–1934.
12. Norgren T, Hiatt L, Dormandy WR, JA. Inter-Society consensus for the management of peripheral arterial disease (TASC II). *J Vasc Surg* 2007; 45:S5.

Chapter 8

Abdominal Aortic Aneurysms

Gerard Stansby, Rob Williams and Vish Bhattacharya

Key Points

- An aneurysm is an abnormal dilatation of a vessel to greater than 50% normal size.
- Smoking, male gender, hypertension and genetics are the main risk factors for abdominal aortic aneurysm (AAA).
- The annual risk of rupture for an AAA of 5–5.9 cm is 5%.
- Contrast enhanced tomography (computed tomography, CT) is the gold standard for measuring the size of an aneurysm and planning intervention.
- The UK small aneurysm trial (UKSAT) helped reach a consensus about the minimal size at which aneurysms should be treated — usually 5.5 cm in the UK.
- The UK endovascular aneurysm repair trial (EVAR) 1 showed better early results for EVAR vs. open surgery, although after 2 years there was no benefit and at 15 years EVAR was inferior.
- The UK EVAR 2 trial in unfit patients showed no difference between endovascular and open repair in unfit patients.
- The IMPROVE, AJAX and the ECAR trials showed similar mortality for endovascular vs. open repair for ruptured aortic aneurysms.

Introduction

The word aneurysm comes from the Greek word *aneurysma* which means "widening". Aneurysms of the abdominal aorta (AAAs) were first described around 100 AD. Despite many advances and improvements in diagnosis and treatment, ruptured AAA still cause around 6000 deaths in England and Wales every year.

Definition

An aneurysm is defined as an abnormal focal dilatation of a vessel with a greater than 50% increase in diameter. About 3 cm is usually considered the minimum diameter of an AAA. Between 2 and 3 cm, the aorta would be described as ectatic. All three vessel layers, the intima, media and adventitia are intact in a true aneurysm as opposed to a false aneurysm where there is a fibrous wall or organised haematoma around the aneurysm with a defect in the true wall. Aneurysms can be fusiform i.e., a symmetrical cylindrical dilatation of the whole vessel, or saccular, when there is a bulge arising eccentrically from the side of the vessel. Ninety percent of AAAs are infrarenal and the remaining 10% are juxtarenal or suprarenal.

Aetiology

Aneurysmal degeneration occurs most commonly in the elderly and is usually associated with atherosclerosis. However, unlike atherosclerosis alone which usually causes narrowing of vessels, dilatation occurs. The most marked histological changes take place in the media and intima. The media is responsible for the majority of the tensile strength of the aortic wall. It is made of multiple layers of structural proteins the bulk of which are collagen and elastin. Over many years, damage and repair and remodelling occur in the normal aortic wall. In AAA formation, the repair processes are thought to be insufficient and damage to the structural components predominates and with time elastin fibre fragmentation occurs and the media degenerates. Collagen makes up about 25% of the wall of an atherosclerotic aorta and only 6–18% in aneurysms. Matrix metalloproteinase 2, 9 and 12 are found in increased amounts in the wall of aneurysms and cause degradation of the collagen and elastin matrix, causing a decreased amount of both in the wall of an aortic aneurysm. The smooth muscle cells in the media also undergo a phenotype change and are unable to maintain and protect the matrix. Changes in the adventitial layer are less marked but inflammatory infiltrates are often present. A combination of genetic predisposition, aging and damage to the aortic wall from risk factors like smoking and hypertension are involved in the pathogenesis. Once the aortic to all weakens, pressure results in increased wall tension and a cycle of progressive dilation and greater wall stress according to the Laplace Law ($P = 2T/R$, where P = pressure, T = wall tension and R = radius).

Aneurysms due to infections are still called *mycotic*, a term coined by Sir William Osler in 1885, although this is a misnomer as they are not due to a fungus as the name suggests. They are usually due to a secondary infection of the aortic wall either from vertebral discitis, haematogenous spread from other sites or rarely from syphilis.

Other causes of aneurysms include trauma, which may be iatrogenic (false aneurysms), arteritis including Behçet Disease and Takayasu's and connective tissue disorders like Marfans, Ehlers–Danlos and Loeys–Dietz syndromes. These are degenerative aneurysms and are often associated with more rapid progression than atherosclerotic aneurysms.

Risk Factors for AAA

Various risk factors have been identified that can predispose to development of an AAA (see Table 1). The most important of these is smoking

Table 1.   Risk factors for AAA.

- Age
- Male gender
- Race — caucasian
- Family history (genetic)
- Smoking
- Hypertension
- Other atherosclerotic risk factors
  (linkage specifically with AAA is not strong)

which causes an eight-fold rise in risk of developing an aneurysm. There is also an important genetic predisposition although the exact association has not been described. This is strongest among men with male siblings having an absolute risk of 20–30%. The third major risk factor is hypertension.

Epidemiology

AAAs are 4 times more common in men than women. The mean age for presentation is between 65 and 70 years with an increase of 2–6% in men over the age of 60. The prevalence of aneurysm increases with age and Caucasian men are more likely to be affected than other groups with AAAs in Asian and African populations.

Natural History

Most AAAs gradually but exponentially increase in size until either the aneurysm ruptures or the patient dies of other causes. The annual rate of growth in diameter is generally around 10% of the sac diameter. Higher rates of growth are frequently related to either infected or inflammatory aneurysms and this is an indication for earlier and more urgent treatment.

The annual risk of rupture is directly related to the aneurysm size. Below 5 cm, the risk is <2% between 5 and 5.9 cm the annual risk of rupture is 5%. This increases to 6.6% for aneurysms from 6 to 7 cm and 19% for aneurysms over 7 cm. Only 15% of patients with an AAA will rupture and the remainder will die of other causes.

Screening for AAA

To be an appropriate condition for screening, the WHO criteria for screening would need to be fulfilled (Table 2).

AAA fulfils all these criteria when applied to older men and using ultrasound scanning.

A Cochrane review identified four controlled trials involving 127,891 men and 9342 women who were randomly assigned to aneurysm

Table 2.   WHO criteria for a worthwhile screening programme.

1. The condition should be an important health problem.
2. There should be a treatment for the condition.
3. Facilities for diagnosis and treatment should be available.
4. There should be a latent stage of the disease.
5. There should be a test or examination for the condition.
6. The test should be acceptable to the population.
7. The natural history of the disease should be adequately understood.
8. There should be an agreed policy on whom to treat.
9. The process should be cost effective.
10. The overall benefits of screening should outweigh the harm.

screening using ultrasound, or no screening [1]. Only one trial included women. Two of these were conducted in the UK [2], one in Denmark [3] and one in Australia. The results provided evidence of benefit from screening in men with a strongly significant reduction in deaths from AAA. The odds ratio for death was 0.6 for men aged 65–83 but was not reduced for women. Screening with ultrasound combined with elective treatment reduces mortality by 42% in the age group 65–74.

The UK Abdominal Aortic Screening Programme was introduced in the NHS in 2009 and fully implemented across the country (England and Wales) in April 2013. Men at the age of 65 are offered a single ultrasound scan. Around 1.58 million men were invited and 1.24 million men screened with an uptake rate of 78%. Over 15760 AAAs >3 cm were detected which give a prevalence rate of 1.3% [4,5].

Around 3653 men were referred for surgery and some 2213 treated with a mortality of 0.8% (seven deaths).

Presentation

About 70–75% of aortic aneurysms are asymptomatic and are found either during routine physical examination or during imaging investigations for another problem. Aneurysms are commonly seen on abdominal ultrasound, US computerised tomography (CT) or magnetic resonance imaging (MRI) studies.

Aneurysms tend to become palpable on abdominal examination when they reach around 5 cm or more in size. The figure varies greatly between patients depending on their body habits. Retroperitoneal masses adjacent to the aorta, unusual tortuosity and lumbar lordosis can cause the aorta to be pulsatile although only a true aneurysm will be expansile.

About 20% of patients with AAA present with rupture. The classic triad of a ruptured AAA consists of mid-abdominal or diffuse abdominal pain radiating to the back or flank, shock and a pulsatile mass. The pain can be quite severe and mimic renal colic. Although a catastrophic event, the rupture can be contained in the retroperitoneum with the contained haematoma tamponading the leaking aorta allowing time for assessment and treatment. Free intra-peritoneal ruptures are normally rapidly fatal. Only a small percent of patients of this group of these patients reach hospitals and have a higher mortality rate. Many elderly patients who die in the community of undiagnosed ruptured AAAs do not have a post-mortem and the deaths are falsely attributed to cardiac causes.

Imaging

Plain radiographs

Plain radiographs are of limited use for diagnosis but incidental vascular calcification on a plain X-ray may be seen. They are useful in the follow-up of patients after endovascular repair of aneurysms, as they allow the detection of graft migration when the stent position is compared against the lumbar vertebrae with standard projection.

Ultrasound

Many AAAs are found as incidental findings on U/S for other problems. With a few exceptions, detection is easy, although obesity and gas within the bowel lumen can obscure the aorta. Abdominal ultrasound suffers from significant interobserver errors and therefore the technique needs to be meticulous and consistent within a unit. The UK AAA screening service specifically measures the AP diameter from the inner wall to the opposite inner wall of the aorta. Due to inherent errors in the transverse measurement on USS, AAAs are measured in the anteroposterior (AP) plane. This rarely causes problems with fusiform aneurysms but can lead to measurement errors with saccular aneurysms.

Abdominal ultrasound is the main stay of aneurysm surveillance for small aneurysms as it is quick, relatively cheap and risk free for the patients. Surveillance should be at 6–12 monthly intervals. Ultrasound is unreliable for investigating ruptured aneurysms as most patients who survive long enough to present with ruptures have a retroperitoneal haematoma which is often obscured by bowel and abdominal viscera.

Computerised tomography

Contrast enhanced CT has become the gold standard for diagnosing aortic aneurysms and assessing the size and morphology. Dedicated arterial phase images acquired on a multi-slice scanner with the slices reconstructed at thicknesses of 3 mm or less provide detailed information that allows treatment to be tailored to the patient. This is particularly important to plan endovascular treatment. CT is also the gold standard for diagnosis of ruptured AAA. Intravenous contrast is not required to visualise the haematoma but is necessary if the patient is being considered for emergency endovascular repair. Some clinicians are concerned that imaging introduces an unnecessary delay in treatment. Certainly, in a shocked and unconscious patient with a rupture, imaging in any form is not necessary and the patient must be taken to theatre immediately.

CT is not without potential problems as the radiation dose is equivalent to around 5 years of normal background radiation which carries a small appreciable risk of malignancy. Repeated imaging increases this risk.

MRA

Magnetic resonance angiography (MRA) protocols require intravenous gadolinium-based contrast media to provide high quality information and care needs to be taken with interpretation as some sequences only display the vessel/aneurysm lumen and may underestimate the true size of the vessel.

The resolution is generally less than that of CT and MRI is not commonly used for treatment planning unless there is a contraindication to contrast enhanced CT.

Magnetic resonance imaging is susceptible to artefacts from metals, particularly ferromagnetic and pacemakers. Some metallic implants are absolute contraindications to scanning. Gadolinium-based contrast media should be used with care in patients with impaired renal function due to the risk of nephrogenic fibrosis.

Elective Treatment of AAA

The aim of elective treatment is to prevent death from future rupture of the aneurysm. Aneurysm repair has a significant surgical mortality and small aneurysms have a low risk of rupture. Surgery should be reserved for patients whose risk of rupture exceeds the risk of surgery and for all others conservative management with aneurysm surveillance is indicated. In the UK, the threshold for treatment is usually at 5.5 cm.

The UK SAT (UK Small Aneurysm Trial) and the ADAM (Aneurysm Detection and Mortality Trial) trials considered the minimum size of an aneurysm at which benefit of treatment outweighs the risks of surgical repair. The UKSAT randomised 1090 patients in 93 centres. About half received early surgery and the other half were under ultrasound surveillance between September 1991 and November 1995. Overall, the 30-day operative mortality was 5.5% in the early surgery group and 7.2% in the surveillance group in which surgery took place when the aneurysm expanded to 5.5 cm or the rate of increase was 1 cm per year or there was a rupture. After 12 years, the mortality was 64% in the early surgery group and 67% in the surveillance group. Sixty percent of all deaths were due to cardiovascular disease. A comparison with age and sex matched population showed a higher risk of death even after successful repair of small aneurysms [6]. Similarly, the US ADAM study showed a lower mortality of 2.7% in the elective group but also did not demonstrate a better survival in the early surgery group.

The National Vascular Registry has shown that in 2008 the mortality rate following elective surgery was 7%. However, by 2012, it had fallen to 2.4%. and the latest report in November 2016 says that vascular units in UK are all performing at a similar standard of care [7].

Patient selection is critical and therefore pre-operative assessment and work up is important. They should all undergo standard risk scoring and have a full assessment by a vascular anaesthetist and increasingly with cardiopulmonary exercise testing as the standard. All patients should be discussed at an MDT and CT used to assess suitability for open or endovascular repair.

Open aneurysm repair

Dubost performed the first successful open repair in 1951 with a homograft [8]. Open repair has evolved over the last six decades but the basic principles remain the same. Blood should be cross-matched pre-operatively, prophylactic antibiotic administered and a bladder catheter inserted and large calibre venous access established. Both central venous catheter and invasive arterial monitoring are normally used. Normothermia is important for coagulation and metabolic function and therefore all IV fluids should be warmed and the patient covered with a forced air warming blanket.

For most infrarenal aneurysms, the aneurysm is approached by an anterior midline approach although favour a transverse incision. A retroperitoneal approach can be used most commonly from the left side for juxtarenal or suprarenal repairs as this allows better access to the suprarenal aorta. Shortly before the proximal aortic clamp is applied, 5000 I.U. of heparin is given. Where possible, the clamp should be placed on the infrarenal aorta in order to maintain kidney perfusion. In some cases with a short neck, clamping above one or both real arteries may be needed. This requires identification of the left renal vein which may need to be ligated. Five percent of people have a retro aortic left renal vein which can be vulnerable to iatrogenic trauma if not appreciated. Supraceliac control requires separation of the diaphragmatic crura and retraction of the left lobe of liver.

Once proximal and distal control has been obtained the aneurysm sac is opened and thrombus removed and lumbar vessels under run. Graft reconstruction is carried out with Dacron or PTFE straight tube grafts, bifurcated aorto iliac or aorto bifemoral grafts depending on the extent of the aneurysm and iliac involvement.

Initial post-operative care requires intense monitoring in the ITU. The major risks in the early stages of recovery include myocardial, renal, visceral or limb ischaemia as well as bleeding or lung infection. Complications should be managed aggressively and there is evidence that this is a feature of the best performing units giving rise to the concept of "failure to rescue" when this isn't the case. Longer term complications include graft infection, incisional hernias, pseudo aneurysms and erectile dysfunction in men. Most patients are discharged within a week.

Endovascular repair

Endovascular repair (EVAR) developed in response to the significant mortality and morbidity with elective open repair. In 1970, Juan Parodi in Argentina proposed the concept of using an endovascular route to insert fabric grafts reinforced with metal stents. The first human implant was performed in 1990 and the operation was a success and the patient lived for 9 years before succumbing to pancreatic cancer.

The early grafts were simple fabric tubes reinforced with stents which relied on radial force to maintain their position within the aorta. These proved vulnerable to migration and sometimes loss of the seal with the aortic wall. Over the next three decades, the grafts have evolved and most are now modular bifurcated tubes with some form of active fixation at the proximal end to reduce the incidence of migration. The active fixation normally consists of a bare metal stent that extends into the suprarenal aorta or barbs and hooks that embed into the aortic wall. Some grafts use a combination of the two methods. The only other mechanism to prevent distal migration involves resting the flow divider of the stent graft directly onto the aortic bifurcation.

Pre-operative workout is generally identical to that required for open repair as very rarely an endovascular repair may need to be converted to open. All patients need a planning CT with contrast and timed for the arterial phase. The images need to be reconstructed at 3 mm maximum slices or 1.5 mm for fenestrated stents. Around 25% of all pre-EVAR CT scans will show an unsuspected abnormality and should therefore always be reported by a radiologist. Three-dimensional reconstruction allows true axial measurements related to the vessel and not the patient. There is a variation of 1–2 mm in the measurement of diameter depending on the phase of the cardiac cycle when the scan was acquired. Length measurement need not be accurate due to significant and unpredictable variability on the confirmation of the grafts. The limb lengths can be measured more accurately during the procedure itself using calibrating catheters.

Aortic morphology is perhaps the biggest limiting factor for EVAR. Most grafts require a portion of the infrarenal aorta called the proximal neck to be at least 10–15 mm long with a diameter of less than 30 mm to provide a proximal sealing zone.

The neck should be angulated by less than 60° and free from atheroma and thrombus. Both common iliac arteries should have normal portions for the distal sealing zones although the grafts can be extended to the external iliac arteries if required. The external iliac arteries and common femoral artery should be large enough to allow the passage of deliver systems. Most grafts require a diameter of 7–8 mm. Iliac tortuosity alone does not to cause any major problems although extensive calcification and tortuosity can cause major difficulties. Strictly following the IFUs (manufacturer's indications for use) of the currently available grafts allows about 40–50% of all infrarenal aortas to be treated with EVAR.

EVAR should be done in a theatre environment to reduce the infection risk which although rare, can be catastrophic. The quality of fluoroscopy use is critical and most units now use a hybrid theatre for this purpose. A hybrid theatre can be defined as a combined operating theatre and radiology suite and as such should have fixed, rather than mobile C-arm imaging as a minimum.

The procedure can be done under general, regional or local anaesthesia although the latter can be uncomfortable for the patient due to lower limb ischaemia when the delivery system occludes the femoral arteries. Most procedures start with surgical exposure of the femoral arteries although a large number of units are using percutaneous techniques like the Proglide systems.

Guidewires are passed into thoracic aorta and angiograms performed to locate the renal arteries. The main body is deployed with the first covered stent placed as close to the lowest renal artery as possible. The contralateral limb is cannulated from the opposite groin and both stent grafts are extended into the level of the iliac bifurcations. The proximal

192 Postgraduate Vascular Surgery (Second Edition)

and distal seals and the junctions of the modular components can be balloon moulded to improve the seal.

A completion angiogram is performed to confirm the patency of the renal and iliac vessels and identify endoleaks (Table 3).

The term endoleak was coined to describe the situation after endovascular repair, where there is blood flow in the aneurysm sac despite the presence of a stent graft. It does not mean that the aneurysm itself has leaked.

Type I

A type I endoleak is a failure of the seal between the stent graft and the arterial wall. They are divided into proximal, where there is a leak between the main body of the stent graft, and the infrarenal aortic neck and distal, where there is a leak between the stent graft and iliac artery. As the blood leaking into the sac is at systolic arterial pressure, it can result in a significant increase in intra-sac pressure which may lead to a significant risk of aneurysm rupture. Although small type I endoleaks may close spontaneously, usually type I endoleaks seen on completion imaging are treated as

Table 3.   Endoleaks.

Type I: Leak at graft attachment site
- Ia   Proximal
- Ib   Distal
- Ic   Occluder

Type II: Leak from sac branch vessel
- IIa   Single vessel
- IIb   Multiple vessels

Type III: Leak through defect in graft
- IIIa   Functional separation
- IIIb   Fracture or holes in endograft

Type IV: Leak through graft from graft porosity

Type V: Expanding sac but no leak seen = endotension

early as possible. The simplest treatment involves using a moulding balloon to improve the contact between graft and aortic wall. If the leak persists, additional bare metal stent(s) can be used. If this fails, an external surgical band may be used. Usually, this requires laparotomy but can also be placed laparoscopically and there is no need to open the sac. The procedure involves tying nylon tapes around the neck of the aneurysm to snug it down onto the stent graft to achieve a seal.

Type II

This is due to filling of the sac from branches off the sac such as from the lumbar arteries with blood filling in a retrograde direction. They are often complex and blood may flow in through one branch and out through another. Around 20% of patients will have a type II endoleak the majority of which are benign as they do not significantly pressurise the sac. Sixty percent will resolve spontaneously in 1 year. A small proportion can cause persistent sac expansion and can be occluded using micro catheters via the translumbar route or via the IMA/SMA or occasionally by direct injection. The cavity can be occluded by a variety of embolic materials including coils or glue. They can also be treated by laparotomy and direct suture of the vessels after opening the sac.

Type III

These leaks are due either to fabric defects in the graft material or dislocation and separation of the stent graft components. The former is normally due to manufacturing defects and are fortunately very rare. The latter tend to occur much later as the aneurysm remodels and distorts the stent graft. Like type I endoleaks, these must be treated as soon as possible endovascularly or by explantation as the sac will be pressurised.

Type IV

Immediately after implantation some grafts are porous especially when patients are anticoagulated with heparin. These are visible as a contrast blush in the aneurysm sac. They resolve spontaneously and have no clinical consequence.

Type V

This is also known as endotension and is due to be transmission of the arterial pulse pressure into the sac without a true leak of blood or flow. This concept is controversial as many believe that this is just an endoleak(s) that is subtle and difficult to identify.

EVAR Trials

The first trials comparing EVAR with open repair was the DREAM Trial (Dutch Randomised Endovascular Aneurysm Management trial) reported in 2004 [8, 9]. The authors randomised 345 patients for both techniques with end points being operative mortality or severe complications [6]. The operative mortality rate was 4.6% in the open-repair group (8 of 174 patients and 1.2% in the endovascular-repair group (2 of 171 patients, resulting in a risk ratio of 3).

Soon afterwards, the UK EVAR trial participants published their results. EVAR I compared open repair with endovascular repair. It demonstrated that 30-day mortality was less than half for EVAR as compared to open repair (1.7% vs. 4.7%).

Patients also recovered more quickly and were discharged from hospital much earlier. However, by 4 years, all-cause mortality was identical at 28% although the EVAR group had a significantly higher reintervention rate.

Eight years' and 15 years follow up of the EVAR trial have been reported and the investigators recorded 9.3 deaths per 1000 person years in the EVAR group and 8.9% per 1000 person years in the open group over mean of 12.7 years.

They have noted that there was early benefit in the first 6 months in the EVAR group, similar mortality for open and EVAR from 6 months to 1 year and a significantly higher mortality in the EVAR group at 12 years. The late divergence in the EVAR group was due to late ruptures (13 deaths vs. 2, respectively) [10, 11].

In the EVAR 2 trial, 404 patients not fit for open surgery were recruited from 33 UK centres. These included 207 patients receiving no intervention and 197 having an EVAR. There was a high 30-day mortality of 7.3% in the stenting group with reduced aneurysm related mortality at 4 years but no overall benefit in terms of all-cause mortality. Thirty percent of the no intervention group crossed over and chose to have an EVAR during follow up [12].

Follow up post-EVAR

After EVAR, patients normally require long-term, usually lifelong, follow up with 10–20% requiring reintervention at some stage.

CT remains the gold standard for follow up but has the disadvantage that the patients are exposed to radiation and iodine contrast media. Some studies have shown that endoleak detection is better with ultrasound although this is largely operator-dependent.

Contrast enhanced ultrasound protocols are now being undertaken in several centres after 1 year and CT only used for patient specific risk adjusted protocols.

Fenestrated and branched repairs

Fenestrated endovascular repair (FEVAR) was developed to allow EVAR of AAAs with little or no normal aorta below the level of renal arteries. These grafts have fenestrations that correspond with the positions of the renal artery and/or the SMA to allow the covered portion of the stent graft to be placed more proximally.

They are reinforced with either small bare metal stents or covered stents which extend into the renal arteries. This helps to prevent migration and maintain alignment between the fenestrations and the renal arteries. The grafts are custom made for each patient and need very accurate planning.

Branched grafts come in two different forms. Iliac branch grafts are relatively simple bifurcated grafts that extend the limb onto a standard stent graft. One branch sits in the internal iliac artery and the other in the external iliac artery. This allows treatment of aneurysms involving the distal CIA while maintain patency of the internal iliac. The other type of branched graft has multiple branches to the visceral vessels.

Laparoscopic AAA repair

This can be done totally laparoscopically or using a midline mini-laparotomy incision as well as several laparoscopic ports for hand-assisted laparoscopic surgery. Clamps are applied above and below the aneurysm, the sac is opened, thrombus removed and lumbar arteries and inferior mesenteric arteries are sutured from the inside of the aneurysm or clipped outside it.

A prosthetic vascular graft is sutured in laparoscopically and the aneurysm wall and the parietal peritoneum are closed to cover the graft. Currently, the evidence for laparoscopic repair is weaker than for EVAR or traditional open repair and more trials are needed.

Inflammatory AAAs

Inflammatory aneurysms are defined by the presence of a thickened aneurysm wall, marked peri-aneurysmal and retroperitoneal fibrosis and dense adhesions to adjacent organs. They represent 3–10% of all AAAs and the triad of abdominal or back pain, weight loss and an elevated ESR in a patient with an AAA is highly suggestive. They tend to occur in a younger age group than other atherosclerotic AAAs and are almost always abdominal and not thoracic. The term periaortitis is used to describe the appearance of inflammatory tissue around the aorta which enhances with intravenous iodinated contrast media and therefore can be picked up on CT scanning.

This condition overlaps with and is a variant of retroperitoneal fibrosis and the precise aetiology remains elusive. An inflammatory response in the aortic wall to unknown antigens is thought to drive the process. Corticosteroids and other immunosuppressive drugs have been found to decrease symptoms and the degree of peri-aortic inflammation and fibrosis but their use prior to surgery remains controversial and surgery remains the treatment of choice.

Operative open repair of a large inflammatory AA is often challenging and operative mortality is 2–3 times greater than the usual open repair. The duodenum may be stuck to the neck of the AA in a dense white sheet of inflammatory tissue and needs dissection in the wall using an 'onion skin peeling' technique, where the duodenum is separated from the aorta by sharp scalpel dissection. If there is associated ureteric involvement and hydronephrosis prior to surgery, ureteric stenting may be required and concomitant ureterolysis can be performed.

Traditionally open repair is preferred to stenting inflammatory AAAs particularly with renal involvement as it is thought that the inflammation in the retroperitoneum is more likely to resolve when the aortic atheroma and thrombus is removed rather than just excluded by EVAR. However, EVAR is now more frequently being used and is associated with improved early survival. There are no randomised trials but the consensus is that open repair by and experienced surgeon remains the treatment of choice in patients who are sufficiently fit.

Treatment of Ruptured AAAs

Ruptured AAA (rAAA) is commonly fatal and many (probably >50%) die before reaching the hospital. Even if they survive surgery, there is a high rate of complications including cardiac, renal, respiratory and gastrointestinal and prolonged ITU and hospital stays are common. They can present with signs and symptoms ranging from abdominal, back or loin pain to shock and coma. Haemodynamically unstable patients will need to go immediately to theatre, stable patients may have time for the diagnosis to be confirmed by CT scan. Occasionally, patients with significant comorbidities should be managed palliatively but most rAAAs require urgent repair, either open or endovascular, as without treatment mortality is 100%. The Hardman index can be used as a supplement to clinical judgement and >3 Hardman variables are said to be associated with a close to 100% mortality rate (Table 4). Other risk prediction models such as the Glasgow aneurysm score and rAAA Possum score can also be used.

The key to successful outcomes is to avoid delay and to get the aneurysm repaired or controlled as rapidly as possible. Although controversial, there is evidence that limited resuscitation with permissive hypotension should be employed initially or for transfer with the aim of keeping the systolic BP at 70–100 mmHg and not greater. The theory is that excessive fluid administration can restart bleeding and deplete clotting factors. Blood should be cross matched (8–10 units) and clotting factors (FFP and platelets) should also be requested.

Table 4.   Hardman Index.

	Score
Age >76 years	1
Creatinine >190 μmol/L	1
Hb <9 d/dL	1
MI on ECG	1
Loss of consciousness in hospital	1

Notes: Score of 2 or more = >80% mortality, 3 or more = 100% mortality.

The most important step in surgery on a patient with a rAAA is the rapid control of the proximal neck to reduce ongoing blood loss. In most cases, this can be done infrarenally but supraceliac control may be required if the hematoma is large. Another method for aortic control is balloon occlusion by placing a balloon in the proximal aorta without supraceliac exposure.

EVAR for ruptured AAA

Advantages of EVAR for rAAA is that it is less invasive, avoids damage to Pre-aortic and abdominal structures, reduces bleeding from surgical dissection and minimises hypothermia. However, despite the development of EVAR and its lower degree of invasiveness, open repair remains the standard treatment for rAAAs in the majority of UK hospitals.

The IMPROVE (Immediate Management of the Patient with Ruptured Aneurysm: Open Versus Endovascular repair) trial in the UK included 613 patients in 29 centres between 2009 and 2013. In this double blinded trial, the mortality from EVAR was 35.4 % as compared to 37.4 % for open repair (not statistically significant). However, the hospital stay was shorter and the quality of life better in the EVAR group [13].

The AJAX (Amsterdam Acute Aneurysm Trial) looked at 116 patients in three centres between 2004 and 2011. This trial showed a mortality of 22% for EVAR vs. 25% for open repair. This trial showed a higher rate of renal insufficiency in the open repair group vs. the EVAR group (30% vs. 11%) [14].

The French ECAR trial in 107 patients in 14 centres between 2000 and 2012 showed a 30-day mortality of 18% for EVAR and 24% for open repair [15]. All three trials showed improvement benefits for women in the EVAR group and also showed that the length of the aneurysm neck but not the diameter appeared to be a predictor of 30-day mortality especially after open repair. In systematic review and meta-analysis, there is a trend to support EVAR over open repair for rAAA but more trials are needed.

When undertaking rAAA repair issues to consider are the use of an aortic occlusion balloon, possible conversion to an aorto-uniiliac graft and the occurrence of abdominal compartment syndrome. An aortic occlusion balloon is useful when severe hemodynamic instability occurs. There are two ways to approach the proximal aorta in such cases: the femoral approach and the brachial approach. The balloon control can be obtained under local anaesthetic in advance of full anaesthesia for the repair.

Abdominal Compartment Syndrome After AAA Repair

After either open or endovascular repair, about 20% of patients can develop abdominal compartment syndrome, which can be defined as raised intra-abdominal pressure sufficient to impair abdominal organ perfusion. Factors key to its development are the presence of significant retroperitoneal haematoma and bowel oedema both of which lead to increased intra-abdominal volume and subsequently pressure.

Intra-abdominal pressure (IAP) can be easily monitored in ITU post-operatively using a pressure transducer attached to a bladder catheter. Normal IAP is <15 mmHg. Decompressive laparostomy should be considered if the pressure is >15 mmHg with associated organ dysfunction (for example, progressive renal dysfunction, difficulty ventilating) or if >20 mmHg otherwise. In high risk patients or where the abdomen is very tight on attempted closure, then a laparostomy approach can be considered from the outset. Despite initial concerns, laparostomy after ruptured AAA repair does not seem to lead to high graft infection rates and commercial vacuum dressing systems are available to aid with wound management.

References

1. Cosford PA, Leng GC, Thomas J. Screening for abdominal aortic aneurysm. *Cochrane Database of Syst Rev* 2007;18(2):CD002945.
2. The Multicentre Aneurysm Screening Study (MASS) into the effect of abdominal aortic aneurysm screening on mortality in men: A randomised controlled trial. *Lancet* 2002;360(9345):1531–1539.
3. Lindholt JS, Sørensen J, Søgaard R, Henneberg EW. Long-term benefit and cost-effectiveness analysis of screening for abdominal aortic aneurysms from a randomized controlled trial. *Br J Surg* 2010;97(6):826–34.
4. Davis M, Harris M, Earnshaw JJ. Implementation of the National Health Service Abdominal Aortic Aneurysm Screening Programme in England. *J Vasc Surg* 2013;57(5):1440e5.
5. https://www.gov.uk/topic/population-screening-programmes/abdominal-aortic-aneurysm.
6. UK Small Aneurysm Trial Participants. Long term outcome of immediate repair compared with surveillance for small abdominal aortic aneurysm. *N Engl J of Medicine* 2002;346:1437–1444.
7. Waton S, Johal A, Heikkila K, Cromwell D. Clinical Effectiveness Unit, The Royal College of Surgeons of England; Loftus I, Vascular Society of Great Britain and Ireland (VSGBI) The National Vascular Registry November 2016.
8. Dubost C, Alary M, Oesconomos N. Treatment of aortic aneurysms; removal of the aneurysms. Reestablishment of continuity by grafts of preserved human aorta. *Mem Acad Chir (Paris)* 1951;77:381–383.
9. Prinssen M, Verhoeven EL, Buth J, Cuypers PW *et al.* A randomized trial comparing conventional and endovascular repair of abdominal aortic aneurysms. (Dutch Randomised Endovascular Aneurysm Management (DREAM) Trial Group. *N Engl J Med* 2004;351:1607–1618.
10. The EVAR Trial participants. Comparison of endovascular aneurysm repair with open repair in patients with abdominal aortic aneurysm (EVAR 1) 30 day operative mortality results; randomised control trial. *Lancet* 2005; 365(9478):2179–2186.
11. Patel R, Sweeting J, Powell JT, Greenhalgh R for the EVAR trial investigators. Endovascular versus open repair of abdominal aortic aneurysm in 15-years' follow-up of the UK endovascular aneurysm repair trial 1 (EVAR trial 1): A randomised controlled trial. *Lancet* 2016;388:2366–2374.
12. The EVAR Trial participants. Endovascular aneurysm repair and outcome in patients unfit for open repair of abdominal aortic aneurysm (EVAR 2): Randomized control trial. *Lancet* 2005;365:2187–2192.

13. IMPROVE trial investigators, Powell JT, Sweeting MJ, Thompson MM, Ashleigh R, Bell R *et al*. Endovascular or open repair strategy for ruptured abdominal aortic aneurysm: 30 day outcomes from IMPROVE randomised trial. *BMJ* 2014;348:f7661.

14. Reimerink JJ, Hoornweg LL, Vahl AC, Wisselink W, vanden Broek TA, Legemate DA *et al*. Endovascular repair versus open repair of ruptured abdominal aortic aneurysms: a multicenter randomized controlled trial. *Ann Surg* 2013;258:248–256.

15. Desgranges P, Kobeiter H, Katsahian S, Boufi M, Gouny Favre J-P *et al*. ECAR (Endovasculaire ou Chirurgiedans lesAnévrysmes aorto-iliaquesRompus): A French randomized controlled trial of endovascular vs. open surgical repair of ruptured aorto-iliac aneurysms. *Eur J Vasc Endovasc Surg* 2015; 50(3):303–10.

Chapter 9

Thoracic, Thoracoabdominal and Suprarenal Aortic Aneurysms

Jennifer Robson and Roderick Chalmers

Key Points

- Aneurysm disease affects the thoracic aorta much less commonly than the infrarenal aorta.
- Most patients are asymptomatic, but may have chest, back or abdominal pain.
- Diagnosis is on computed tomography (CT) angiogram and the Crawford classification is used to describe the extent of the aneurysm.
- Intervention is recommended if the aneurysm is >6 cm (or 5 cm in the presence of a connective tissue disorder or a family history of rupture).
- Open surgery remains the standard treatment for complex suprarenal, thoracic and thoracoabdominal aneurysms.
- Specific complications include risks of paraplegia and renal and visceral ischaemia.
- Endovascular repair is suitable for descending thoracic aneurysms.

Epidemiology

The incidence of aneurysmal disease affecting the suprarenal aorta and the thoracic aorta is difficult to estimate since it is a condition that is usually asymptomatic and rupture, which is often rapidly fatal, is commonly misattributed to other causes such as myocardial infarction or pulmonary embolism. The incidence is approximately 6 per 100,000 people per year. Males are affected about twice as commonly as females, but interestingly the gender difference is less than for infrarenal aortic aneurysms, where the ratio is up to 7:1.

Natural history data are scarce, typically involving retrospective observation of patients not fit for open repair. In a series of 1600 cases, the rupture risk for a 6 cm aneurysm of the thoracic aorta was 3.6% per year and for the composite endpoint of rupture/dissection/death, the annual risk was 14.1%.

Aetiology and Pathophysiology

The causes of descending thoracic aortic aneurysm (DTAA) and thoraco-abdominal aortic aneurysm (TAAA) overlap significantly with those of infrarenal aortic aneurysm (described in Chapter 6). Whilst atherosclerotic disease is still the most common cause of thoracic aneurysms, other causes, including chronic dissection and connective tissue disease (e.g., Marfan's, Ehlers–Danlos and Loeys–Dietz syndromes) as well as infection, trauma and arteritis, account for a higher percentage of cases of thoracic than abdominal aneurysms. Aneurysmal tissue is characterised by deficiency of the tunica media of the vessel wall. Neovascularisation, inflammation and proteolytic digestion of the extracellular matrix are important processes, and biomechanical factors are also involved.

Presentation

The majority of DTAA and TAAA are asymptomatic. Those presenting to the vascular surgeon have either ruptured or have been detected as an incidental finding during an investigation for another indication. Patients may complain of chest, back or abdominal pain and if the aneurysm extends into the abdominal aorta may be detectable as an expansile mass on examination. Distal embolisation can occur and usually manifests as 'trashing' of the lower limbs giving rise to the so-called 'blue toe syndrome'. Other symptoms such as hoarseness, stridor, haemoptysis, haematemesis, nerve root pain and dysphagia aortica can result from compression or erosion of surrounding structures. The small proportion of aneurysms that are inflammatory can cause ureteric, bowel or venous obstruction, and occasionally a low-grade temperature and weight loss. Patients with a ruptured aneurysm will have sudden onset of severe chest, back or abdominal pain with syncope or profound cardiovascular collapse, and mottling of the lower limbs, in particular. A retroperitoneal haematoma may be evident in a TAAA and superficial bruising is sometimes seen if the diagnosis is delayed.

Imaging and Classification

A CT angiogram of the entire thoracic and abdominal aorta is required to define the extent of the aneurysm and its relationship to the key aortic branches. Computed tomography (CT) is also the investigation of choice for suspected rupture.

DTAAs commence beyond the left subclavian artery and terminate above the level of the diaphragm. TAAAs affect a variable length of the thoracic and abdominal aorta and are described according to the Crawford classification (Fig. 1).

This practical classification system is useful for planning the surgical approach and for predicting complications. For example, a laparotomy is often appropriate for type IV TAAA whilst an extensive thoracolaparotomy is required for aneurysms extending into the chest. Regarding complications, aneurysms affecting the visceral aorta carry a higher risk of renal and visceral ischaemia, and the risk of paraplegia is highest for the most extensive aneurysms and lower for those starting below the level of T6.

Management

Based on what is known of the natural history of TAAA and DTAA, intervention is generally considered in medically fit patients when the descending thoracic component reaches 6 cm or the ascending aorta

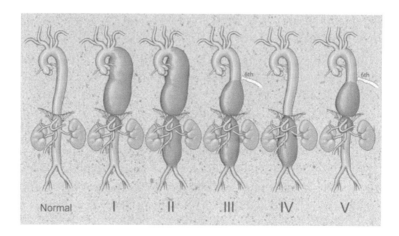

Figure 1.   Modified Crawford classification of thoracoabdominal aneurysms.

Source: Safi HJ *et al*. Evolution of risk for neurologic deficit after descending and thoracoabdominal aortic repair. *Ann Thorac Surg* 2005;80:2173–9; discussion 2179. Reproduced with permission.

reaches 5 cm. A lower threshold of 5 cm may also be considered appropriate in patients with Marfan's syndrome or a familial tendency to rupture. Open surgical management of DTAA and TAAA is a major undertaking which, even with recent advancements in peri-operative care and surgical technique, is associated with a significant morbidity and mortality. There is an emerging and increasing role for the use of endovascular techniques in certain patients, which can reduce the surgical insult. Comprehensive pre-operative assessment is essential.

Management of DTAA and TAAA disease is complex, but the frequency of cases is relatively low. Centralisation of services is essential and there is evidence that outcome is significantly better when patients are managed by high volume surgeons in high volume centres with dedicated vascular anaesthetists.

Non-operative management

Patients with an aneurysm below the diameter-threshold for intervention should remain in a surveillance programme with CT scans at appropriate intervals. These patients should receive standard cardiovascular, best medical treatment including an antiplatelet agent and a statin (regardless of cholesterol) unless contraindicated, with careful control of blood pressure and blood sugar levels in diabetic patients. Patients who are not fit for surgical intervention can generally be discharged from the surveillance programme and are treated with best medical therapy in the community.

Pre-operative assessment

The extent of the aneurysm and the relationship to key aortic branches is determined using CT scanning, which may also reveal surgically impor-tant anomalies such as a retro-aortic left renal vein, multiple renal arter-ies or a horseshoe kidney. From this information, the nature of the operation and the risk of important complications can be gauged. The other side of the equation, how fit the patient is to withstand surgical intervention, is evaluated on the basis of a number of investigations.

It is important to obtain a full medical history and perform a thor-ough physical examination. In the assessment of cardiac function, the information available from a standard electrocardiogram (ECG) and echocardiogram is supplemented by some form of stress testing, either an exercise tolerance test or a stress echocardiogram. Whilst an exercise bicycle or treadmill may be used for exercise testing, a treadmill is gener-ally preferred since most patients are unused to cycling and quadriceps fatigue may limit exercise capacity. With continuous ECG monitoring, the Bruce protocol involves up to 12 min of walking on a treadmill during which the speed and elevation are increased every 3 min, aiming to achieve 85% of the patient's maximum predicted heart rate. A positive test involves the development of angina-related symptoms, a fall in blood pressure or ECG changes including ventricular dysrhythmias or ST changes. Stress echocardiography may be preferred in patients with mobility difficulties and where motion affects data interpretation. During this examination, echocardiography is performed during the infusion of a pharmacological agent such as dobutamine, which has positive inotropic and chronotropic effects. The focus of this test is the detection of wall motion abnormalities and assessment of their relationship to cardiac exertion, and is a sensitive way to detect stress-induced myocardial ischaemia. Cardiac catheterisation and angiography are performed selectively following non-invasive investigations. An assessment of pulmonary function is made using spirometry (FEV1, FVC and FEV1/FVC ratio). In addition, a functional assessment, such as asking a patient to walk up a flight of stairs, is often informative. Cardiopulmonary exercise (CPX) testing is now available in a number of centres and gives detailed global information on the patient's cardiopulmonary performance during exercise. Whilst exercising on a static bicycle ergometer, a closed breathing circuit is used to measure inspired and expired volumes and pO2 and pCO2 breath by breath. As the intensity of exercise increases, the ECG is observed for ischaemic changes, and the anaerobic threshold and oxygen consumption are calculated.

Renal function and hepatic function are assessed using standard blood laboratory measures. The patient's current level of mobility, independence and mental resilience, although hard to assess objectively, are also important in their ability to rehabilitate following major surgery.

The results of all these investigations should be considered by a team of surgeons and anaesthetists with additional input from a radiologist in order that an appropriate management plan can be recommended to the patient. The patient's medications should be reviewed and consideration given to whether they can be optimised in advance of any surgical or endovascular intervention. In particular, consideration is given to antiplatelet, β-blocker and statin therapy.

Open surgical management

Types I, II, III and V thoracoabdominal aortic aneurysms

With the patient in the right lateral position, an extensive thoracolaparotomy is made through the left 6th intercostal space with partial division of the anterior muscular part of the diaphragm, partial division of the left crus of the diaphragm and posterior division of the sixth rib to facilitate access. The left lung is partially deflated using a double lumen endotracheal tube and the aorta is exposed behind the left lung by division of the parietal pleura allowing control of the proximal aorta to be secured. The dissection is continued into the abdomen with medial visceral rotation of the left colon, left kidney and spleen being performed through the left paracolic gutter to expose the entire length of the aorta in the abdomen. The iliac arteries are dissected out and the left femoral artery is exposed through a separate incision to accommodate the bypass circuit. Following full heparinisation, left heart bypass is established with the afferent limb in the left pulmonary vein or left atrium and the efferent limb in the femoral artery. For a type II TAAA, the aorta is cross-clamped distal to the left subclavian and in the mid-descending aorta (above T6). The aorta is opened longitudinally between the clamps and transected proximal to the aneurysm. The proximal end of a Dacron graft of appropriate diameter is anastomosed using a continuous 3-0 prolene suture, and Teflon pledgelets and cyanoacrylate glue can be used to reinforce this suture line. The graft is clamped just beyond the anastomosis and the aortic clamp is replaced in a supraceliac position. The thoracic aorta is opened along its length and large intercostals arteries, usually between T8 and L1, are selected for anastomosis to the graft on a patch. Occasionally, a jump graft is required if vessels are widely spaced. Remaining small intercostal arteries are oversewn. The graft clamp is replaced beyond the intercostal patch restoring inline flow to the spinal artery for the remainder of the procedure. The infrarenal aorta is then clamped and the renal, supraceliac and superior mesenteric arteries are anastomosed to the graft on a patch using a jump graft to incorporate the left renal artery if necessary. Flow to the visceral vessels is restored whilst the distal anastomosis is performed.

By using a serial clamping technique, the ischaemic insult to the spinal cord and viscera is minimised compared to clamping the entire aorta for the duration of the procedure. Prior to closing, the patient is actively warmed since normothermia is important for achieving haemostasis. The surgical techniques and adjuncts that can be used to reduce the complication rate are discussed below.

Descending thoracic aneurysms

An aneurysm of the descending thoracic aorta is repaired through a left-sided thoracotomy without the need to open the abdomen. Otherwise, the technique for open repair is similar to that described for the thoracic component of an extensive TAAA. As discussed below, DTAA are readily amenable to endovascular repair, which has now largely superseded open repair in this setting.

Aneurysms involving the aortic arch

Complete replacement of the ascending aorta and arch mandates deep hypothermic cardioplegic circulatory arrest and cardiopulmonary bypass, and lies within the remit of the cardiothoracic surgeon. However, the vascular surgeon is frequently faced with an aneurysm of the descending aorta, which also involves part of the aortic arch or which allows insufficient space to clamp the aorta distal to the left subclavian artery. Endovascular stenting of the arch would interrupt the blood supply to the brain if the proximal landing zone were to occlude the left carotid artery and the left vertebral artery, which is a branch of the left subclavian artery. In this situation a staged procedure should be performed involving a carotid-carotid bypass and a carotid-subclavian bypass before the aneurysm is repaired endovascularly. Alternatively, a custom-made branched endograft can be used.

Type IV thoracoabdominal and suprarenal aneurysms

The surgical approach for type IV and suprarenal aneurysms is similar and generally involves a midline laparotomy or 'roof-top' incision, although some surgeons prefer a thora-colaparotomy through the 8th, 9th or 10th interspace. The retroperitoneal space is accessed though the left paracolic gutter and the viscera (descending colon, spleen and left kidney) are mobilised and rotated medially to reach the aorta. The left crus of the diaphragm is partially divided, but the diaphragm itself is left intact. A Dacron graft is used to replace the abdominal aorta. A bevel at the proximal end allows the incorporation of the renal and visceral vessels on a patch. The size of the patch should be minimised to reduce the chance of further aneurysm formation, so if the vessels are widely spaced any outlying vessels are anastomosed using a jump graft. Cerebrospinal fluid (CSF) drainage and other adjuncts are not generally considered to be necessary for the repair of type IV and suprarenal aneurysms.

Type IV and suprarenal aneurysms are less amenable to endovascular repair than infra-renal and descending thoracic aneurysms due to the difficulty in preserving the visceral vessels (see below). A hybrid approach can be used, but does not offer improved outcomes in most patients compared to standard open surgery. In a hybrid approach, the coeliac, superior mesenteric and renal arteries are revascularised in a retrograde fashion using a graft from one of the iliac arteries prior to the placement of an endovascular stent-graft to exclude the aneurysm.

Endovascular management

Endovascular strategies offer a minimally invasive alternative to open surgical management with the particular advantage of reducing cardiorespiratory complications. Descending thoracic aneurysms are particularly amenable to a wholly endovascular approach since there is no involvement of the arch or visceral vessels. Branched and fenestrated grafts open up the possibility of treating aneurysms involving the arch and visceral vessels, but these techniques are still being evaluated and currently are only available in a small number of centres with a particular interest in endovascular aneurysm treatment. Encouraging mid-term outcomes have been achieved for BEVAR and FEVAR at five high volume European centres, with 95% and 99% technical success rates, respectively, and 73.4% and 81.8% 2-year survival rates. However, whilst early technical success rates are high, target vessels remain at risk from stent migration, fracture and kinking [1]. Endografts manufactured with fenestrations rather than branches seem to yield more favourable outcomes in terms of renal artery patency (2.3% vs. 9.6% renal occlusion rate). Such grafts are individually made for elective patients, but cannot be obtained in time for patients requiring urgent intervention. Wholly endovascular techniques undoubtedly reduce the cardiopulmonary complications associated with open repair, but the risk of paraplegia remains, reintervention may be necessary, long-term durability results are awaited and annual post-procedure CT surveillance is required [1]. The stent graft industry is continuously developing improved devices that make increasingly complex lesions accessible to endovascular approaches. Hybrid procedures, combining endovascular exclusion of the aneurysm with open surgical revascularisation of aortic branches covered by the stent, have also been advocated, but again accrual of outcome data is ongoing. Hybrid procedures have been used with particular success to treat arch aneurysms when accompanied by an open debranching procedure of the arch.

Complications and Adjuncts

The morbidity and mortality associated with repair of extensive aneurysms has been reduced to acceptable levels over recent years with a better understanding of the pathophysiology of complications leading to modifications to the peri-operative strategy [2]. Despite this, however, it is unsurprising that the complication rate, as a product of the magnitude of the operation and the level of comorbidity present in the DTAA/TAAA patient population, remains significant. Table 1 shows the incidence of the major complications associated with thoracic and thoracoabdominal aneurysm repair reported in two large contemporary case series.

Reducing the overall risk

Pre-operative assessment is necessary to stratify the risk of complications on an individual patient basis and to select patients suitable for intervention. Centralisation of services for managing DTAA and TAAA is vital in order that experienced surgical, anaesthetic, critical care and

Table 1.   Contemporary results of open repair of thoracoabdominal aneurysms.

	Conrad *et al.* [4]	Coselli *et al.* [3]
Number of patients (dates)	445 (1987–2005)	2286 (since 1986)
Crawford extent I/II	41.8%	64.2%
Ruptured	11.4%	6.1%
Death (< 30 day)	8.3%	6.6%
Major paraplegia	9.5%	3.8%
Renal failure (requiring dialysis)	4.6%	5.6%
Cardiac complications	14.7%	7.9%
Pulmonary complications	49%	32.1%

theatre teams can be assembled along with the wide range of facilities and equipment that they require.

Intra-operatively systemic heparinisation is preventative against myocardial infarction, minimises the risk of embolisation, preserves the microcirculation and reduces the risk of thrombosis of key branches, particularly intercostal arteries, during clamping. Moderate permissive hypothermia (32–34°C) reduces the metabolic demands of the viscera and the spinal cord, thereby increasing their tolerance to ischaemia. Unlike repair of the ascending aorta and aortic arch, full hypothermic circulatory arrest is rarely required for DTAA and TAAA repair. Left heart bypass is used for extensive repairs (Crawford extent I and II) enabling retrograde aortic perfusion, facilitating cooling/rewarming and reducing spinal cord and visceral ischaemia. Left heart bypass also allows patients with cardiac disease to tolerate proximal aortic clamping more readily by offloading the left side of the heart. Serial aortic clamping (as described above) involves moving the clamps distally along the aorta as the operation progresses and reduces the ischaemic insult and subsequent reperfusion injuries. Additional strategies are directed at reducing the incidence of specific complications.

Reducing cardiac and respiratory complications

The aetiology of cardiac and respiratory complications following DTAA and TAAA repair is multifactorial involving, in particular, existing comorbidities, a large surgical incision involving the thoracic cavity and fluid replacement to compensate for significant blood loss. Unfortunately, there is limited potential to modify these factors, which is the reason that cardiopulmonary complications remain problematic in extensive aortic surgery and is why the possibility of endovascular repair is so attractive. Nonetheless, identification of risk and optimisation of function pre-operatively are important. Limitation of the incision to a laparotomy for type IV repair avoids the need to enter the thorax. Chest drains are placed routinely when the chest has been entered. Prompt extubation reduces ventilator-associated pneumonia and respiratory muscle wasting, and early tracheostomy placement in selected patients facilitates weaning.

Reducing the risk of paraplegia

The risk of paraplegia was much higher (in the region of 16%) before the introduction of modern adjuncts, but remains higher for type II aneurysms (6.3–14.5%) than for less extensive type IV aneurysms (2.9–3.8%) [3]. This is directly related to the length of aorta that is replaced and the risk of paraplegia is also increased following previous aortic surgery or dissection. The blood supply to the spinal cord is from multiple sources including the vertebral arteries, anterior segmental medullary arteries (intercostal and lumbar) and the internal iliac arteries, all of which contribute to the anterior spinal artery. The artery of Adamkiewicz is the largest contributor to the anterior spinal artery and is generally a left-sided intercostal artery, but may sometimes arise from the right or from a lumbar artery.

Reimplantation of the major segmental arteries, ideally including the artery of Adamkiewicz, is thought to be important in reducing the risk of paraplegia. Whilst some surgeons advocate pre-operative mapping of the spinal cord blood supply using MRI, most would select one to three large pairs of intercostal vessels (usually between T6 and T12) intra-operatively for reattachment. Serial clamping and left heart bypass reduce spinal cord ischaemia during extensive repair, but despite this, some degree of spinal cord ischaemia is inevitable. Placement of a CSF drain allows monitoring of CSF pressure during the operation and post-operatively. CSF is drained actively during aortic cross-clamping and then passively for 48 h post-operatively allowing decompression of the vertebral foramen in the event of spinal cord swelling. Since CSF drainage carries the risks of infection and haematoma formation, it is reserved for extensive aneurysm repairs. Spinal cord perfusion is optimised further by maintaining the mean arterial pressure >80 mmHg and avoiding hypotensive, vasodilating drugs where possible. Motor-evoked potentials can be used to detect spinal cord ischaemia during cross-clamping and following reimplantation of vessels. Post-operatively, rather than being fully sedated, even intubated patients are nursed in a reusable state to facilitate assessment of the neurological function of the lower limbs and detection of signs of delayed-onset spinal cord ischaemia.

Reducing the risk of renal and gastrointestinal tract ischaemia

Left heart bypass, moderate systemic hypothermia, heparinisation and serial clamping all contribute to a reduced risk of visceral ischaemia. Additionally, a trial of renal cooling comparing renal perfusion with normothermic blood and 4C crystalloid fluid found the latter to be advantageous in reducing renal complications. Retrograde aortic perfusion on left heart bypass maintains the blood supply to the abdominal viscera during surgery on the proximal aorta. When the clamps are replaced on the infrarenal aorta, selective visceral perfusion can be maintained using individual balloon perfusion catheters in the ostia of the visceral vessels. Some surgeons use renal cooling and selective visceral perfusion routinely whilst others use these measures selectively in patients perceived to have a higher than average risk of complications.

Reducing complications of blood loss and coagulopathy

Significant blood loss occurs during the repair of extensive aneurysms and massive heterologous transfusion is associated with a number of complications including coagulopathy, hypothermia and transfusion reactions. The use of a cell saver and autologous transfusion reduces heterologous transfusion requirements. Near-patient testing of coagulation, such as thromboelastography, can be used to detect impending coagulopathy before it becomes evident clinically. It also enables identification of the specific part of the coagulation cascade that is deficient so that treatment can be targeted and timely before bleeding complications become problematic.

References

1. Greenberg RK, Lytle B. Endovascular repair of thoracoabdominal aneurysms. *Circulation* 2008;117:2288–2296.
2. Coselli JS, LeMaire SA. Tips for successful outcomes for descending thoracic and thoracoabdominal aortic aneurysm procedures. *Semin Vasc Surg* 2008;21:13–20.

3. Coselli JS, Bozinovski J, LeMaire SA. Open surgical repair of 2286 thoracoab-dominal aortic aneurysms. *Ann Thorac Surg* 2007;83:S862–S864; discussion S890–S892.

4. Conrad MF, Crawford RS, Davison JK, Cambria RP. Thoracoabdominal aneu-rysm repair: A 20-year perspective. *Ann Thorac Surg* 2007;83:S856–S861; discussion S890–S892.

Chapter 10

Aortic Dissection

Jennifer Robson and Roderick Chalmers

Key Points

- Aortic dissection may be defined according to the time since onset of symptoms as hyperacute (<24 h), acute (2–7 days), subacute (8–30 days) or chronic (>30 days).
- Acute aortic dissection is associated with hypertension and pre-existing disease of the aortic wall.
- Patients usually present with severe, tearing chest and back pain.
- Diagnosis is with transoesophageal echocardiogram and computed tomography (CT) angiogram.
- The Stanford or DeBakey classifications are used to describe the pattern of dissection.
- Type A dissections require early surgical treatment. The in-hospital mortality is high, but the prognosis is very good in patients surviving to discharge from hospital.
- Type B dissections are treated medically in the first instance. The in-hospital mortality is much lower compared to type A, but complications may occur following discharge.
- Chronic type B dissection may result in aortic dilatation and rupture, so surveillance is required.
- There is an expanding role for early endovascular intervention.

Epidemiology

Acute aortic syndrome, comprising aortic dissection (85–90%) and intramural haematoma (10–15%), occurs with an incidence of approximately 3 per 100,000 per year. Accurate estimates are difficult due to the high out-of-hospital mortality for this condition and the low post-mortem rate in most countries. It affects males twice as commonly as females and the risk increases with age. Interestingly, as with a number of other cardiovascular conditions, it demonstrates circadian variation with a peak incidence early in the morning and during the winter. This pattern correlates with times of peak blood pressure.

Aetiology

Factors predisposing to aortic dissection involve pre-existing degenerative, genetic or inflammatory conditions that weaken the aorta and primary or secondary causes of hypertension. Table 1 shows the factors that have an association with aortic dissection.

Pathophysiology

Aortic dissection involves a breach in the aortic intima that allows blood to track within the media of the vessel wall, creating a true lumen and a

Table 1.   Factors associated with aortic dissection.

- Increasing age
- Male sex
- Diabetes mellitus
- Pre-existing aortic disease, e.g., aneurysmal disease, atherosclerosis, arteritis
- Connective tissue disorders, e.g., Marfan's syndrome, Ehlers–Danlos syndrome
- Congenital anomalies, e.g., bicuspid valve, aortic hypoplasia
- Hypertension primary or secondary, e.g., pregnancy, cocaine use, weightlifting
- Iatrogenic, e.g., cardiac catheterisation and intervention, coronary artery bypass grafting, valve replacement
- Trauma, e.g., deceleration injury
- Previous aortic surgery
- Family history

false lumen. This entry tear usually lies in the ascending aorta, aortic arch or just distal to the left subclavian artery. Dissection results from a combination of the stress applied to the aortic wall due to high, fluctuating blood pressure and disease processes, which damage and weaken the vessel wall. A breach in the intima may also be caused by a penetrating atherosclerotic ulcer that erodes the intima. In a smaller number of patients, the intimal injury is traumatic or iatrogenic.

Disruption of vasa vasorum within the aortic wall leads to the formation of an intramural haematoma. Intramural haematoma may precede aortic dissection if the haematoma continues to expand and reptures into the aortic lumen. Although initially benign, intramural haematoma regresses in only 10% of patients, whilst 28–45% progress to aortic dissection and 20–45% rupture, with more proximal lesions being particularly prone to complications [1].

Intimal disruption initiates the dissection. Proximal and/or distal propagation follows and is facilitated if the media has been weakened by enzymatic (e.g., matrix metalloproteinases) degradation of the extracellular matrix. Blood may travel within the false lumen along a variable length of the aorta and its branches. The exit tear may re-enter the true lumen connecting it with the false lumen or it may rupture outwards, with the latter generally resulting in rapid death.

Presentation

The classical presentation of acute aortic dissection is with sudden onset of extremely severe chest pain, often described as 'tearing' in nature, radiating to the neck or back and migrating as the dissection propagates. Whilst pain is prominent in the majority of patients, a proportion will complain of less severe pain or no discomfort at all and, in fact, lack of pain is a predictor of poor outcome, perhaps because diagnosis is delayed. Where chest pain is present the diagnosis is often confused with acute myocardial infarction or pulmonary embolism although, if a detailed history is taken, the nature of the symptoms may be used to distinguish the true cause. It should be noted that myocardial ischaemia/ infarction may also occur concurrently if the coronary arteries are affected by the dissection. The integrity of the aortic valve may be disrupted causing acute aortic regurgitation and, if the dissection communicates with the pericardium, tamponade may result. Patients with a type A dissection are often hypotensive whilst hypertension is typical in type B dissection.

As the false lumen extends, it may compromise some of the key branches of the aorta, impairing end-organ perfusion and precipitating organ dysfunction or failure. Symptoms include myocardial ischaemia (coronary arteries), cerebrovascular accident (carotid and vertebral arteries), spinal cord ischaemia (vertebral, intercostal and lumbar arteries), renal dysfunction (renal arteries), mesenteric ischaemia (coeliac and mesenteric arteries) and limb ischaemia (subclavian and iliac arteries), which often become evident in serial fashion as the dissection extends. On examination, pulses may be weak, asymmetrical or absent, and again may disappear serially with progression of the dissection.

Diagnosis and Classification

Sudden death may occur, but in those surviving to present to the emergency department, rapid diagnosis is important to plan treatment. Plain radiography and electrocardiography (ECG) are commonly performed in patients presenting with acute chest pain. Neither is diagnostic in this setting, but they may show some non-specific features associated with dissection and may also identify complications. A plain radiograph of the chest may [2] reveal mediastinal widening, an abnormal contour of the aortic arch or a haemothorax/effusion, but is normal in a third to a half of patients, especially in those with type B dissections. ECG is often normal, but may show signs of myocardial ischaemia or left ventricular strain/hypertrophy.

An echocardiogram and cross-sectional imaging (either magnetic resonance imaging, MRI or computed tomography, CT) are needed to confirm the diagnosis and the extent of the dissection proximally and distally. Whilst transthoracic echocardiography (TTE) has the advantage of being rapid and non-invasive in unstable patients, transoesophageal echo (TOE) has a higher sensitivity and specificity (90% and 95% respectively) compared to TTE (80% and 85%, respectively). CT and magnetic resonance angiography offer comparable sensitivities and specificities of 95–100%. Compared to echocardiography, they yield additional information about organ perfusion and the relative flow in the true and false lumens, and also have the advantage of imaging the entire thoracic cavity if an alternative diagnosis is possible. The performances of CT and MRI are comparable in diagnosing and excluding aortic dissection. The advantage of CT is that it is more widely available and the scanning time is short. The use of MRI for long-term surveillance to avoid an accumulating ionising radiation dose is beneficial.

Dissection has traditionally been defined as being acute within 2 weeks of the onset of symptoms, and chronic beyond that time. However latterly, data from the IRAD database have suggested an updated classification is more useful in terms of predicting complications and mortality at different timepoints: hyperacute (<24 h), acute (2–7 days), subacute (8–30 days) and chronic (>30 days). The Stanford and DeBakey classifications are useful for stratifying risk, predicting complications and planning treatment. The Stanford classification distinguishes dissections affecting the ascending aorta (type A) with or without involvement of the descending aorta, from those which affect only the descending aorta (type B). The DeBakey classification further subdivides dissections affecting the ascending aorta into those affecting the descending aorta as well (type I) and those only affecting the ascending aorta (type II). DeBakey type III is equivalent to Stanford type B (Fig. 1).

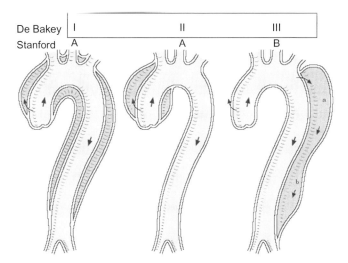

Figure 1.   Stanford and DeBakey classification of aortic dissections.

Source: From Ref. [2]. Reproduced with permission.

If the ascending aorta is affected, the patient may experience cardiac, cerebral and upper limb complications since the coronary, carotid and subclavian arteries are at risk. Dissections of the descending and abdominal aorta cause complications related to spinal cord as well as visceral and limb ischaemia. Considering treatment, type A dissections generally require early surgical intervention whilst type B dissections can be managed medically initially in the majority of patients, with consideration given to early endovascular intervention.

Management

The management of aortic dissection depends upon the extent and location of the dissection and the stability and comorbidities of the patient [6]. Due to the nature of this condition, there is a paucity of high-level evidence to support practice, but the International Registry of Aortic Dissection (IRAD) has gathered valuable information about the trends and outcomes of recent practice [1, 4]. In addition, the European Society of Cardiology taskforce produced guidelines for the management of aortic dissection [2].

Type A

Type A dissections account for around two thirds of all cases of dissection [4]. Urgent surgery is almost always required for type A dissections, unless the patient is moribund or has significant pre-existing comorbidities. Untreated type A dissections have a mortality in the region of 1–2% per hour for the first 24 h, amounting to 50–75% by 2 weeks. With medical management alone the mortality of type A dissections in the IRAD database was 56% [1]. Surgical management involves sealing off the entry point to decompress the false lumen and reduce the risk of propagation of the dissection. Since the entry tear usually lies in a diffusely diseased part of the aorta, this generally involves resection of the aorta at the site of the entry tear and reconstruction using a short graft (e.g., Dacron) through a median sternotomy approach with cardiopulmonary bypass, and in some patients deep hypothermic cardioplegic circulatory arrest. When the entry tear lies in the arch, reconstruction or reimplanation of the innominate, carotid and subclavian vessels will be necessary. If there is incompetence of the aortic valve, this may have to be reconstructed or, more commonly, replaced with a prosthesis. The ostia of the coronary arteries may also require reconstruction or coronary artery bypass grafting. The operative mortality for dissections of the ascending aorta is in the region of 16%, higher (31.4%) if the patient is shocked before surgery [1].

The false lumen may extend for a variable distance into the descending aorta, but due to the morbidity associated with replacing long segments of the aorta, including the visceral vessels, this is usually avoided in the first instance where possible. The operation on the ascending aorta effectively converts this situation into a type B dissection, which can then be managed medically as described below. Whilst there is not yet an established role for endovascular management of type A dissections, there is interest in using a hybrid approach combining open surgery for the ascending aorta and arch with endovascular stenting of the descending aorta. This approach may be useful for patients with malperfusion syndromes, intractable pain, uncontrolled hypertension or continued propagation or expansion of the false lumen.

An elephant trunk procedure is used when it is anticipated that the descending aorta will need to be replaced subsequently. The ascending aorta and the arch are replaced with a tube graft. The arch vessels are re-implanted into the graft on a single patch. Rather than cutting the graft to length, the distal end is left long and projects into the descending aorta enabling a staged procedure to be performed. At a later date, an open surgical approach to the descending aorta can be used with the proximal anastomosis being made to the elephant trunk, or the elephant trunk can be used as the proximal landing zone for an endovascular stent graft. The advantage of this is that it avoids the need to graft directly onto diseased and fragile aortic wall.

Type B

Type B — Uncomplicated

The early outcomes for type B dissection are much more favourable than for type A dissection with a 30-day survival rate of 89% [1]. However, data suggest that the longer-term outlook is less benign with three quarters of dissected aortas in medically-treated patients becoming aneurysmal by 5 years, and a 30% mortality rate in the same group at 5 years.

Surgical management is extremely hazardous and is avoided if possible [5]. In-hospital mortality in the region of 30% has been reported, although this is undoubtedly biased by the more complicated presentation of the patients selected for surgery. Aggressive medical management involving analgesia and control of hypertension and heart rate is essential. Patients should be admitted to a critical care unit for close monitoring of blood pressure, end-organ function and any evidence of progression such as escalating or intractable pain, or development of new symptoms. Intravenous short-acting beta-blockers (e.g., esmolol, labetalol), unless contraindicated, are used in the first instance to reduce both heart rate and blood pressure, with a target heart rate of 50–60 beats per minute, systolic blood pressure of 100–120 mmHg and MAP <80 mmHg. Peripherally-acting calcium channel blockers (e.g., nicardipine) may be added as second-line agents or in patients intolerant of beta blockers. Whilst vasodilators cause a reflex tachycardia when used in isolation, hydralazine may be used in addition to the previously listed agents. Adequate opioid analgesia is essential to control heart rate and blood pressure further. End-organ function (e.g., urine output) should be monitored since blood pressure lowering may cause organ dysfunction in these usually hypertensive patients, and dynamic changes in blood flow can precipitate malperfusion syndromes. Once blood pressure is well-controlled and symptoms are stable, the patient is converted to oral anti-hypertensives. Angiogenesis-converting enzyme (ACE) inhibitors may have the additional advantage of promoting remodelling of the aortic wall, but the evidence for this has not yet been accumulated.

Endovascular intervention may be considered in patients with type B dissection that is uncomplicated at presentation (see below).

Type B — Complicated

In the International Registry of Acute Aortic Dissection (IRAD) database, 17.2% of patients with type B dissection required surgical intervention during the acute phase [6]. Indications for surgery were rupture (23%), further propagation of the dissection (52%), uncontrolled hypertension

(15.5%), intractable pain (14.1%), malperfusion of the viscera (23.9%) or limbs (15.5%) or a combination of these factors. The exact procedure is tailored to the anatomy of the dissection for a given patient. Graft replacement of the descending aorta is the most common open surgical procedure (69.3% of surgically managed acute type B dissections in the IRAD series) [9], which may be performed in conjunction with replacement of the arch as well as fenestration of the dissection flap, stenting or bypass for compromised vessels. The requirement for surgical intervention was associated with high mortality (29.3%), particularly if required during the first 2 days [6] and there has therefore been considerable interest in the possibility of employing endovascular techniques in the management of complicated acute type B dissection.

In the IRAD database, endovascular treatment was associated with better short-term outcomes than open surgical treatment for complicated acute type B dissection [1]. Long-term follow-up data are awaited. In this context, a stent graft may be used to occlude the entry tear and bare metal stents to hold the true lumen open and compress the false lumen, which may improve dynamic malperfusion phenomena. Compromised vessels may also be targeted directly with bare metal stents to restore flow.

Type B — Chronic

Accurate data on the outcome of patients with chronic dissection are sparse and 5-year mortality is estimated at 30%, suggesting that medical management alone is suboptimal. The European Society of Cardiology recommends regular surveillance at 1 month, 3 months, 6 months, 12 months and annually thereafter to monitor for expansion of the affected aorta [2]. Thresholds for intervention are recommended at 5 cm for the ascending aorta and 5.5–6 cm or an expansion rate of >1 cm/year for the descending aorta in patients with spontaneous sporadic dissection [2]. In patients with an arteriopathy (e.g., Marfan's syndrome, Loeys–Dietz syndrome), a lower threshold of 5.0 cm is recommended for the descending aorta as the risk of rupture is higher. Furthermore, patients with arteriopathies should be managed by open surgery rather than endovascular repair as there is continued dilatation of the remaining aorta which compromises the long-term durability of endovascular stent grafts.

Surgical management involves graft replacement of the entire aorta as described for open thoraco-abdominal aneurysm repair. The evidence supporting endovascular repair of chronic type B dissection is currently limited, but early results do not appear to be as encouraging as for acute dissection. This is partly because the aortic wall has limited capability to remodel at this late stage.

Endovascular repair

Endovascular repair has an established role in the management of patients with complicated type B dissection with indications including refractory pain, malperfusion syndromes and impending rupture (increasing false lumen or total diameter, increasing thrombus size or increasing pleural effusion volume). However, the role in uncomplicated type B dissection remains unclear. The high long-term mortality of type B dissection of 30–50% suggests that medical management alone may be inadequate.

The INSTEAD trial randomised patients ($n = 140$) with uncomplicated acute type B dissection >14 days from onset of symptoms to optimal best medical therapy alone or optimal best medical therapy plus elective TEVAR (Medtronic TALENT at a median of 57 days following onset of symptoms). There was no difference in all-cause mortality or aorta-related mortality at 2 years, although the trial was underpowered to detect a difference. Using a controversial landmark analysis, the investigators were able to demonstrate that in patients surviving for more than 2 years, all-cause mortality, aorta-specific mortality and disease progression were improved in the TEVAR group.

The ADSORB trial randomised 61 patients with uncomplicated type B dissection within 14 days of onset of symptoms to optimal medical therapy or optimal medical therapy plus TEVAR (Gore Tag at a median of 5.5 days from onset of symptoms). The study was powered to look at favourable aortic remodelling (not mortality) and demonstrated that patients in the TEVAR group had a higher rate of false lumen thrombosis, lower false lumen diameter, higher true lumen diameter and lower total aortic diameter at 1 year.

Whilst there is inadequate level 1 evidence to make a clear recommendation, it would appear that at least a proportion of patients with initially uncomplicated type B dissection benefit from early endovascular repair. Optimum timing of intervention is unclear, but very early intervention carries a high risk of rupture and retrograde dissection. Certain factors that predict increased risk of disease progression may be used to stratify patients and select those who would benefit from intervention. These include aortic diameter >44 mm, false lumen diameter >22 mm, age >60 years, longer length of dissection, multiple vessels coming off false lumen, partial (vs. no or complete) false lumen, thrombosis, large entry tear and multiple entry tears.

The initial endovascular approach is to cover the entry tear using a stent graft to promote false lumen thrombosis and encourage aortic remodelling. The optimal length of stent graft is not clear, with longer stents providing a more comprehensive repair but carrying a higher risk of spinal cord ischaemia, especially if it is necessary to cover the left subclavian in order to achieve a proximal seal. If this is not feasible, the dissection flap may be fenestrated using a balloon. Where major aortic branches are compromised to the extent that they are causing end-organ ischaemia, they may be opened using a bare metal stent.

Complications of Intervention

The main complications of type A dissection repair are myocardial ischaemia, stroke and death. The complications of intervention for type B aortic dissection are similar to those described for open repair of extensive TAAA, but patients with a history of dissection are at higher risk of paraplegia, renal failure and death.

Whilst acute type A dissection has a high in-hospital mortality (33%) amongst patients who survive to discharge, the 1- and 3-year survival rates are 96% and 91%, respectively [1]. In contrast, 90% of patients with acute type B dissection survive to discharge, but amongst those surviving to be discharged from hospital the 1–3- and 5-year survival rates are 78%, 76% and 70%, respectively [1].

References

1. Tsai TT, Trimarchi S, Nienaber CA. Acute aortic dissection: Perspectives from the International Registry of Acute Aortic Dissection (IRAD). *Eur J Vasc Endovasc Surg* 2009;37:149–159.
2. Erbel R *et al.* Diagnosis and management of aortic dissection. *Eur Heart J* 2001;22:1642–1681.
4. Trimarchi S *et al.* Contemporary results of surgery in acute type A aortic dissection: The International registry of acute aortic dissection experience. *J Thorac Cardiovasc Surg* 2005;129:112–122.
5. Akin I, Kische S, Ince H, Nienaber CA. Indication, timing and results of endovascular treatment of type B dissection. *Eur J Vasc Endovasc Surg* 2009;37:289–296.
6. Trimarchi S *et al.* Role and results of surgery in acute type B aortic dissection: Insights from the International Registry of Acute Aortic Dissection (IRAD). *Circulation* 2006;114:357–364.
7. Leurs LJ *et al.* Endovascular treatment of thoracic aortic diseases: Combined experience from the EUROSTAR and United Kingdom Thoracic Endograft registries. *J Vasc Surg* 2004;40:670–679; discussion 679–680.

Chapter 11

Femoral Artery Aneurysm

Robert Davies and Rajiv Vohra

Key Points

- The majority of femoral artery aneurysm (FAA) present with local symptoms or thigh pain or claudication.
- Type I aneurysms involves the CFA only and type II involves the CFA and SFA.
- The majority can be repaired using straight or bifurcated interposition grafts.
- Pseudo aneurysms form as a result of IV drug abuse or iatrogenic injury from catheterisation.
- Most small pseudo aneurysms less than 3 cm have an indolent course and can be managed conservatively.
- Symptomatic ones can do treated with ultrasound guided compression or thrombin injection.

True Femoral Aneurysms

Introduction

Femoral artery aneurysm (FAA) is the second most common peripheral artery aneurysm after popliteal artery aneurysms (PAAs). They predominantly occur in male patients over 65 years of age with an age adjusted incidence of combined femoral and PAAs of 7.39 per 100,000 population in the USA; male to female ratio of 10:1 [1]. Patients with FAAs demonstrate a high incidence of cardiovascular disease and associated risk factors including hypertension, smoking and hypercholesterol-aemia. Diabetes mellitus appears to be protective for FAA. Although FAAs predominantly occur in association with atherosclerotic disease, reports suggest an association with vasculitides and connective tissue disorders [2,3].

FAAs rarely occur in isolation and are frequently associated with a contralateral aneurysm or/and aneurysmal disease affecting the aorta or other peripheral arteries. In a cohort of one hundred patients with FAAs, Graham *et al.* reported 72% were bilateral, 85% were associated with aorta-iliac aneurysms and 44% were associated with PAAs [4]. Alternatively, Diwan *et al.* reported the incidence of FAAs in 313 consecutive patients with abdominal aortic aneurysms as 6%, all of which were men. Furthermore, an extra 4% had demonstrable femoral artery ectasia [5].

Pathophysiology

The pathophysiological conditions predisposing to the development of FAAs are poorly understood. It has been postulated that in conjunction with weakening of the arterial wall by atherosclerosis, turbulent flow plays an important part. Constriction at the level of inguinal ligament may promote the development of post-stenotic dilatation with resultant turbulent flow and pressure fluctuations affecting the common femoral artery (CFA). This localised change in flow dynamics causes the arterial segment to vibrate, clinically evident as a bruit, weakening the arterial wall predisposing it to aneurysmal change [4,6]. This would be consistent with the clinical finding that FAAs classically affect the CFA in isolation without extending proximal to the inguinal ligament.

Signs and symptoms

Around 30–40% of patients with FAAs are asymptomatic at the time of diagnosis with an incidental finding of a smooth, fusiform and pulsatile mass. However, the majority of patients with FAAs present with localised symptomatology or lower limb claudication/rest pain. In 20% of patients, localised pain in the groin or anterior thigh is the sole symptom.

Slowly enlarging FAAs may cause chronic compression of the adjacent neurovascular structures. Up to 10% of patients demonstrate changes attributable to lower limb chronic venous hypertension secondary to chronic femoral vein compression. However, chronic dysesthesia or paraesthesia resulting from femoral nerve compression is uncommon unless associated with spontaneous FAA rupture.

FAAs may be complicated by acute or chronic thromboembolism or rupture in as many as 50% of cases at the time of initial presentation [7]. The incidence of FAA thrombosis varies in the literature although the incidence of chronic and acute thrombosis appears to be similar. Acute thrombosis complicates up to 16% of FAAs at the time of presentation [8]. Patients present with an acutely ischaemic lower limb (Rutherford Classification IIb or III) clinically mimicking a femoral artery embolus. Inflow into both the superficial femoral artery and PFA is disrupted thereby dramatically reducing any potential source of collateral flow. Chronic thrombosis may mimic peripheral occlusive disease in presentation particularly as a high number of patients have concomitant atherosclerotic cardiovascular disease.

Symptomatic distal embolisation is less common with a reported incidence of 2–8% [1,4,9]. This may not reflect the true incidence as it is thought a large proportion of distal emboli are clinically silent. The majority of reports cite FAA rupture as occurring less frequently than thrombosis or distal embolisation with an incidence of 0–14%. This may partly reflect the 'protective' nature of the tough femoral sheath [4,6,8].

Investigations

Only 20% of FAAs are reliably identified on clinical examination alone. Those measuring <2 cm are particularly unlikely to be identified by routine physical examination [5]. As such, a high index of suspicion is required depending on the circumstances in which the patient presents. All patients with abdominal aortic aneurysms or peripheral artery aneurysms should undergo formalised imaging assessment of their lower limb vasculature. Conversely, all patients with FAAs should undergo formalised assessment of their abdominal aorta and popliteal arteries.

Duplex Doppler ultrasonography (DUS) is an adequate screening tool in both the emergency and elective setting. High quality images can be obtained of the aneurysm sac size, thrombus content and morphology whilst other vascular beds can be screened for aneurysmal or occlusive disease.

Upon confirmation of the diagnosis, a suitable imaging modality is required to accurately quantify the extent of thromboembolic disease locally and distally as well as any concomitant aneurysmal disease identified by DUS. This should be dictated by the patients' clinical picture. Computed tomography angiography (CTA) and magnetic resonance angiography (MRA) provide accurate assessment of the femoral artery complex, inflow and outflow vessels. Crural vessels with a heavy burden of calcification or pedal vessels with poor flow may not be adequately assessed with a CTA or MRA; these patients should undergo a percutaneous angiogram to further assess these arterial trees when in doubt.

In the patient with an acutely ischaemic limb a lengthy pre-operative investigation should not prevent a limb saving operation from being performed expeditiously. In these situations, a hybrid procedure combining open surgical revascularisation with on-table angiography/angioplasty is key to limb salvage.

Classification

FAAs can be classified into type I and type II according to the involvement of the superficial femoral artery (SFA) and profunda femoris artery (PFA). Type I involves the CFA in isolation, type II involves the CFA and one or both of the SFA and PFA.

Treatment

All medically fit patients with symptomatic aneurysms or aneurysms complicated with thromboembolism or rupture should be offered primary surgical repair. Aneurysms that are enlarging on serial imaging should also be considered for elective surgical repair.

The treatment of asymptomatic aneurysms remains controversial. Conflicting evidence regarding the safety of conservative management exists in the literature. Proponents of a conservative management strategy cite the lack of evidence between the aneurysm size and the development of ischaemic complications. Furthermore, the risk of developing limb threatening complications in an asymptomatic aneurysm with conservative treatment at 2 years follow-up is less than 5% [4]. When taken into account with the significant cardiovascular morbidities these patients often suffer with, a non-operative strategy is attractive. Alternatively, proponents of an aggressive operative strategy cite rates of limb loss >15% secondary to the development of complications in asymptomatic aneurysms [10]. In practice, the authors consider any FAA measuring >3 cm or enlarging on serial imaging for elective repair.

The majority of type I femoral aneurysms are best repaired with a straight interposition graft anastomosed proximally at the external CFA junction and distally to the CFA bifurcation. This is performed from within the aneurysm with the redundant sac plicated over the graft. Conduit utilised is dependent on individual surgeon preference, but unless there is a suspicion of infection autologous conduit offers no benefit over prosthetic. A variety of configurations have been utilised for type II femoral aneurysms often based around the concept of an interposition graft extending distally into either the SFA or PFA with reimplantation of the remaining artery with or without an interposition graft. Peri-operative mortality rates following FAA repair are low although they rise to 5% when undertaken concomitantly with other aneurysm repairs [4]. The 5-year patency rates in asymptomatic patients approach 90% [8]. Patients presenting with lower limb claudication or rest pain/gangrene have less good patency rates at 5 years [4].

Endovascular repair can be performed in isolation or as part of a hybrid repair for patients with associated iliac artery aneurysms or SFA aneurysms. Access can either be obtained percutaneously from the contralateral groin or from a cut-down under local anaesthetic onto the SFA distal to the aneurysmal change. Sufficient 'normal' artery is required proximally and distally in order to obtain an adequate seal when exclud-ing an FAA with a stent-graft and is often not available. In these patients where the FAA extends to the CFA bifurcation, the option of extending the stent-graft into the SFA, with or without PFA chimney/snorkel revas-cularisation, to maintain a purely endovascular solution has been described. However mid- and long-term outcomes remain unknown and this technique remains purely investigational and not currently recom-mended by the authors. Alternatively, those patients with adverse fea-tures for a formal groin incision; a limited CFA exposure can be performed at the level of the bifurcation through a transverse incision and a stent-graft can be deployed through the FAA and sealed proximally. The distal end is then physically anastomosed to the CFA bifurcation maintaining flow into both the PFA and SFA. This technique abates the need for an extensive groin incision and dissection and has been employed success-fully by the authors.

Often, femoral aneurysms occur in conjunction with aortoiliac and popliteal aneurysmal or occlusive disease. In these situations, the type of repair needs to be tailored to the anatomy of the presenting pathology. In particular, the most pressing disease needs to be dealt with first whilst simultaneously planning for any second- or third-stage procedures.

Profunda femoris artery aneurysms

Isolated Profunda femoris artery aneurysms (PFAa) are rare and account for <3% of femoral aneurysms [11]. Three quarters of patients have con-comitant aneurysmal disease affecting one other vascular bed, most often the popliteal artery [12]. Due to the difficulty in identifying isolated PFAa at clinical examination, spontaneous rupture rates are higher than for other peripheral aneurysms with up to 45% of patients presenting with rupture [13]. Diagnosis is predominantly by DUS and formal assess-ment of the aorta-iliac and popliteal arteries is recommended to identify concomitant aneurysms.

There is no current evidence regarding the optimal size at which PFAa should be repaired, however, many surgeons recommend considering repair for those >2 cm in an otherwise fit patient. Those medically unfit for repair should be evaluated regularly with DUS to assess for aneurysm expansion. The primary aim of the treatment is to prevent rupture. However, one series reports ipsilateral SFA occlusion in 45% of cases, therefore maintaining that the PFA blood flow is important [12].

The treatment of PFAa primarily consists of vessel reconstruction with an interposition graft or aneurysm ligation and autologous bypass. Few reports describe an endovascular approach with coil embolisation and/or stent-graft occlusion. Both these techniques risk loss of important collaterals when PFAa is associated with concomitant femoral-popliteal arterio-occlusive disease.

Femoral Artery Pseudoaneurysms

Pathophysiology

Femoral artery pseudoaneurysms (FApA) develop as a result of high pressure blood flow through an arterial wall defect that becomes constrained by the perivascular soft tissue or surrounding haematoma. Unlike a true aneurysm, the wall consists of thin fibrous tissue and not all three tunica layers.

Iatrogenic, post-catheterisation pseudoaneurysm formation is the commonest cause with a reported incidence of 1–6% in prospective sonographic studies [14,15]. Factors predisposing to post-catheterisation pseudoaneurysm formation include anticoagulation, hypertension, obesity, sheath size >7 fr, cannulation of superior femoral/PFA, simultaneous puncture of artery and vein, heavily calcified arteries, haemodialysis and short vessel compression time post-catheterisation [16]. Infection, particularly in the drug abuser population and anastomotic leakage may lead to FApA formation. About 2.5% of all femoral anastomosis and 8% of aortobifemoral bypasses at a median follow-up of 8 years are complicated by FApA formation [17,18].

Signs and symptoms

FApAs may present as a pulsatile groin mass that may or may not be painful. Enlargement may cause compression of the adjacent femoral nerve or vein with resultant paraesthesia/dysesthesia or symptoms/signs of venous hypertension, respectively. Mycotic aneurysms present as a painful, erythematous groin mass with or without purulent/sanguineous discharge.

Investigations

DUS is the initial investigation of choice with a reported sensitivity and specificity of 94% and 97%, respectively [19]. Computed tomographic angiography may be utilised as an adjunct to USS, particularly in the assessment of patients with anastomotic pseudoaneurysms in whom complex reconstructive surgery may be required.

Treatment

Most small post-catheterisation pseudoaneurysms lead to an indolent clinical course with the majority undergoing spontaneous thrombosis. Pseudoaneurysm size and anticoagulation status of patients are the two most important predictors of spontaneous thrombosis. Toursarkissan *et al.* reported 87% of FApAs ≤ 3 cm undergoing spontaneous thrombosis at a mean follow up of 23 days [20]. Thus, it is acceptable to initially treat a small pseudoaneurysm (<3 cm) conservatively with serial DDU evaluation. However, the economic burden of such an approach can be prohibitive and many institutions advocate active treatment of all FApA irrespective of size.

The advent of minimally invasive percutaneous treatment methods has limited the indications for open surgical repair to those FApAs that are either rapidly expanding, infected, causing neurovascular compression, skin necrosis, or have undergone failed percutaneous treatment. The presence or absence of infection dictates the surgical technique. For mycotic pseudoaneurysms, the surgery is aimed at excising infected tissues whilst endeavouring to preserve the distal circulation. This may require the use of autologous arterial bypasses routed outside the field of infection. In cases of gross suppurative infection, the primary ligation of the femoral vessels may become necessary with a 30% risk of subsequent amputation widely quoted in the literature, although in the authors experience the risk is considerably lower. Non-infected pseudoaneurysms are repaired primarily with interrupted non-absorbable sutures or with a vein patch-angioplasty depending on the size of the arterial defect.

In recent years, minimally invasive methods of treating FApAs and particularly post-catheterisation FApAs, have been trialled. Ultrasound, guided compression was the first to gain widespread acceptance with success rates between 63% and 100% [16]. Patients undergoing anticoagulation and pseudoaneurysm size > 3 cm are predictors of failure of ultrasound-guided compression. Complications including rupture, femoral vein thrombosis and acute limb ischaemia have been reported in 2–4% of patients [16].

Ultrasound-guided percutaneous thrombin injection into the pseudoaneurysm sac is in widespread usage with reported success rates of >90% and is the gold standard of practice. This may be performed in combination with an intra-arterial balloon protection device to prevent spillage of thrombin into the native vessels, particularly in pseudoaneurysms with wide necks. Thrombin (IIa) directly converts fibrinogen (I) to fibrin (Ia) circumventing the uphill coagulation cascade activation normally required for the conversion of prothrombin (II) to thrombin (IIa). This direct thrombin activation means that unlike the ultrasound-guided compression, the patients' anticoagulation status does not adversely affect the outcome. The procedure is relatively painless being performed under local anaesthetic and complications including distal embolisation and anaphylaxis are reported in ≤4% of cases [21]. Best results are achieved for FApAs measuring <3 cm, but the technique has been widely extended to treat larger FApAs in isolation or as part of a combined approach with open surgery for patients with compression symptomatology with encouraging results.

References

1. Lawrence PF, Lorenzo-Rivero S, Lyon JL. The incidence of iliac, femoral, and popliteal artery aneurysms in hospitalized patients. *J Vasc Surg* 1995; 22(4):409–415.
2. Hatrick AG, Malcolm PN, Burnand KG, Irvine AT. A superficial femoral artery aneurysm in a patient with Marfan's syndrome. *Eur J Vasc Endovasc Surg* 1998;15(5):459–460.

3. Sasaki Sh, Yasuda K, Takigami K, Shiiya N, Matsui Y, Sakuma M. Surgical experiences with peripheral arterial aneurysms due to vasculo-Behçet's disease. *J Cardiovasc Surg (Torino)* 1998;39(2):147–150.

4. Graham LM, Zelenock GB, Whitehouse WM Jr, Erlandson EE, Dent TL, Lindenauer SM, Stanley JC. Clinical significance of arteriosclerotic femoral artery aneurysms. *Arch Surg* 1980;115(4):502–507.

5 Diwan A, Sarkar R, Stanley JC, Zelenock GB, Wakefield TW. Incidence of femoral and popliteal artery aneurysms in patients with abdominal aortic aneurysms. *J Vasc Surg* 2000;31(5):863–869.

6. Gow BS, Legg MJ,Yu W, Kukongviriyapan U, Lee LL. Does vibration cause poststenotic dilatation *in vivo* and influence atherogenesis in cholesterol-fed rabbits? *J Biomech Eng* 1992;114:20–25.

7. Baird RJ, Gurry JF, Kellam J, Plume SK. Arteriosclerotic femoral artery aneurysms. *Can Med Assoc J* 1977;117(11):1306–1307.

8. Cutler BS, Darling RC. Surgical management of arteriosclerotic femoral aneurysms. *Surgery* 1973;74(5):764–773.

9. Adiseshiah M, Bailey DA. Aneurysms of the femoral artery. *Br J Surg* 1977; 64(3):174–176.

10. Pappas G, Janes JM, Bernatz PE, Schirger A. Femoral aneurysms. Review of surgical management. *JAMA* 1964;190:489–493.

11. Roseman JM, Wyche D. True aneurysm of the profunda femoris artery. Literature review, differential diagnosis, management. *J Cardiovasc Surg (Torino)* 1987;28(6):701–705.

12. Harbuzariu C, Duncan AA, Bower TC, Kalra M, Gloviczki P. Profunda femoris artery aneurysms: Association with aneurysmal disease and limb ischemia. *J Vasc Surg* 2008;47(1):31–34.

13. Tait WF, Vohra RK, Carr HM, Thomson GJ, Walker MG. True profunda femoris aneurysms: are they more dangerous than other atherosclerotic aneurysms of the femoropopliteal segment? *Ann Vasc Surg* 1991;5(1): 92–95.

14. Katzenschlager R, Ugurluoglu A, Ahmadi A, Hülsmann M, Koppensteiner R, Larch E, Maca T, Minar E, Stümpflen A, Ehringer H. Incidence of pseudoaneurysm after diagnostic and therapeutic angiography. *Radiology* 1995; 195(2):463–466.

15. Lumsden AB, Miller JM, Kosinski AS, Allen RC, Dodson TF, Salam AA, Smith RB 3rd. A prospective evaluation of surgically treated groin complications following percutaneous cardiac procedures. *Am Surg* 1994;60(2):132–137.

16. Morgan R, Belli AM. Current treatment methods for postcatheterization pseudoaneurysms. *J Vasc Interv Radiol* 2003;14(6):697–710.

17. Marković DM, Davidović LB, Kostić DM, Maksimović ZL, Kuzmanovic IB, Koncar IB, Cvetkovic DM. False anastomotic aneurysms. *Vascular* 2007; 15(3):141–148.
18. Biancari F, Ylönen K, Anttila V *et al.* Durability of open repair of infrarenal abdominal aortic aneurysm: A 15-year follow-up study. *J Vasc Surg* 2002; 35:87–93.
19. Coughlin BF, Paushter DM. Peripheral pseudoaneurysms: Evaluation with duplex US. *Radiol* 1988;168(2):339–342.
20. Toursarkissian B, Allen BT, Petrinec D, Thompson RW, Rubin BG, Reilly JM, Anderson CB, Flye MW, Sicard GA. Spontaneous closure of selected iatrogenic pseudoaneurysms and arteriovenous fistulae. *J Vasc Surg* 1997;25(5): 803–808.
21. Corriere MA, Guzman RJ. True and false aneurysms of the femoral artery. *Semin Vasc Surg* 2005;18(4):216–223.

Chapter 12

Popliteal Artery Aneurysm

Robert Davies and Rajiv Vohra

Key Points

- Popliteal artery aneurysm (PAA) is the most common lower limb aneurysm.
- PPAs rarely occur in isolation.
- The majority present either as an incidental finding or as lower limb ischaemia.
- Aneurysm rupture is rare, but life and limb threatening when it occurs.
- All symptomatic PAAs should undergo repair.
- Asymptomatic PAAs >2 cm in maximum diameter should be considered for repair.
- Adequate imaging of the proximal and distal vasculature is vital for successful repair.
- Endovascular repair has promising results but the evidence base is still relatively weak.

Introduction

Popliteal artery aneurysms (PAAs) are the second most common peripheral arterial aneurysm after abdominal aortic aneurysm (AAA). Although multifactorial in aetiology, most occur in men with associated atherosclerotic risk factors. They frequently occur in association with other arterial aneurysms, including aortic and femoral, and are often identified as an incidental finding during routine examination or radiological imaging. They may present with acute ischaemia or chronic lower limb thromboembolism or occasionally with pressure on adjacent structures or rarely rupture. For emergency presentations, limb salvage can be challenging and thus their identification and subsequent elective management is important.

Pathophysiology

The majority of PAAs develop secondary to atherosclerosis and are often associated with aneurysms elsewhere. In early retrospective studies in which PAAs were detected clinically or with the use of angiography rather than duplex scanning, the incidence of PAAs in patients with aortic aneurysms was <4%. However, more recent prospective studies have suggested the incidence to be 2–3 times greater than this. Conversely, if a PAA is detected, then concomitant aortic and femoral aneurysms are present in up to 50% and 40% of cases, respectively. It is also important to examine and image the contralateral popliteal artery, as 30–70% are bilateral [1–3].

Causal explanations for the preponderance of the popliteal artery to become aneurysmal include fixation at the adductor hiatus and exposure to repetitive trauma with use of adductor magnus or extrinsic compression from knee flexion and extension. Uncontrolled hypertension is also associated with aneurysm expansion. Non-atherosclerotic causes of aneurysmal change are rare and include inflammatory and connective-tissue disorders such as Marfan's syndrome and Bechet's disease as well as mechanical causes such as post-stenotic dilatation after popliteal artery entrapment and both blunt and penetrating trauma. Mycotic aneurysms in the popliteal fossa have also been reported.

Symptoms and Signs

Most occur in men with a median age of 60–65 years at the time of diagnosis and a male to female ratio of 20:1. Approximately, two-thirds (see Table 1) are symptomatic at presentation with asymptomatic aneurysms

Table 1.   Presentation of popliteal aneurysms.

Presentation	%
Limb ischaemia	55
Asymptomatic	37
Rupture	1.4
Local compression	6.5

detected on palpation or surveillance duplex Doppler ultrasound (DUS) of the popliteal fossae in patients with diagnosed aortic, iliac, femoral or contralateral PAAs.

A pulsatile mass on palpation of the popliteal fossa must be differentiated from other vascular lumps such as psedoaneurysm following trauma. Venous aneurysm and non-vascular lumps with transmitted pulsation arising from soft-tissue such as Baker's cyst, bursae, tumours and lymph nodes are also included in the differential diagnoses.

The most common complication of PAA is thrombosis, embolism or a combination of both. This may present as an emergency with acute limb ischaemia requiring complex revascularisation to prevent limb loss. Because of the need for aneurysm ligation during surgery and greater risk of embolism during intra-arterial thrombolysis, it is important to differentiate acute ischaemia secondary to PAA from ischaemia related to other causes of thrombosis and embolism [4].

A more insidious presentation is that of a gradual onset of claudication or chronic critical limb ischaemia with rest pain and tissue loss secondary to gradual embolisation and occlusion of pedal and/or crural vessels; this is an indication for urgent repair. Large aneurysms may also compress neighbouring structures such as the popliteal vein and/or tibial nerve. The former may be mistaken for other causes of lower limb oedema and venous hypertension whilst the latter may be misdiagnosed as a primary neurological disorder. Rupture is unlikely rare presentation of popliteal aneurysms but if it occurs may threaten life as well as limb.

Investigations

Investigations are predominantly aimed at providing information relating to (a) the size and extent of the aneurysm and presence of thrombus, (b) the patency of inflow and run-off vessels and (c) presence of a suitable autologous venous conduit [5–7]. Information about the effect on neighbouring structures is also important if there are compression related symptoms.

Duplex DUS provides excellent information regarding inflow, outflow, diameter and presence of sac thrombus. Computed tomography angiography (CTA) or magnetic resonance angiography (MRA) accurately demonstrates the morphology of the PAA and its relation to surrounding structures. Percutaneous angiography remains the gold standard for assessing the run-off although with the widespread availability of CTA and/or MRA, it is reserved for cases in which doubt remains as to the state of the distal circulation following non-invasive imaging. Fusiform aneurysms tend to involve the whole length of the popliteal artery and may have stenotic or occluded segments in addition to the aneurysmal disease and may also affect the superficial femoral artery. Saccular aneurysms, on the other hand, are more localised, affecting mainly the mid-popliteal artery (see Figs. 1(a) and 1(b)).

Management

When to repair

All patients with symptomatic PAAs require intervention for the relief of symptoms and prevention of limb loss. The indications for surgery in asymptomatic popliteal aneurysm remain controversial with no randomised controlled trials available to establish clear indications for intervention. Enthusiasts of surgery argue that since up to 100% of asymptomatic aneurysms will develop thromboembolic complications within 5 years without surgery, with an associated amputation rate <67%, intervention is always recommended [8,9]. In one prospective study, 18 of 58 aneurysms that had been treated conservatively developed complications [2]. This argument is strengthened by better graft patency and limb salvage rates with reconstruction for asymptomatic as compared to symptomatic aneurysms. The results for reconstruction for PAA are better than for occlusive disease and may relate to better run-off, use of shorter length grafts or reduced thrombogenicity of blood in these patients compared with occlusive disease. In contradiction, Schellack *et al.* showed that only 2 of 26 (8%) aneurysms

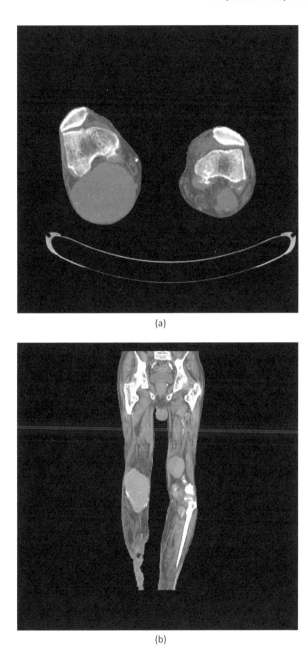

(a)

(b)

Figure 1.   (a) Cross-sectional view of bilateral popliteal aneurysms. (b) Coronal view of bilateral popliteal aneurysms.

developed thromboembolic complications at a mean follow-up of 37 months [10]. Furthermore, Bowyer *et al.* reported good results with intra-arterial thrombolysis for asymptomatic aneurysm presenting with acute ischaemia [11]. Thus, some surgeons favour an expectant policy with asymptomatic PAAs, sometimes with anticoagulation to reduce thrombosis risk.

Many authors have tried to quantify the risk of thromboembolism in asymptomatic aneurysms. The majority of these studies have been retrospective with risk factors for complications being a diameter greater than 2 cm, presence of aneurysm sac thrombus and signs of silent embolism i.e., loss of pedal pulses or lowering of ABPI. Varga *et al.* attempted to identify indications for management of asymptomatic aneurysm in a prospective multi-centre study but the numbers with small aneurysm (<2 cm) were insufficient to establish risk of complications with conservative treatment in this group [2]. In another prospective study, Galland *et al.* showed that those with a diameter of less than 3 cm were unlikely to thrombose [12]. Conversely, it has been shown that enlarging the diameter of the sac does not increase the risk of thromboembolism [13]. Also, some small aneurysms (<2 cm diameter) may have disproportionate amounts of thrombus in the sac with a greater risk of embolism [14]. Thus, we advocate elective surgical repair for all asymptomatic PAAs ≥2 cm in maximum diameter or those PAAs ≥1.8 cm with high thrombus content in suitable patients or those with evidence of run-off embolisation on imaging.

Surgical approaches

The most widely utilised surgical technique for repair of PAA is proximal and distal aneurysm ligation combined with long saphenous vein bypass through a medial approach [2]. The advantages of this approach are the ability to expose the crural vessels and harvest the long saphenous vein from the same incision. However, the disadvantage is the potential for continued sac expansion post-repair and the need for a longer graft than for posterior repair. One large series reported 15% of PAA repairs treated by ligation and bypass demonstrated sac perfusion at a median of 75 months after primary PAA repair. About 40% of these patients presented with symptoms, including one rupture [15]. This complication of the ligation and bypass technique has been reported by others and is thought to be secondary to patent collaterals, similar in endovascular terms to a type II collateral endoleak. This imparts near systemic arterial pressure within the excluded sac causing expansion with the possibility of subsequent rupture or neurovascular compression [16–18].

Some authors advocate a posterior approach with interposition grafting in the presence of compressive features or focal PAAs [14,19,20]. This involves an 'S' shaped incision in the popliteal fossa with dissection of the aneurysm from other popliteal structures followed by inlay grafting (Figs. 2(a) and 2(b)). The advantage of this approach is the direct visualisation of the sac which can be opened and the ligated geniculate arteries prevent aneurysm sac reperfusion. Furthermore, the sac may be excised which is especially important in cases of neurovascular compression. This technique is not generally suitable for PAAs extending proximal to the adductor hiatus or where crural vessel exposure is required. It may be associated with improved patency. Thus, the authors advocate interposition grafting through a posterior approach as the operation of choice for focal, large PAAs that do not extend above the adductor hiatus.

Conduits

Although autologous vein is the conduit of choice, the conduit for grafting depends on the availability of suitable vein, the presence of infection and the length of the graft required. For mycotic aneurysms, prosthetic conduits should be avoided.

Inlay grafting requires a small length of graft and as such prosthetic conduits such as PTFE have been shown to produce adequate results although a venous conduit is recommended if the distal anastomosis is on to distal below-knee popliteal artery [21]. A pre-marked upper arm basilic vein can be harvested in the prone position and in the experience of authors is a better size match for the popliteal artery than the short saphenous vein and the long-term results using this approach are comparable to ligation and bypass with a trend for superior primary patency rates [15].

For bypass grafts below the knee, a thorough search for vein using a combination of pre-operative vein mapping and on-table exploration of

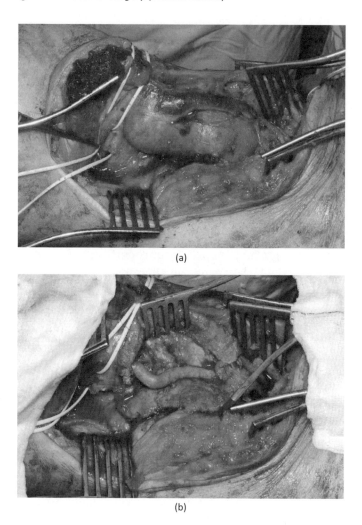

(a)

(b)

Figure 2.   (a) Posterior approach to large popliteal aneurysm. (b) Vein inlay graft repair of large popliteal aneurysm.

the leg veins (saphenous trunks) usually allows several segments of composite spliced vein to be anastomosed together to form a suitable conduit if a single length of vein is not available. Arm vein can be utilised instead of saphenous vein if an autologous conduit is required. The second best option is the use of a composite-sequential conduit with above-knee prosthetic conjoined by a 3-panelled anastomosis to above-knee popliteal artery and vein traversing the knee [22]. A prosthetic graft with the addition of a venous cuff or fistula remains the least attractive option due to the relatively poor results in terms of graft patency, limb salvage and risk of infection.

Management of thromboembolism

The acutely ischaemic leg from PAAs remains a challenge associated with relatively poor limb salvage rates. A multi-disciplinary approach involving a vascular surgeon and interventional radiologist is optimal. Treatment options include intra-arterial thrombolysis alone, thrombolysis to remove clot in the aneurysm sac and run-off followed by surgery or intra-operative lysis with thromboembolectomy followed by reconstruction. The choice of treatment depends on the degree and duration of ischaemia and comorbidities. In a chronically ischaemic leg, it is unlikely that lysis or embolectomy will clear a well packed clot in the run-off and therefore a crural or pedal bypass remains the most realistic option. Interventional radiological techniques include pre-operative intra-arterial thrombolysis and aspiration embolectomy. First described by Schwarz *et al.* in 1984, thrombolysis can be successfully used as the primary intervention [22]. In a unit favouring conservative treatment of all asymptomatic aneurysms, Bowyer *et al.* reported successful thrombolysis in 6 of 9 patients with acute thromboembolic complications [11]. Limb salvage was achieved in all the nine patients including those with failed lysis requiring additional procedures such as lumbar sympathectomy and angioplasty. The combination of pre-operative lysis followed by surgery was shown to be effective by Carpenter *et al.* who reported a limb salvage rate of 100% for combination treatment in comparison to 57% for surgery alone [23]. However, details of run-off clearing procedures were not given for the latter technique. Pre-operative intra-arterial thrombolysis should not be considered in every case, especially in the presence of neurological signs. Immediate surgery is required in this situation. Pre-op lysis is also associated with a risk of distal embolism of 13% in PAAs compared to 2% in patients with acute ischaemia due to occlusive disease [4]. Not all cases are successful and lysis may not be effective in dislodging well-packed clot or cholesterol emboli ('trash') with clearance rates of only 58–66%.

The theoretical risk of stroke as well as systemic bleeding has been reduced when a low dose lytic agent has been used in the on-table technique. Intra-operative thrombolysis may be delivered either transfemoral, via the popliteal artery or from the ankle routes with the latter two routes being favoured in cases of a threatened limb with more rapid clearance of run-off being achieved with the catheter being closer to the run-off [24–26]. Isolated limb perfusion may also give good results and limit side effects by reducing the dosage of lytic agent reaching the systemic circulation.

Methods for improving the removal of distal thrombus include popliteal trifurcation embolectomy and ankle-level micro-embolectomies. The embolectomy catheter may not pass easily from the popliteal artery all the way down the calf vessels for mechanical reasons such as angulations or due to the nature of occlusive disease. In these circumstances, embolectomy of the crural and pedal vessels via arteriotomy at the ankle may successfully retrieve clot in the crural or pedal vessels that is otherwise inaccessible. In this technique, the anterior tibial, posterior tibial or both arteries are exposed by small separate ankle incisions and opened transversely using loupe magnification and a micro-knife [27]. Proximal and distal embolectomy can be carried out using a size 2 fogarty balloon catheter, directed proximally to the popliteal trunk and distally into and around the pedal arch. Adjunctive thrombolysis may also be used in cases of incomplete embolectomy.

In our series, of the 17 patients with acute ischaemia, aneurysm thrombosis alone accounted for the presentation in four cases, embolism alone in 1 with a combination of both thrombosis and distal embolism in 12. Thirteen cases had severe ischaemia with 12 of these undergoing thromboembolectomy (trifurcation alone in eight and together with microtibial embolectomy in four) and bypass grafting, with fasciotomy in six. Four patients received intra-arterial thrombolysis initially with two of these being successful, requiring elective bypass procedures to the below-knee popliteal artery; the other two required immediate crural bypass grafting. Five of the grafts in patients with acute ischaemia occluded early with another two patients requiring major limb amputation during the first year. Acutely ischaemic limbs had a cumulative 5-year secondary patency of 80% and a 30-day mortality of 11.8%. Of the 17 with acute ischaemia, limb salvage was achieved in 14. Such an aggressive surgical approach can achieve results comparable to combinations of pre-operative or intra-operative thrombolysis with or without surgery [24–26].

Endovascular Popliteal Aneurysm Repair (EPAR)

EPAR relies on the exclusion of the PAA from the systemic circulation by the deployment of a stent-graft to seal proximally and distally in normal artery. The use of EPAR is limited by the patient's anatomy and in order to ensure good outcome, EPAR should be reserved for those patients with: (a) adequate (>20 mm)proximal and distal landing zones, (b) at least two good quality outflow vessels in the lower leg and (c) <4 mm discrepancy in the diameter between the proximal and distal landing zones. Other relative contraindications are the presence of a stenosis at the edge of the PAA as this may increase the risk of stent-graft collapse and thrombosis, large PPAs with compression related symptomatology, and involvement of the origin of the anterior tibia artery.

The Viabhan (WL Gore and associates, Flagstaff, Arizona) stent-graft system is preferred by the authors and is deployed in an antegrade fashion through either a percutaneous puncture or a proximal superficial femoral artery cut-down depending on patient related factors e.g., obesity, vessel calcification, etc. The stent-graft is oversized by 1 mm compared to the diameter of the artery; minor discrepancies (<4 mm) in diameter of proximal and distal landing zones can be managed with overlapping stents. Completion of angiography with the knee in full extension and 90° flexion should be performed to confirm stent-graft patency. Post-procedure dual antiplatelet (aspirin and clopidogrel) for 3 months followed by single therapy has been reported to reduce stent-graft thrombosis and is routine in author's practice.

Stent-graft related complications following EPAR are not infrequent. Endoleak may occur in up to 20% of EPAR at 4-year follow-up [28]. All type I and type III endoleaks require re-intervention, but 50% of type II endoleaks are not associated with sac expansion and thus can be treated conservatively. Due to the repetitive flexion and extension nature of the knee joint EPAR is also at risk of stent fracture, intimal hyperplasia at the stent-graft artery interface resulting in stent-graft stenosis/occlusion. Therefore the authors advocate a stent-graft surveillance programme to ensure durability of this procedure.

Improvement in stent-graft technology has seen an increase proportion of PAAs treated with EPAR. The Swedvasc registry reported a four-
fold increase in the proportion of patients treated by EPAR over the last
decade with 17% of all PAAs now treated endovascularly; the Vascunet
registry reports similar results [29]. The perceived advantages of EPAR
relate to its lower level of invasiveness compared to open surgical repair;
this translates to a reduced length of hospital stay, shorter recovery and
less wound complications. However, there remains a distinct lack of high
quality studies comparing EPAR with open surgical repair (OSR). A recent
meta-analysis identified only five studies comparing OSR to EPAR of
which only one was a randomised controlled trial [30]. Thirty-day graft
occlusion (ER vs. OS: 9% vs. 2%) and reintervention (ER vs. OS: 9% vs. 2%)
rates were significantly greater following EPAR. Over a 4-year period,
there was no significant differences in the risk of graft thrombosis
between EPAR and OSR, primary patency rates ranged from 54% to 86%
for EPAR and 63% to 8% for OSR. A separate meta-analysis reporting the
outcome of Gore Viabahn/Hemobhan for the treatment of PAA reported
pooled 5-year primary and secondary patency rates for ER to be similar
to those for OSR registries [28].

Despite these encouraging results for EPAR, the lack of randomised
clinical trials comparing EPAR and OSR and the heterogeneous nature of
large series reporting the outcomes of EPAR prevent strong recommendations about the best treatment for PAA. In younger, more active
patients, OSR may still be preferred.

References

1. Dawson I, Sie RB, van Bockel JH. Athersclerotic popliteal aneurysm. *Br J Surg* 1997;84(3):293–299.
2. Varga ZA, Locke-Edmonds JC, Baird RN. A multicenter study of popliteal aneurysms. Joint Vascular Research Group. *J Vasc Surg* 1994;20:171–177.
3. Lowell RC, Gloviczki P, Hallett JW Jr, Naessens JM, Maus TP, Cherry KJ Jr, Bower TC, Pairolero PC. Popliteal artery aneurysms: The risk of nonopera-tive management. *Ann Vasc Surg* 1994;8(1):14–23.
4. Galland RB, Earnshaw JJ, Baird RN, Lonsdale RJ, Hopkinson BR, Giddings AEB, Dawson KJ, Hamilton G. Acute limb deterioration during intra-arterial thrombolysis. *Br J Surg* 1993;80:1118–1120.

5. Lilly MP, Flinn WR, McCarthy WJ 3rd, Courtney DF, Yao JS, Bergan The effect of distal arterial anatomy on the success of popliteal aneurysm repair. *J Vasc Surg* 1988;7(5):653–660.

6. Ascher E, Hingorani A, Markevich N, Costa T, Kallakuri S, Khanimoy Y. Lower extremity revascularization without preoperative contrast arteriography: Experience withduplex ultrasound arterial mapping in 485 cases. *Ann Vasc Surg* 2002; 16(1):108–114.

7. Piccoli G, Gasparini D, Smania S, Sponza M, Marzio A, Vit A, Bazzocchi M. Multislice CT angiography in the assessment of peripheral aneurysms. *Radiol Med (Torino)* 2003; 106(5–6):504–511.

8. Dawson 1, van Bockel JH, Brand R, Terpstra JL. Popliteal artery aneurysms. Long-term follow-up of aneurysmal disease and results of surgical treatment. *J Vasc Surg* 1991;13:398–407.

9. Shortell CK, DeWeese JA, Ouriel K, Green RM. Popliteal artery aneurysms: A 25-year experience. *J Vasc Surg* 1991;14(6):771–776.

10. Schellack J, Smith RB, Perdue GD Jr. Non-operative management of selective popliteal aneurysms. *Arch Surg* 1987;122:372–375.

11. Bowyer RC, Cawthorn SJ, Walker WJ, Giddings AEB. Conservative management of asymptomatic popliteal aneurysm. *Br J Surg* 1990;77:1132–1135.

12. Galland RB, Magee TR. Management of popliteal aneurysm. *Br J Surg* 2002;89(11):1382–1385.

13. Inahara T, Toledo AC. Complications and treatment of popliteal aneurysms. *Surgery* 1978;84:775–783.

14. Mahmood A, Salaman R, Sintler M, Smith SRG, Simms MH, Vohra RK. Surgery for popliteal artery aneurysms: A 12-year experience. *J Vasc Surg* 2003;37:586–593.

15. Davies RS, Wall M, Rai S, Simms MH, Vohra RK, Bradbury AW, Adam DJ. Long-term results of surgical repair of popliteal artery aneurysm. *Eur J Vasc Endovasc Surg* 2007;34(6):714–718.

16. Ebaugh JL, Morasch MD, Matsumura JS, Eskandari MK, Meadows WS, Pearce WH. Fate of excluded popliteal artery aneurysms. *J Vasc Surg* 2003;37(5):954–959.

17. Kirkpatrick UJ, McWilliams RG, Martin J, Brennan JA, Gilling-Smith GL, Harris PL. Late complications after ligation and bypass for popliteal aneurysm. *Br J Surg* 2004;91(2):174–177.

18. Mehta M, Champagne B, Darling RC 3rd, Roddy SP, Kreienberg PB, Ozsvath KJ, Paty PS, Chang BB, Shah DM. Outcome of popliteal artery aneurysms after exclusion and bypass: Significance of residual patent branches mimicking type II endoleaks. *J Vasc Surg* 40(5):886–890.

19. Beseth BD, Moore WS. The posterior approach for repair of popliteal artery aneurysms. *J Vasc Surg* 2006;43(5):940–944.
20. Ouriel K. Posterior exposure for popliteal-crural bypass: A useful approach. *Semin Vasc Surg* 1997;10(1):23–30.
21. Mahmood A, Garnham A, Sintler M, Smith SRG, Vohra RK, Simms NM. Composite-sequential grafts for femoro-crural bypass reconstruction: Experience with a modified technique. *J Vasc Surg* 2002;36(4): 772–778.
22. Schwarz W, Berkowitz H, Taormina V, Gatti J. The preoperative use of intra-arterial thrombolysis for a thrombosed popliteal artery aneurysm. *J Cardiovasc Surg (Torino)* 1984;25(5):465–468.
23. Carpenter JP, Barker CF, Roberts B, Berkowitz HD, Lusk EJ, Perloff LJ. Popliteal artery aneurysms: Current management and outcome. *J Vasc Surg* 1994;19:65–73.
24. Thompson JF, Beard J, Scott DJA, Eamshaw JJ. Intra-operative thrombolysis in the management of thrombosed popliteal aneurysm. *Br J Surg* 1993;80:858–859.
25. Greenberg F, Wellander E, Nyman U, Uher P, Lindh M, Lindblad B, Ivancev K. Aggressive treatment of acute limb ischaemia due to thrombosed popliteal aneurysms. *European J Radiol* 1998;28:211–218.
26. Steinmetz, E, Bouchot O, Farroy F, Charmasson L, Ter-riat B, Becker F, Cercueil JP, Krause D, Brenot R, David M. Pre-operative intra-arterial thrombolysis before surgical revascularization for popliteal artery aneurysm with acute ischaemia. *Ann Vasc Surg* 2000;14:360–364.
27. Mahmood A, Hardy R, Gamham A, Samman Y, Sintler M, Smith SRG, Vohra PK, Simms MH. Microtibial Embolectomy. Eur *J Vasc Endovasc Surg* 2003;25(I):35–39.
28. Patel SR, Hughes CO, Jones KG, Holt PJ, Thompson MM, Hinchliffe RJ, Karthikesalingam A. A Systematic review and meta-analysis of endovascular popliteal aneurysm repair using the hemobahn/viabahn stent-graft. *J Endovasc Ther* 2015;22(3):330–337.
29. Cervin A, Tjärnström J, Ravn H, Acosta S, Hultgren R, Welander M, Björck M. Treatment of popliteal aneurysm by open and endovascular surgery: A contemporary study of 592 procedures in Sweden. *Eur J Vasc Endovasc Surg* 2015;50(3):342–350.
30. von Stumm M, Teufelsbauer H, Reichenspurner H, Debus ES. Two decades of endovascular repair of popliteal artery aneurysm — A meta-analysis. *Eur J Vasc Endovasc Surg* 2015;50(3):351–359.

Chapter 13

Carotid, Subclavian and Vertebral Disease

A. Ross Naylor

Key Points

- The extracranial arteries are prone to involvement with a number of important atherosclerotic and non-atherosclerotic conditions.
- The provision of best medical therapy should not be delegated to the most junior member of the team. It is an essential component of care.
- Patients with symptomatic carotid disease benefit from very rapid intervention. Investigative strategies and rapid access to the operating theatre should be geared to ensuring all patients are treated within 2 weeks of suffering their index symptom.
- Relatively few patients with asymptomatic carotid disease benefit from intervention (especially females and patients aged >75 years). It is essential that trials identify high-risk subgroups.
- The role of several technical aspects of carotid surgery have been guided by large randomised trials.
- Patients with symptomatic vertebral stenoses may have a much worse prognosis than was previously thought, but there is no compelling evidence that stenting confers significant benefit over medical therapy.

Radiation Arteritis

Demographics

Despite the widespread use of radiotherapy in the treatment of head and neck cancers, there is still insufficient data regarding the incidence of symptomatic radiation arteritis.

Pathology

Acute phase: Fibrin deposition/endothelial swelling followed by intimal necrosis.

Subacute phase: Endothelial regeneration with destruction of the internal elastic lamina. Inflammatory cell infiltration of the media and adventitia.

Chronic phase: Intima becomes thickened with a tendency towards accelerated atherosclerosis. The media and adventitia become fibrotic.

Clinical features

These include false aneurysm or vessel rupture (acute/subacute phase), stroke due to carotid/vertebral thrombosis, or upper limb ischaemia following subclavian thrombosis (subacute phase). In the chronic phase (where radiation arteritis coexists with atherosclerosis), thrombo-embolic stroke/TIA or upper limb claudication (subclavian stenosis/occlusion) can occur.

Investigation

First line is duplex ultrasound (DUS). Computed tomography angiography (CTA) or magnetic resonance imaging (MRI)/contrast-enhanced MRA (CEMRA) should be performed to evaluate the full extent of the arteritic process (proximally and distally) and the status of the circle of Willis and to exclude recurrent malignant disease.

Management

Management decisions should take account of patient comorbidities and whether there is ongoing malignant disease. Management decisions will be influenced by the acute/chronic nature of the arteritic process, patient age, mode of presentation, presence of a tracheostomy, likelihood of cranial nerve injury (CNI), likelihood of compromising skin flaps and whether there is ongoing embolisation using transcranial Doppler (TCD). In general, asymptomatic stenoses should probably be treated conservatively, unless there is a non-functioning circle of Willis. Symptomatic lesions should be considered for intervention (autologous reconstruction/carotid stenting). Stenting is currently the preferred option (especially in patients with a tracheostomy), although surgery may be preferable in patients with crescendo symptoms and evidence of embolisation on TCD.

Prognosis

There is little quality data regarding the prognosis in untreated patients.

Fibromuscular Dysplasia [1]

Demographics

Fibromuscular dysplasia (FMD) affects 0.5% of patients undergoing angiography for symptomatic cerebral vascular disease, while 10% of patients suffering a carotid dissection (CD) will have FMD in the contralateral internal carotid artery (ICA). FMD is bilateral in up to 60%, 25% with carotid involvement will have renal artery FMD. One quarter of FMD cases involve the vertebral arteries (VAs), while up to 50% of patients with carotid/vertebral FMD will have an intra-cranial aneurysm.

Pathology

FMD is a non-inflammatory, non-atheromatous segmental disorder. Three main subtypes are based upon involvement of media, intima or adventitia. Intimal fibroplasia (<10% of FMD cases) causes band-like narrowing or long smooth stenoses and carries a poorer prognosis. Medial dysplasia (90% of FMD cases) causes a 'beading' appearance and is subdivided into medial fibroplasia (75–85%), perimedial fibroplasia (<10%) and medial hyperplasia (<5%). Adventitial fibroplasia is only seen in <1% of cases and is characterised by dense collagen formation.

Clinical features

Wide spectrum ranging from asymptomatic (the majority) to subarachnoid haemorrhage, embolic TIA/stroke, neurovascular hypertension or features suggestive of CD (see later).

Investigation

Duplex is the first line investigation, but it cannot image the distal ICA/vertebral arteries. If there is any suspicion of FMD, CTA/CEMRA should be performed (preferably including the renal vasculature). The intracranial circulation should be imaged to exclude an aneurysm.

Management

There is no level I evidence to guide practice. Asymptomatic patients should probably be treated conservatively and kept in surveillance. Carotid/vertebral angioplasty is now the first line treatment for patients with symptomatic FMD, with stenting being reserved for patients with a poor technical result or secondary dissection.

Prognosis

Multi-focal intimal fibroplasia carries the worst prognosis; medial dysplasia carries a reasonably good prognosis. It is important to remember that more than one vascular bed can be affected by FMD and not ignore the possibility of a concurrent intracranial aneurysm.

Carotid Artery Dissection

Demographics

CD causes few strokes, but traumatic CD complicates 1% of all head injuries and 25% of trauma patients with an unexplained focal neurological deficit will have a dissection.

Pathology

CD occurs spontaneously (Marfan's/FMD), it can follow iatrogenic injury (cannulation, angioplasty) or trauma (forced lateral rotation and hyper-extension which causes the ICA to be crushed between the skull base and the transverse process of C2). The dissection usually starts 2–3 cm beyond the ICA origin and then extends over a variable distance towards the skull base. Type I lesions cause a minor intimal irregularity or stenosis <50%. Type II lesions involve either false aneurysm formation or a stenosis >50%. In type III lesions, CD is associated with complete vessel occlusion through compression of the true lumen by a thrombosed false lumen.

Clinical

Ipsilateral headache and/or neck pain affects 80% of patients. Ocular signs/symptoms are present in 60% (miosis, painful Horner's syndrome, hemianopia, ischaemic optic neuropathy) along with III, IV or VI cranial nerve palsies. Stroke/TIA may complicate a dissection (thrombosis or embolisation from the false lumen). False aneurysms tend to be asymp-tomatic and rarely cause a stroke/TIA.

Investigation

Awareness of the diagnosis is integral to instituting effective treatment. Duplex is limited by its inability to image the upper ICA and VAs. Here, CTA or CEMRA is the investigation of choice and is also useful for serial surveillance of small false aneurysms.

Management

There is no level 1 evidence to guide practice. Traditionally, the majority of patients with CD have been managed conservatively with anticoagulation (heparin followed by warfarin), but meta-analyses suggest that dual antiplatelet therapy offers similar outcomes [2]. Most dissections will recanalise spontaneously and clinically improve. A few symptomatic patients have undergone attempts at surgical revascularisation, but this has now been replaced by endovascular technology (covered stents, etc.), which also lessens the likelihood of CNI.

Prognosis

Stroke following undiagnosed CD carries a high morbidity and mortality. The key to minimising stroke risk is awareness and early institution of dual antiplatelet therapy or anticoagulation. In a recent systematic review of 166 distal false aneurysms after acute CD, >95% neither increased in size nor gave rise to late cerebrovascular symptoms suggesting that they have a good prognosis and can be managed conservatively [3].

Giant Cell Arteritis (GCA) [4]

Demographics

GCA is the commonest vasculitis in the western world and predominantly affects women aged >50 years (mean age at presentation is 75). One-third will have polymyalgia rheumatica at the time of diagnosis. GCA predominantly affects large (thoracic aorta) and medium-sized vessels (extracranial carotid branches, subclavian, axillary and vertebral).

Pathology

This shows panarteritis involving predominantly lymphocytes and macrophages, together with multi-nucleated giant cells in up to 5%. There is sparing of the intracerebral arteries.

Clinical features

Three syndromes co-exist:

(i) **Systemic Inflammatory Syndrome:** Non-specific constitutional symptoms including arthralgias, myalgias, anorexia, weight loss and night sweats.

(ii) **Cranial Arteritis:** Localised vasculitis of the carotid and VAs causing headache/facial pain, scalp tenderness, jaw claudication, hoarseness and visual loss.

(iii) **Large Vessel Vasculitis:** Symptoms secondary to stenotic/occlusive disease of the subclavian and axillary arteries (arm claudication, Raynaud's phenomenon). GCA involvement of the thoracic aorta predisposes to aneurysm formation. Cerebrovascular events (stroke/TIA) occur in 3–4% of GCA patients and follow inflammatory occlusion of the vertebral/carotid arteries. Episodes of transient visual loss precedes permanent visual loss in 50% of untreated patients within seven days and is usually due to inflammatory occlusion of the short posterior ciliary arteries causing ischaemia of the optic disc and choroids.

Investigations

Temporal artery biopsy should be performed as soon as possible (negative in 50% of patients with large vessel vasculitis). DUS will identify stenoses/occlusions and possibly a 'halo' sign around the temporal artery, but CEMRA or CTA is preferred in order to evaluate aortic arch and major branch vessels (looking for bilateral patterns of disease, thoracic aneurysm) as well as excluding intracranial vasculitis. Laboratory investigations should include ESR (85% of GCA patients will have ESR >50 mm/h), CRP (98% sensitivity for active GCA), thrombocytosis (present in 48% of biopsy positive patients) and normocytic normochromic anaemia.

Management

High dose steroid therapy (intravenous or oral), which is gradually reduced over 6–12 months with titration against CRP and other inflammatory markers is suggested.

Prognosis

Visual loss >24 h tends to be permanent. High dose steroid therapy is then aimed at preventing visual loss in the other eye. Patients with thoracic aneurysm require serial monitoring.

Takayasu Arteritis (Ta) [5]

Demographics

Panarteritis of unknown aetiology affecting aorta and its main branches and seen predominantly in young females, especially from the Orient. Incidence is about 2.6 cases per million per year.

Pathology

The inflammatory process starts with infiltration (lymphocytes plus occasional giant cells) around the vasa vasorum, extending transmurally. If disease progression is rapid, aneurysm formation becomes more likely. In the latter stages of the condition, there is progressive fibrosis leading to occlusion (hence the term 'pulseless' disease). The common carotid arteries (CCAs) are involved in 65–75% of the cases, the subclavian arteries in 50–75%, while the VAs are involved in 6–10%.

Clinical features

The American College of Rheumatology advises that a diagnosis of TA requires at least three of the following six criteria to be present: (i) age at onset <40 years, (ii) claudication of extremities, (iii) decreased brachial artery pulse, (iv) BP difference >10 mmHg between arms, (v) bruit over subclavian arteries or aorta and (vi) arteriogram abnormality. Given the large number of arteries that are liable to aneurysm formation, stenosis or occlusion, the mode of presentation varies considerably. In the early stages, most complain of constitutional symptoms (fatigue, malaise). In the second stage, symptoms are related to the increasing inflammatory reaction: (i) systemic inflammatory response (fatigue, fevers, extremity pain, headache, rashes), (ii) vascular insufficiency (claudication, arm numbness, TIA/stroke/amaurosis fugax) or a combination of (i) and (ii). In the final 'burned out' stage, the inflammatory reaction is replaced by transmural fibrosis.

Investigations

Lab investigations (ESR, thrombocytosis, anaemia) indicate an underlying inflammatory reaction and enables monitoring of treatment. Conventional angiography has been replaced by CTA/CEMRA for evaluating the anatomical extent of the inflammatory process. These imaging modalities also permit evaluation of aneurysm formation and measurement of arterial wall thickness and extent of oedema, which is used for monitoring treatment.

Management

High dose steroid therapy (intravenous then oral), which is reduced over 6–12 months with titration against CRP and other inflammatory markers. If it proves difficult to reduce the steroid dose or side effects occur, Methotrexate, Cyclophosphamide and Azathioprine are alternatives. Patients with renovascular hypertension require aggressive treatment and patients should receive antiplatelet therapy unless contraindicated. There is relatively limited experience with angioplasty or stenting in TA and surgical revascularisation of the carotid, subclavian and VAs is rarely required. If revascularisation becomes necessary, avoid this in the acute phase of the condition. It is also important to perform an inflow from the aorta rather than the subclavian artery.

Prognosis

Provided medical treatment is initiated early, approximately 90% of patients will survive 5 years.

True and False Aneurysms

Incidence

Aneurysms of the carotid, VA and subclavian arteries comprise <2% of all arterial aneurysms.

Pathology

The prevalence of true/false aneurysms will reflect differing patient populations. South African studies tend to describe aneurysms in young men with infection (HIV, tuberculosis). In metropolitan areas, many will be secondary to trauma (gunshot, knife), while in urban populations, the majority of true aneurysms are classed as 'atherosclerotic'. The commonest cause of a false aneurysm is prosthetic patch infection after carotid endarterectomy.

Clinical features

The commonest presentation is a pulsatile neck mass. Aneurysm rupture is extremely rare, but TIA/stroke is a relatively common presentation (presumably secondary to thromboembolism), as are cranial nerve signs/symptoms due to direct compression. Patients with false aneurysms will present with related symptoms/signs (e.g., history of trauma, evidence of patch infection, etc.).

Investigation

The majority presenting with a 'pulsatile neck mass' will be found to have coiling/ectasia of the CCA or innominate arteries (i.e., no aneurysm). Accordingly, the first line investigation is DUS. Thereafter, investigations are directed towards determining the underlying cause (FMD, trauma, etc.), as management strategies will vary. Second line investigations include CTA/CEMRA, which can rapidly image other arteries (e.g., renal arteries in suspected FMD). They will also provide information regarding the feasibility of endovascular treatment.

Management

Management depends upon the underlying aetiology, urgency of symptoms and the level/distal extent of the aneurysm. Operative strategies include (i) proximal/distal ligation, (ii) open reconstruction (venous bypass, partial aneurysm excision, patch angioplasty, prosthetic bypass, resection and end-to-end bypass) and (iii) endovascular repair (stent-graft exclusions, carotid stenting augmented with coil exclusions, endovascular balloon occlusion). In the carotid and VA circulations, ligation should only be considered if reconstructive options have been excluded. Inflation of an endovascular balloon within the artery under local anaesthesia may assist in determining whether ligation will be tolerated.

Prognosis

Most patients with carotid or vertebral true aneurysms will become symptomatic with time. Surgery, however, carries the risk of procedural stroke and CNI in 5–7% of patients. Management decisions must therefore balance the risks and benefits associated with intervention, which may mean adopting a more conservative strategy in selected asymptomatic patients with small distal ICA aneurysms.

Carotid Body Tumour [6]

Demographics

The carotid body is a collection of chemoreceptor cells responsible for detecting changes in blood oxygen/carbon dioxide levels and pH and is located within the adventitia of the bifurcation. Carotid body tumours (CBTs) may be sporadic or familial. Familial CBTs (10% of all CBTs) are more common in females and are more likely to be bilateral. CBTs represent <1% of all neck tumours.

Pathology

CBTs are highly vascular and derived from the neural crest ectoderm. They are the commonest type of cervical paraganglioma (glomus vagale, glomus jugular, glomus tympanicum). Most present in the fourth to fifth decades and cause splaying of the bifurcation. By contrast, glomus vagale tumours (second commonest) cause splaying of the ICA and ECA above a normal bifurcation. Up to 5% of CBTs are bilateral, 5% will be locally malignant and 5% systemically malignant.

Clinical features

Asymptomatic neck swelling (commonest). Larger lesions cause pain, cranial nerve palsies (XII, IX, X) and rarely, Horner's syndrome. Stroke/ TIA are unusual, while some will present with a neuroendocrine-mediated syndrome with flushing, dizziness, arrhythmias and hypertension.

Investigations

Consider CBT in all patients with lateral cervical swellings and definitely before any decision is made to undertake an open biopsy. DUS will show the characteristic blush of hypervascularity within a splayed carotid bifurcation. Cross-sectional imaging provides information regarding the upper and lower limits of the lesion, which is useful in planning surgical strategies. CT/MRI are useful in excluding bilateral lesions. Radionuclide imaging and conventional angiography are not routinely necessary.

Management

Resection is the main treatment strategy and is typically described as being performed in a subadventitial plane. A conservative approach is indicated in elderly patients with small lesions. Occasionally, it may be preferable to resect the tumour and carotid bifurcation (adherent tumour, carotid injury, suspicion of malignancy) and perform an inter-position bypass. Peri-operative bleeding may be reduced by pre-operative embolisation of ECA branches or insertion of a covered stent within the ECA. The latter strategy is probably only necessary in large lesions.

Prognosis

Resection carries a 1% mortality and a 2–3% risk of stroke. Cranial nerve injuries are not uncommon, but tend to be transient. Provided a macroscopically complete excision has been performed, the risk of recurrence is <5%.

Carotid Occlusive Disease

Demographics

Stroke (causing 12% of UK deaths) is defined as a focal (occasionally global) loss of cerebral function which lasts for >24 h and which has a vascular cause. A TIA carries a time scale of <24 h. The incidence of first-ever stroke is 2.4/1000, but increases with age. The annual incidence of TIA is 0.5/1000.

Pathology

Approximately 80% of all strokes are ischaemic (20% are haemorrhagic), while approximately 80% of ischaemic strokes affect the carotid territory. The main causes of carotid territory ischaemic stroke include thrombo-embolism of the ICA and/or middle cerebral artery (50%), small vessel occlusion of penetrating end-arteries (25%), cardiac embolism (15%), haematological disorders (myeloma, polycythaemia, thrombocytosis) in 5%, whilst 5% have a miscellany of causes (tumour, arteritis, oral contraceptive, etc.). Risk factors include hypertension, ischaemic heart disease, smoking, hyperlipidaemia, TIA, diabetes and hyperfibrinogenemia. The commonest single cause of ischaemic, carotid territory stroke is thrombo-embolism from an atherosclerotic plaque at the origin of the ICA. The carotid bifurcation is prone to atherosclerosis, particularly on the outer aspect of the bulb. Some plaques then undergo acute change (plaque rupture, intraplaque haemorrhage), which predisposes towards thrombus formation and embolisation to the brain.

Clinical features

(i) **Asymptomatic disease:** About 10% of the population will have an asymptomatic >50% ICA stenosis, but only 1% will have a stenosis >70%. Asymptomatic stenoses are usually detected by auscultation of a bruit or by ultrasound. However, the term 'asymptomatic' may be misleading as many patients do not consider a transient episode of hand paraesthesia or weakness to be important and it could go unreported. Similarly, because 33% of our lives are spent sleeping, nocturnal TIAs go unreported. Approximately 25% of 'asymptomatic' patients will have ischaemic brain injury on CT/MR.

(ii) **Symptomatic disease:** Carotid territory symptoms include hemisensory/ motor signs, higher cortical dysfunction (dysphasia, visuospatial neglect) and monocular blindness. There has previously been a tendency to ascribe a diagnosis of 'non-hemispheric' symptoms to patients with blackouts, isolated diplopia, isolated vertigo, isolated dizziness, presyncope and syncope. In practice, these should never be considered to be carotid (or VA in origin) unless they coexist with more typical symptoms.

Investigations

Baseline investigations include biochemistry, lipids, glucose, full blood count, plasma viscosity, chest X-ray and ECG. More specialised investigations (thrombophilia screening, autoantibodies, homocysteine levels, echocardiography and 24-h tapes) should be reserved for selected cases. Routine catheter angiography (previously the gold standard) is not now indicated (radiation exposure, 1–2% stroke risk), having been replaced by non-invasive alternatives. Table 1 summarises the sensitivity and specificity for duplex, CTA (excluding multi-slice CT), MRA and CEMRA from a systematic review [7]. Overall, CEMRA emerged as the best investigation, but is limited by accessibility and the potential for gadolinium induced nephrogenic systemic fibrosis. In practice, each imaging modality has an important role because investigations in patients being worked up for CEA are different to those for carotid artery stenting (CAS).

Duplex is the first line investigation. In centres with internal validation, CEA can be performed on the basis of ultrasound alone, provided the first scan is corroborated by a second (using a different technologist) [7]. Elsewhere, duplex findings are corroborated by CTA/MRA, especially if

Table 1.   Results of a meta-analysis of the accuracy of non-invasive imaging for all stenosis groups and imaging modalities.[a]

Stenosis group (%)	Imaging	Sensitivity (%)	Specificity (%)
70–99	US	89	84
	CTA	77	95
	MRA	88	84
	CEMRA	94	93
50–69	US	36	91
	CTA	67	79
	MRA	37	91
	CEMRA	77	97
0–49, 100	US	83	84
	CTA	81	91
	MRA	81	88
	CEMRA	96	96

Source: [a]Reproduced with permission from Ref. [7], "Accurate, practical and cost-effective assessment of carotid stenosis in the UK". Health Technology Assessment 2006;Vol 10:No. 30. Department of Health Crown copyright material is reproduced with the permission of the Controller of the HMSO and Queen's Printers for Scotland. Document available at: http://www.hta.ac.uk/fullmono/mon1030.pdf.

there is any question of inflow/outflow disease or excessive calcification. The main advantage of CEMRA/CTA is the ability to image the arch, great vessel origins, distal ICA and intracranial circulation (essential for CAS). The main disadvantage of CEMRA/CTA is that neither are as accessible as duplex.

Management

Table 2 summarises American Heart Association guidance regarding 'optimal medical therapy' in patients presenting with symptomatic and asymptomatic carotid disease [8,9]. In addition to risk factor control and medical therapy, selected patients will benefit from CEA or CAS.

Table 2.   American Heart Association recommendations for 'best medical therapy' in patients with asymptomatic and symptomatic carotid disease [8,9].

Treatment	Level of evidence	
	Asymptomatic	Symptomatic
BP <140/90 mmHg or <130/80 mmHg in diabetics	Level I/Grade A	Level I/Grade A
Glycaemic control to prevent other diabetic complications		Level I/Grade B
Statin therapy	Level I/Grade A	Level I/Grade A
Stop smoking	Level I/Grade C	Level I/Grade C
Avoid heavy consumption of alcohol	Level I/Grade C	Level I/Grade C
Regular physical activity	Level I/Grade B	Level IIa/Grade C
Low salt, low saturated fat, high fruit and vegetable diet rich in fibre	Level I/Grade B	Level IIa/Grade C
HRT should not be used for stroke prevention in women	Level III/Grade A	Level III/Grade A
Aspirin	Level IIa/Grade A	Level I/Grade A
Aspirin and dipyridamole		Level I/Grade B
Clopidogrel		Level IIb/Grade B

Symptomatic carotid disease

Table 3 summarises the 5-year findings from the Carotid Endarterectomy Trialists Collaboration (CETC) who combined data from the ECST, NASCET and VA trials (>6000 patients), having remeasured the pre-randomisation angiograms using the NASCET method [10]. CEA conferred no benefit in patients with 0–50% stenoses. A small but significant benefit was seen in patients with 50–69% stenoses, while maximum benefit was present in those with 70–99% stenoses [10].

Secondary analyses from ECST, NASCET and the CETC have provided information regarding which patients gain most benefit from CEA. Markers of increased benefit include (i) males vs. females, (ii) increasing age, especially >75 years, (iii) hemispheric vs. ocular symptoms (iv) cortical vs. lacunar stroke, (v) increasing medical comorbidity, (vi) very recent symptoms, especially the first 2 weeks, (vii) irregular vs. smooth plaques,

Table 3.   Five-year prevention of 'any' stroke in the symptomatic and asymptomatic randomised trials comparing CEA with medical therapy.

Trial	Stenosis	n	30-day CEA risk	Surgery	Medical	ARR	RRR	NNT	Strokes prevented per 1000 CEAs
					5-year risk				
(1) Symptomatic trials[a]									
CETC	<30%	1746	No data	18.36%	15.71%	−2.6%	n/b	n/b	None at 5 years
CETC	30–49%	1429	6.7%	22.80%	25.45%	+2.6%	10%	38	26 at 5 years
CETC	50–69%	1549	8.4%	20.00%	27.77%	+7.8%	28%	13	78 at 5 years
CETC	70–99%	1095	6.2%	17.13%	32.71%	+15.6%	48%	6	156 at 5 years
CETC	string	262	5.4%	22.40%	22.30%	−0.1%	n/b	n/b	None at 5 years
(2) Asymptomatic trials[b]									
ACAS	60–99%	1659	2.3%	17.5%	12.4%	+5.1%	29%	20	51 at 5 years
ACST	60–99%	3120	2.8%	11.8%	6.4%	+5.4%	46%	19	54 at 5 years

Notes: [a]Data derived from the CETC [10] which combined data from ECST, NASCET and the VA trial. All pre-randomisation angiograms were remeasured using the NASCET method. [b]The ACAS data cited here are for the 5-year risk of 'any' stroke, in order to permit direct comparison with ACST.
n/b = no benefit conferred by CEA, ARR = Absolute Risk Reduction, RRR = Relative Risk Reduction, strokes prevented per 1000 CEAs = number of strokes prevented at 5 years by performing 1000 CEAs, NNT = number of operations to prevent one stroke at 5 years.

(viii) increasing degrees of stenosis (not subocclusion), (ix) contralateral occlusion, (x) tandem intracranial disease and (xi) a failure to recruit intracranial collaterals. Patients with subocclusion (string sign) derived no apparent benefit from CEA [11].

One of the most striking predictors of benefit was speed to treatment. It had previously been taught that the 7-day risk of stroke after TIA/minor stroke was 1–2% (2–4% at 30 days). These data, along with a perception that procedural risks increase the quicker one intervenes, made surgeons reluctant to intervene quickly. However, recent evidence suggests that the 7-day risk of stroke may be as high as 8–10% [11]. Table 4 summarises CETC data regarding outcomes stratified for delays to surgery and show (unequivocally) that delay significantly reduces the long-term benefit accruing to the patient [8].

There has also been controversy about how long CEA should be delayed after suffering a stroke (traditionally 6–8 weeks). Evidence suggests that expedited CEA can be safely undertaken in patients meeting the following criteria: rapid neurological recovery/neurological plateau, no carotid occlusion, Rankin score 0–2, area of infarction <1/3 of the

Table 4. Effect of delay to surgery on overall benefit conferred by carotid endarterectomy.[a]

Stenosis group (%)	Delay (wks)	ARR (%)	NNT	Strokes prevented per 1000 CEAs at 5 years
50–69	<2	14.8	7	148
	2–4	3.3	30	33
	4–12	4.0	25	40
	>12	−2.9	nil	nil
70–99	<2	30.2	3	302
	2–4	17.6	6	176
	4–12	11.4	9	114
	>12	8.9	11	89

Note: [a]Data recalculated from the CETC [10] and excludes patients with 'near occlusion'. ARR = Absolute Risk Reduction in 5-year risk of ipsilateral stroke conferred by CEA over best medical therapy. NNT = Number Needed to Treat to prevent 1 ipsilateral stroke at 5 years. Strokes prevented = number of ipsilateral strokes prevented at 5 years by performing 1000 CEAs.

middle cerebral territory, no intracranial haemorrhage and patients should be lucid and able to give informed consent.

CAS has emerged as an alternative to CEA in the management of symptomatic carotid disease. Seventeen RCTs have now published outcomes comparing CEA with CAS since 1998 [12]. When all RCTs were combined (including symptomatic and asymptomatic patients), CAS was associated with significantly higher rates of any stroke, death/stroke and death/stroke/MI in the peri-operative period [13]. However, all of the very large randomised trials have consistently shown that once the peri-operative period has elapsed, long-term rates of ipsilateral stroke are no different between CEA and CAS [14,15]. At present, CEA remains the first choice intervention for most recently symptomatic patients (especially in the first 14 days after symptom onset where CAS is associated with higher risks), but provided experienced CAS practitioners can perform CAS with 30-day death/stroke rates of <6% that is acceptable [12]. Interventions should not, however, be delayed in order to reduce procedural risks.

Asymptomatic carotid disease

Table 3 summarises outcomes from ACAS and ACST who compared CEA with best medical therapy in asymptomatic patients with 60–99% stenoses. The 'headline' news was that CEA conferred a significant reduction in the 5-year risk of 'stroke'. ACST showed that CEA conferred a significant reduction in fatal/disabling stroke and that CEA was not beneficial in patients aged >75 years. Neither ACAS nor ACST showed any relationship between stenosis severity or bilateral severe disease and 5-year stroke risk. Note that the data published in Table 3 are slightly different to what is normally published as it specifically refers to the 5-year risk of 'any stroke'. The 5-year risks of ipsilateral stroke in ACAS were 11.0% (medical) and 5.9% (surgical).

The management of patients with asymptomatic carotid disease attracts considerable controversy, largely because it is not possible to identify who benefits most from intervention. There is emerging evidence that the natural history risk of stroke is diminishing with time [16], presumably due to improvements in 'optimal medical therapy'. It is imperative, therefore, that we identify high-risk cohorts in whom to target therapy. At present, it is not appropriate to offer CAS to otherwise normal risk asymptomatic patients without participation in ongoing randomised trials (ACST-2, CREST-2, ECST-2, ACTRIS).

The performance of CEA

CEA has been subject to more scientific scrutiny than any other surgical procedure, including a number of RCTs aimed at evaluating different aspects of the procedure.

- The ACE trial showed that low dose aspirin (75–300 mg) conferred significant reductions in early and late death/stroke compared with higher doses (650–1300 mg).
- The GALA trial showed no evidence that performing CEA under general or locoregional anaesthesia influenced outcome, quality of life, hospital stay, ITU stay or costs. Surgeons and anaesthetists may use either anaesthetic technique according to their preference.
- A Cochrane meta-analysis of six randomised trials showed that routine patching conferred a three-fold reduction in the 30-day risk of death/stroke and thrombosis and a similar reduction in late stroke/restenosis compared with routine primary closure. No trial has compared selective with routine patching. The evidence favours a policy of routine patching over routine primary closure and there is no evidence that patch type (vein/prosthetic) influences outcome.
- A meta-analysis of five RCTs showed that provided the arteriotomy is patched, eversion endarterectomy does not confer any additional benefit over traditional endarterectomy.
- A meta-analysis of two randomised trials showed that routine shunting conferred a non-significant 25% reduction in the 30-day risk of death/stroke compared with no shunting. These studies were, however, methodologically flawed. It is intuitively hard to defend a policy of 'never shunting'. Unless surgeons are prepared to perform CEA under locoregional anaesthesia, there is no safe or reliable way of predicting who needs a shunt.

Subclavian Occlusive Disease

Pathology

The commonest cause of occlusive/stenotic disease of the subclavian artery is atherosclerosis, usually at its origin. Other important conditions include arteritis (GCA and TA), thoracic outlet compression, occasionally FMD and rarely aneurysms of the subclavian artery.

Clinical features

Acute obstruction (embolus/thrombosis) of the subclavian artery may cause acute ischaemia of the upper limb, as well as a posterior circulation stroke due to compromised flow in the ipsilateral VA. The more common presentation is pain in the forearm with exercise (claudication) or dizziness while using the ipsilateral limb. The latter condition (subclavian steal syndrome) follows a temporary reduction in flow in the posterior circulation due to reversed flow in the ipsilateral VA during arm exercise. A related condition (coronary steal) is now being reported with the increasing use of the internal mammary artery as a conduit for coronary bypass. In the presence of a proximal subclavian stenosis/occlusion, there may be reversed flow in the internal mammary graft during arm exercise, which can be sufficient to precipitate angina or breathlessness.

Investigations

Duplex is the first line investigation (accessible and cheap), supplemented by CTA/CEMRA. Patients suspected of having arteritis, FMD require additional investigations (see earlier).

Management

Risk factor modification and institution of statin/antiplatelet therapy. A significant proportion of patients with subclavian occlusive disease can be managed conservatively, especially if it is an incidental asymptomatic finding. The decision to intervene should be based on mode of presentation and extent of disability (pain, employment, etc.) in the context of the potential risks (surgery and angioplasty carry a small but significant risk of stroke). Compelling indications include severe arm pain with exercise that compromises employment, vertebrobasilar symptoms at presentation, subclavian steal syndrome and coronary steal syndrome. Less compelling indications include mild dizziness with head movement and minor forearm claudication (especially in the non-dominant limb). In the past, surgical revascularisation was the cornerstone of management (carotid-subclavian bypass, transposition), but many centres now increasingly use angioplasty +/− stenting as the first line option. There is no level I to guide practice. Surgery carries a slightly higher initial risk, but probably offers better long-term durability. Conversely, endovascular interventions are less invasive (and less risky), but long-term patency rates may be slightly poorer.

Vertebral Occlusive Disease

Demographics

Approximately 20% of all ischaemic strokes are vertebrobasilar.

Pathology

The commonest aetiology is atherosclerosis, but dissection, arteritis and FMD must be considered. In a recent population-based study of CEMRA imaging in 151 patients presenting with vertebrobasilar symptoms, 26% were found to have significant disease (>50% stenosis) in the vertebral or basilar arteries [17]. Of those with demonstrable disease, 62% were located in the extracranial VA, 11% in the intracranial VA, while 8% of lesions were found in the basilar artery. Interestingly, in those patients presenting with vertebrobasilar symptoms and who had a significant with extracranial VA stenosis, 69% had their stenoses either at the origin or near to the origin of the VA, while 31% had lesions in the upper third of the VA.

Clinical features

Vertebrobasilar symptoms include bilateral sensory/motor symptoms and signs, hemisensory/motor symptoms and signs (seen in 10% of vertebrobasilar events), bilateral visual loss (cortical blindness), dysarthria, nystagmus and problems with gait and stance. Patients with isolated non-hemispheric symptoms (without definite vertebrobasilar symptoms) should not be considered to have suffered posterior circulation symptoms. Similarly, it has become conventional to make a diagnosis of 'positional' vertebrobasilar ischaemia in patients who develop (dizziness, vertigo) on lateral or flexed head movements. Recent evidence suggests that the vast majority of these patients do not have a vertebrobasilar cause for their symptoms. Such a diagnosis should only be made after comprehensive investigation, as most will have inner ear pathology.

Investigations

DUS is the first line investigation, but is limited by its inability to fully evaluate the extracranial VA. Transcranial Duplex can image the intracranial VA and basilar arteries, but it is preferable to undertake CEMRA/CTA, which provides comprehensive information regarding the arch, subclavian/vertebral origins as well as the circle of Willis. The other advantage of CT/MR is that it provides valuable information about structural cranial abnormalities (tumour, infarction, A-V malformation). However, extracranial and transcranial Duplex can determine whether head movements cause any change in flow in the extracranial VA or posterior cerebral artery.

Management

In the past, the mainstay of management was medical therapy or surgery (vertebral patch angioplasty, transposition to the carotid artery and proximal/distal bypass). Modern endovascular advances now offer an alternative means of treatment (angioplasty, stenting), which is emerging as the new first line intervention in most centres. All patients will, of course, require optimisation of risk factors and antiplatelet/statin therapy. The VAST randomised trial was stopped prematurely (and lacked statistical power), but showed no evidence that stenting conferred benefit over medical therapy alone in recently symptomatic patients. Pending publication of ongoing RCTs, most would only advocate VA stenting for patients with recurrent symptoms despite medical therapy [12].

Prognosis

It was previously thought that patients with vertebrobasilar symptoms faced a lower risk of late stroke than those with carotid artery disease. However, data from population-based studies suggest that this assumption may be erroneous. The Oxford group has shown that 46% of patients with a recently symptomatic VA stenosis suffered either a recurrent TIA or stroke in the first 90 days after presentation [17]. This compares with only 21% in patients with no VA stenosis.

References

1. Olin JW. Recognizing and managing fibromuscular dysplasia. *Cleveland Clin J Med* 2007;74:273–282.
2. Kennedy F, Lanfranconi S, Hicks C, Reid J, Gompertz P, Price C, Kerry S, Norris J, Markus HS; CADISS Investigators. Antiplatelets vs. anticoagulation for dissection: CADISS non-randomized arm and meta-analysis. *Neurology* 2012; 79:686–689.
3. Paraskevas KI, Batchelder AJ, Naylor AR. Fate of distal false aneurysms complicating internal carotid artery dissection: A systematic review. *Eur J Vasc Endovasc Surg* 2016;52(3):281–286.
4. Kawasaki A, Purvin V. Giant cell arteritis: An updated review. *Acta Ophth* 2009;87:13–32.
5. Johnston SL, Lock RJ, Gompels MM. Takayasu arteritis: A review. *J Clin Pathol* 2002;55:481–486.
6. Sajid MS, Hamilton G, Baker DM. On behalf of the Joint Vascular Research Group. *Eur J Vasc Endovasc Surg* 2007;34:127–130.
7. Wardlaw JM, Chappell FM, Stevenson M *et al.* Accurate, practical and cost-effective assessment of carotid stenosis in the UK. *Health Technology Assessment* 2006;10(30). Available at: http://www.hta.ac.uk/fullmono/mon1030.pdf.
8. Meschia JF, Bushnell CB, Boden-Albala B, Braun LT, Bravata DM, Chaturvedi S *et al.* Guidelines for the primary prevention of stroke. A statement for healthcare professionals from the American Heart Association/American Stroke Association. *Stroke* 2014;45:3754–3832.
9. Kernan WN, Ovbiagele B, Black HR, Bravata DM, Chimowitz MI, Ezekowitz MD *et al.* Guidelines for the prevention of stroke in patients with stroke and transient ischemic attack. A guideline for healthcare professionals from the

American Heart Association/American Stroke Association. *Stroke* 2014; 45:2160–2236.

10. Rothwell PM, Eliasziw M, Gutnikov, Warlow CP, Barnett HJM for the Carotid Endarterectomy Trialists Collaboration. Endarterectomy for symptomatic carotid stenosis in relation to clinical subgroups and timing of surgery. *Lancet* 2004;363:915–924.

11. Naylor AR, Sillesen H, Schroeder TV. Clinical and imaging features associated with an increased risk of early and late stroke in patients with symptomatic carotid disease. *Eur J Vasc Endovasc Surg* 2015;49:513–523.

12. Naylor AR *et al*. European Society of Vascular Surgery Guidelines on the management of atherosclerotic carotid and vertebral artery disease guidelines. *Eur J Vasc Endovasc Surg* 2018;55:3–81.

13. Luebke T, Brunkwall J. Carotid artery stenting versus carotid endarterectomy: Updated meta-analysis, meta-regression and trial sequential analysis of short term and intermediate to long term outcomes of randomised trials. *J Cardiovasc Surg* 2016;57:519–539.

14. Brott TG, Howard G, Roubin GS, Meschia JF, Mackey A, Brooks W *et al*. on behalf of CREST Investigators. Long-term results of stenting versus endarterectomy for carotid-artery stenosis. *NEJM* 2016;374:1021–1031.

15. Bonati LH, Dobson J, Featherstone RL *et al*. Long-term outcomes after stenting versus endarterectomy for treatment of symptomatic carotid stenosis: The International Carotid Stenting Study (ICSS) randomised trial. *Lancet* 2015;385:529–538.

16. Naylor AR, Sillesen H, Schroeder TV. Clinical and imaging features associated with an increased risk of late stroke in patients with asymptomatic carotid disease. *Eur J Vasc Endovasc Surg* 2014;48:633–640.

17. Markus HS, van der Worn H, Rothwell PM. Posterior circulation ischaemic stroke and transient ischaemic attack: Diagnosis, investigation, and secondary prevention. *Lancet Neurol* 2013;12:989–998.

Chapter 14

Diagnosis and Management of Thoracic Outlet Syndrome

Hassan Badri and Vish Bhattacharya

Key Points

- Thoracic outlet syndrome (TOS) is caused by compression on neuro-vascular bundle in the thoracic outlet tunnel.
- TOS can be neurogenic (90%), venous (5%), arterial (1%), or any combination of the above three.
- Physical examination is more reliable in the venous and arterial forms but is not straightforward in the neurologic form where more objective tests are required.
- Provocative tests have high false positive rates.
- Dynamic imaging has more diagnostic value than standard imaging.
- Neurologic TOS should be referred to physiotherapy for postural correction and muscle exercise.
- Venous and arterial TOS are treated with surgical decompression and blood vessel reconstructive procedures. The rule is 'the sooner, the better'.

Introduction

Thoracic outlet syndrome (TOS) is one of the most controversial clinical entities in medicine. Its incidence has been estimated at 5:100 000 per year in the UK, although the true figure is still unknown [1].

The thoracic outlet is the region at the top of the rib cage between the base of the neck and the axilla through which the brachial plexus and the subclavian vessels travel. It encompasses three channels. The proximal one is the interscalene triangle, which is bordered by scalenus anterior, scalenus medius and the medial border of the first rib (Fig. 1). The second channel is the costoclavicular space, composed of middle part of the clavicle anteriorly and the first rib and scapula posteriorly. The distal channel is the subcoracoid space below the coracoid process and posterior to the pectoralis minor.

TOS refers to a variety of complex disorders in the upper extremity caused by damage of the brachial plexus, subclavian artery and vein, as they pass through the thoracic outlet tunnel described above. Thoracic outlet is more common in women and in age group between 30 and 50 years, but it has been reported in children as well.

Pathophysiology/Causes

Any factor that causes compression on the neurovascular structures in the narrow thoracic outlet tunnel is a potential cause. However, in many cases, no specific anatomical factor can be identified.

Patients with chronic repetitive arm movements such as overhead reaching or extending the arm can be at increased risk. Professional swimmers, typists, and musicians are examples.

Fibrous bands which traverse the thoracic outlet are the most common congenital anomaly that causes TOS. Cervical ribs are seen in 0.1% of adults and 50% are bilateral but only 5–10% are symptomatic (Fig. 2). Malunion and formation of large callus after clavicle fractures have been reported as a cause of the TOS. Anomalous muscular insertion and muscle hypertrophy have been described. Pancoast tumour and rarely enlarged regional lymph nodes may represent as TOS.

Postures and developmental changes in the cervical spine and shoulder girdle bones and muscles, which might elongate the tunnel and tense the neurovascular bundle, have been accused as etiological factors in the TOS [2].

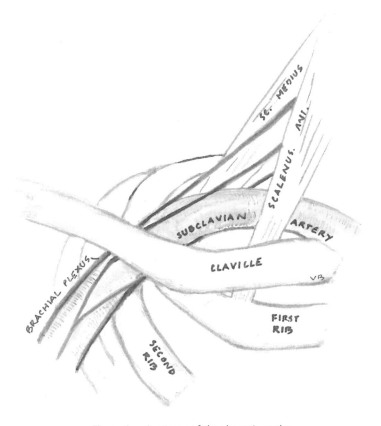

Figure 1.   Anatomy of the thoracic outlet.

Classification of TOS

Clinical features differ according to the compressed structure/s in the thoracic outlet tunnel. Hence, three main clinical syndromes are described as follows:

(1) *Neurogenic TOS (NTOS) (90% of TOS)*

Clinical presentation

Pain is a common presentation and it usually occurs in the back of the neck, supraclavicular region, and shoulder region going down to the arm.

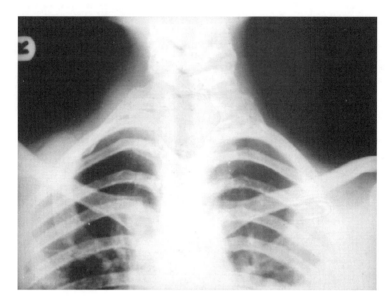

Figure 2.   Right sided cervical rib seen on a plain X-ray.

Paraesthesia is usually felt on the medial aspect of the arm, forearm, hand, and fourth and fifth digits. These symptoms are aggravated by many activities e.g., carrying heavy loads, combing hair, reaching towards shelf and usually affect the lower trunk (C8-T1 roots) distribution (ulnar and median nerves). Motor weakness is most noticed in the intrinsic muscles and might cause clumsiness in fine hand movement and hand grip and in extreme, late presentation, intrinsic muscle wasting has been noted. Vasospastic-type disturbances, such as coldness or Raynaud's, are often present and may lead to an erroneous suspicion of the existence of arterial involvement [2].

Diagnosis of NTOS

Diagnosis of NTOS is difficult, subjective and variable. Patients usually have tenderness over the scalene muscles. Often, the symptoms can be reproduced by the provocative manoeuvres as mentioned below. Many tests have been described but we will mention the most used ones in clinical practice.

Roos test (elevated arm stress test, EAST): The patient is asked to elevate and abduct both arms with the elbows bent at 90° (surrender position). They are then asked to open and close the hands repeatedly for three minutes. A positive test is noted when the patient's symptoms are reproduced, often with disappearance of the radial pulse. The sensitivity and specificity of this test in various studies has been shown to be around 84% and 30%, respectively, with high false positive rates [3,4].

Adson test: The patient is asked to take a deep breath and then extend the neck and rotate the head towards the side being examined. The test is positive if the radial pulse is abolished and the patient's symptoms replicated. Adson test was the most reliable one of 79% sensitivity and 76% specificity [3,4].

Investigations

Cervical spine film and chest radiograph can exclude any bony abnormalities of TOS and cervical disease. MRI and CT scan of the cervicothoracic area are more helpful in detecting the non-bony anomalies (fibrous bands, muscular abnormality, tumours). MRI findings in patients in a provocative position (placing the hand behind the head) (i.e., dynamic MRI) are more valuable in the diagnosis of TOS. Success after anterior scalene muscle blocks with local anaesthesia appears to correlate well with surgical outcomes (94%). The performance measurement of medial antebrachial cutaneous nerve stimulation is a new reliable diagnostic technique for confirming the diagnosis of NTOS [5].

Another simple, diagnostic tool is a dynamic neuromusculoskeletal ultrasound that can confirm the brachial plexus compression during arm elevation in patients with NTOS [6].

Treatment of NTOS

This is usually conservative, with postural correction and physical therapy showing good results at reducing symptoms and improving function. This method involves improving patient's posture by strengthening exercises and stretching/lengthening of the shoulder girdle muscles.

Although controversial, selective botulinum toxin injection of the scalene muscles is also described for short-term treatment of neurogenic TOS with improvement rates reaching 90% [7].

Surgery is indicated in NTOS in case of severe symptoms that interfere with work or daily activities and failure of conservative treatment. Surgical outcome for NTOS reached success rate of up to 90% and is preferred in young patients with short period of symptoms and very importantly before they became dependent on strong analgesics, in particular narcotics [8].

(2) *Venous TOS (VTOS) (5–10%)*

Clinical presentation

Compression and, hence, thrombosis of the subclavian vein occur mostly at the venous triangle in the thoracic outlet. The roof of this is the clavicle, the floor is the first rib with the subclavius/costoclavicular ligament medially and the anterior scalene muscle laterally. Venous TOS is more common in the right arm of males in their 30s and usually occurs after strenuous activity to the upper limb. This is referred to as effort thrombosis or Paget–Schroetter syndrome. Athletes , swimmers, weightlifters and golfers are at increased risk. It is thought that repeated extrinsic compression of the subclavian vein may cause fibrosis, stenosis and eventually thrombosis. It may also be due to a sudden hyper-abduction injury causing intimal damage and thrombosis of the subclavian vein. Patients present acutely with arm swelling, cyanosis, and pain on exertion. Dilated superficial veins (collaterals) are not infrequently seen around the shoulder and upper chest. Chronic intermittent obstruction/ symptoms aggravated by exercise is called McCleery syndrome [9].

Diagnosis of VTOS

Venous duplex ultrasound (DUS) of the upper extremity is the first-line investigation and it is specific in 96% with sensitivity of 94% compared to the gold standard venography. MR and CT venography are certainly helpful in more proximal thrombosis not fully seen on duplex, but they are difficult to interpret in short or non-occlusive thrombus (9).

Treatment of VTOS

Therapeutic protocols now include thrombolysis, surgical correction of the anatomical abnormalities contributing to the thrombosis i.e., cervical/first rib resection, and maintaining patency of the axillo-sub-clavian veins by patch-plasty or balloon venoplasty. There is strong evidence suggesting that the sooner the above protocol is started, the better the outcome for patients. Venous stenting is not recommended in this young group of patients and if balloon venoplasty fails, surgical correction with a patch or interposition graft is a more desired approach [9].

(3) *Arterial TOS (ATOS) (1%)*

Clinical presentation

The rare arterial form of TOS is almost always associated with bony abnormality such as cervical rib, prominent transverse process of C7, large callus of the first rib or clavicle. Repetitive trauma to the subclavian artery can lead to intimal damage and cause stenosis, occlusion, thrombosis, and aneurysm/post-stenotic aneurysm formation. Patients may present with attacks of pallor, pain, paraesthesia and coolness of the hand. Embolisation may occur in acute ATOS and patients present with acute ischaemia of the hand with multiple infarcts of the hand and fingers [10].

Diagnosis of ATOS

In ATOS, an absent radial pulse at rest is common. Although not diagnostic, radial pulse might disappear on arm abduction in some of the provocative tests for TOS. Measurement of bilateral arterial blood pressure will demonstrate the difference, if present.

Investigations for ATOS

Arterial DUS of the upper extremity is non-invasive, first-line investigation. Computed tomography angiography (CTA) and magnetic resonance angiography (MRA) are useful for aneurysm diagnosis and treatment planning. Arteriography is used for treatment or to confirm reconstruction plan. Dynamic tests of the above imaging modalities are useful in chronic cases.

Treatment of ATOS

Surgical correction of all symptomatic ATOS is recommended. This includes removal of the bony anomaly followed by arterial repair which could be a patch, or a bypass [10]. Occasionally, thoracic sympathectomy is required for severe digital ischaemic changes.

There are many surgical approaches for TOS, namely, transaxillary supraclavicular, combined supraclavicular and infraclavicular, and posterior subcapsular. Success rate after surgery ranged from 43% to 88% [11]. Predictive factors of negative outcomes were acute ischaemia, sensory or motor deficit, extended resection of the first rib, and severe postoperative complications [12].

Transaxillary approach has been shown to be associated with recurrence in 20–30% of patients. The exposure via the axilla makes it difficult to release the upper and middle trunks of the brachial plexus. Overlooked fibromuscular bands, long posterior stump of the first rib and reattachment of the anterior and middle scalene muscle to scar tissue have been noted to be the cause of recurrence. The supraclavicular approach provided easier access to the upper and middle trunks as well as a complete anterior and middle scalenectomy [13]. It is also more useful for recurrent TOS.

Conclusion

TOS can present with neurological, venous or arterial symptoms. The neurological presentation is the most complex to diagnose. Treatment includes first rib or cervical rib resection, division of fibrous bands and anterior and medial scalenectomy. Earlier surgical management is useful especially in younger patients with vascular symptoms.

References

1. Thompson JF, Jannsen F. Thoracic outlet syndromes. *Br J Surg* 1996; 83(4):435–436.
2. Sheth RN, Belzberg AJ. Diagnosis and treatment of thoracic outlet syndrome. *Neurosurg Clin N Am* 2001;12(2):295–309.

3. Gillard J, Pérez-Cousin M, Hachulla E, Remy J, Hurtevent JF, Vinckier L, Thévenon A, Duquesnoy B. Diagnosing thoracic outlet syndrome: Contribution of provocative tests, ultrasonography, electrophysiology, and helical computed tomography in 48 patients. *Joint Bone Spine* 2001;68(5): 416–424.

4. Rayan GM, Jensen C. Thoracic outlet syndrome: provocative examination maneuvers in a typical population. *J Shoulder Elbow Surg* 1995;4(2): 113–117.

5. Machanic BI, Sanders RJ. Medial antebrachial cutaneous nerve measurements to diagnose neurogenic thoracic outlet syndrome. *Ann Vasc Surg* 2008;22(2):248–254.

6. Scott M. Fried, Levon N. Nazarian. Dynamic neuromusculoskeletal ultrasound documentation of brachial plexus/thoracic outlet compression during elevated arm stress testing. *HAND* 2013;8:358–365.

7. Jordan SE, Ahn SS, Gelabert HA. Combining ultrasonography and electromyography for botulinum chemodenervation treatment of thoracic outlet syndrome: Comparison with fluoroscopy and electromyography guidance. *Pain Phys* 2007;10(4):541–546.

8. Likes K, Orlando M, Serene Mirza QS, Cohen A, Reifsnyder T, Lum YW, Freischlag JA. Lessons Learned in the Surgical Treatment of Neurogenic Thoracic Outlet Syndrome Over 10 Years. *Vasc Endovasc Surg* 2015;49(1–2): 8–11.

9. Moore R, Lum YW. Venous thoracic outlet syndrome. *Vasc Med* 2015; 20(2):182–189.

10. Hussain MA, Aljabri B, Al-Omran. Vascular thoracic outlet syndrome. *Sem Thoracic Cardiovas Surg* 2016;28(1):151–157.

11. Bhattacharya V, Hansrani M, Wyatt MG, Lambert D, Jones NA. Outcome following surgery for thoracic outlet syndrome. *Eur J Vasc Endovasc Surg* 2003;26(2):170–175.

12. Degeorges R, Reynaud C, Becquemin JP. Thoracic outlet syndrome surgery: Long-term functional results. *Ann Vasc Surg* 2004;18(5):558–565.

13. Terzis JK, Kokkalis ZT. Supraclavicular approach for thoracic outlet syndrome. *Hand* 2010;5(3):326–337.

Chapter 15

Chronic Mesenteric Ischaemia

Arunagiri Viruthagiri, Mohamed Abdelhamid,
Robert Davies and Rajiv Vohra

Key Points

- Chronic mesenteric ischaemia (CMI) is a rare condition, accounting for less than 5% of all intestinal ischaemic events.
- More than 90% of the cases are due to atherosclerotic occlusion or severe stenosis.
- Classic symptoms include post-prandial abdominal pain, sitophobia, and weight loss.
- At least two of the three main splanchnic arteries must be significantly compromised to result in CMI.
- Duplex ultrasonography is non-invasive and expedient, but may miss up to 20% of vascular lesions in celiac artery.
- Computed tomography angiography (CTA) and magnetic resonance angiography (MRA) are equally excellent non-invasive modalities with highly accurate diagnosis.
- Digital Subtraction angiography should be reserved for the diagnosis of CMI only when other modalities have been unhelpful or if intervention such as percutaneous transluminal angioplasty (PTA) is planned.

- Surgical vascular bypass is the definitive therapy for CMI with an overall 5-year graft patency of 78%. It is preferred in younger patients with less comorbidities.
- Endovascular therapy is optimal in short segment atherosclerotic lesions <2 cm from the ostia of coeliac and superior mesenteric artery. Angioplasty and stenting have a significantly lower rate of complications although the intervention rate is higher.

Background

Chronic mesenteric ischaemia (CMI) is an uncommon cause of abdominal pain. It accounts for 5% of all intestinal ischaemic events with acute ischaemia being much more common. Atherosclerotic occlusion, or severe stenosis of the mesenteric arteries, is the most common aetiology and the incidence of atherosclerotic lesions affecting the mesenteric arteries in a person >65 years is 17.5% [1]. In patients with peripheral arterial disease and renal artery stenosis, 25% of the individuals examined had greater than 50% stenosis in either the CA or SMA, but only 3.4% had significant occlusion of both arteries [2].

Symptoms of CMI such as intestinal angina, weight loss and sitophobia (i.e., fear of eating) usually only occur when at least two of the three main splanchnic arteries are affected, out of which one is most commonly SMA. This is because the mesenteric arterial circulation is rich in collaterals. The mesenteric collateral pathway is illustrated in Fig. 1.

Pathophysiology

The majority of those affected are elderly patients with generalised atherosclerosis. Atherosclerotic occlusion or severe stenosis of the mesenteric arteries accounts for more than 90% of the causes of CMI [3]. Hyperlipidemia, diabetes and smoking contribute to the occurrence of CMI. Thrombotic occlusion or stenosis usually occurs at the origin of the artery adjacent to the ostium. Diffuse atherosclerosis of the whole vessel is seen in fewer patients. The CA and SMA are more commonly affected than the inferior mesenteric artery (IMA). Other causes of CMI and differential diagnosis are listed in Table 1. Takayasu arteritis can present as mid-aortic syndrome with involvement of visceral segment of aorta and

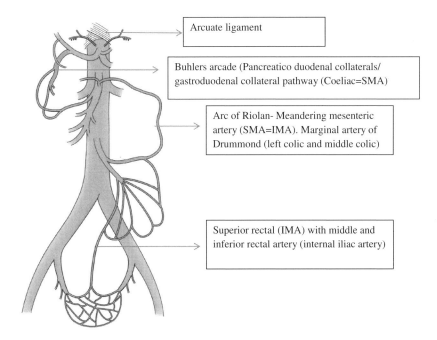

Figure 1.   Diagram of collateral pathways for the mesenteric vessels. The clinical significance of meandering mesenteric artery is it is often encountered along with Inferior mesenteric vein. Ligating it during aortic surgeries could potentially precipitate mesenteric ischaemia.

Notes: SMA — Superior mesenteric artery; IMA — Inferior mesenteric artery.

Table 1.   Aetiology and differential diagnosis of CMI.

Aetiology	Differential diagnosis
Atherosclerosis (90%)	Abdominal malignancy
Takayasu arteritis	Chronic pancreatitis
Fibromuscular dysplasia	Chronic cholecystitis
Aortic dissection	Peptic ulcer
Giant cell arteritis/PAN	Inflammatory bowel disease
Median arcuate ligament syndrome	Spastic colon
Drug-induced (Ergot, Cocaine)	
Radiation-induced arteritis	
Buerger's disease	

these patients may present with renovascular hypertension also. Median arcuate ligament syndrome, caused by dynamic compression of celiac artery by arcuate ligament, is more common in women.

Relative ischaemia occurs after eating when there is an increased demand for flow within the mesenteric circulation while the arteries are unable to dilate due to the fixed occlusive lesions. This results in transient ischaemic pain, known as intestinal angina.

Clinical Presentation

The typical patient is a female with a median age of 65 years. Most of the available literature quote a female to male ratio of 3:1 to 4:1. Pain is dull in nature and typically post-prandial, 30 min after eating, and occurs in the periumbilical region. It may last 1–4 h and fades gradually. The patients develop fear from eating, resulting in the reduction of the size of meals in order to avoid the pain, which eventually leads to weight loss [3]. CMI involving the coeliac artery may result in disorders such as gastroparesis, gastric ulceration and gall bladder dyskinesia.

Physical examination is usually unremarkable except for abdominal pain that is out of proportion to examination. These patients have obvious signs of malnutrition, muscle wasting, and a scaphoid abdomen. Sometimes, an epigastric bruit may be audible.

Diagnosis

Diagnosis requires careful history-taking and exclusion of other illnesses such as malignancy, chronic pancreatitis, and gastric ulcer (Table 1). Investigative modalities to diagnose CMI include visceral Duplex ultrasound, computed tomography angiogram and magnetic resonance angiogram.

Duplex Ultrasound

Visceral duplex ultrasound (VDU) evaluation of the mesenteric arteries is non-invasive. It has been used successfully to document occlusive disease in the proximal SMA and, to a lesser extent, in the CA. The IMA is rarely imaged by transabdominal ultrasound due to its anatomic location. Overall, VDU has a 90% accuracy in identifying significant proximal SMA stenosis and 80% accuracy for coeliac trunk lesions [4].

Diagnostic criteria:

(1) Peak systolic velocity (PSV) of greater than 200 cm/s and an end-diastolic velocity exceeding 55 cm/s have been shown to have high correlation with CA stenosis (2).
(2) PSV greater than 275 cm/s with end diastolic velocity greater than 45 cm/s is specific to lesions of the proximal SMA.

However, limitations of duplex include effects of respiration, obesity, food ingestion, bowel gas, anatomic variations and operator. If screening ultrasonography detects vascular stenosis or occlusion, further detailed imaging is usually indicated.

CT Angiogram

Computed tomography angiography (CTA) is most often the investigation of choice with high sensitivity and specificity to identify significant splanchnic vascular stenosis. The availability of 3D image reconstruction can diagnose significant atherosclerotic lesions of all the three major mesenteric arteries and many of their main branches. In addition to providing 3D images, this modality has faster scanning time. Thinner collimation of 0.5–1.0 mm thickness facilitates better visualisation of small vessels and branches. In suspected intestinal angina, a negative CTA study of the mesenteric arteries makes the diagnosis of CMI virtually unlikely. It also has an advantage of providing imaging of the bowel to rule out other causes.

MR Angiogram

In recent years, MRA has become a valuable tool for diagnosing CMI, particularly since its cost and image acquisition times have substantially decreased. MRA images provide high-resolution mesenteric angiograms with sensitivity greater than 90% of SMA and CA lesions, 81–88% of portal vein disease, and 25% of lesions affecting the IMA vessels [6]. However, small peripheral arterial branches are less well visualised.

Digital Subtraction Angiography

Diagnostic angiography is reserved when other non-invasive imaging modalities are inconclusive, especially in patients with heavy calcific disease at the ostium, patients with prior stents as they cause an artefact and in patients with small vessels. Lateral projection is mandatory to visualise celiac axis and SMA origin.

Endoscopy

Both upper gastointestinal endoscopy and colonoscopy are often done to rule out other pathologies and in 40% of the patients, it may show evidence of ischaemic lesions in stomach or colon.

The advantages and disadvantages of the various diagnostic modalities are listed in Table 2.

Table 2.   Diagnostic methods of CMI.

Modality	Advantages	Disadvantages
Duplex Ultrasound	Non-invasive, low cost, 90% and 80% sensitivity for SMA and CA, respectively	Operator-dependant, not for IMA, limited by obesity, respiration, bowel gas and food ingestion
CTA	Non-invasive, 96% sensitive for celiac and SMA, operator-independent	Renal impairment, contrast allergy
MRA	Non-invasive, 90% sensitive for celiac and SMA, operator-independent	Low sensitivity for IMA, cost, claustrophobia, patients with Implants
DSA	Useful in patients with heavy calcific disease, prior stent placement, small arteries, 100% sensitive for all three arteries	Invasive, renal impairment, contrast allergy

Notes: CTA — Computed tomography angiography; MRA — magnetic resonance angiography; DSA — digital subtraction angiography; SMA — superior mesenteric artery; CA — celiac artery; IMA — inferior mesenteric artery.

Treatment

There is no role for a conservative approach in symptomatic patients with chronic mesenteric ischaemia. The therapeutic goal in patients with CMI is to revascularise the mesenteric arterial circulation to improve the blood supply for increased demand and prevent the development of bowel infarction. Mesenteric vascular stenosis or occlusion usually requires open surgical repair or endovascular therapy.

In asymptomatic patients with all three vessel involvement, revascularisation would be indicated in those who undergo concomitant aortic reconstruction.

Surgical repair

Surgical repair has been the standard treatment for CMI since the first successful repair reported by Shaw in 1958. The surgical options include the following:

A Transaortic endarterectomy

This is indicated for ostial lesions of patent CA and SMA. This can be achieved by left medial visceral rotation to expose the aorta and its mesenteric branches. Transaortic endarterectomy is also beneficial in patients with concomitant renal artery stenosis and CMI due to atherosclerosis. It is rarely performed now. It is useful in previous abdominal surgery, multiple abdominal wall hernia surgeries as it is a retroperitoneal approach and in perforated gut where avoiding a prosthetic material would be beneficial.

B Surgical bypass

This is indicated for occlusive lesions located 1–2 cm from the origin of the mesenteric arteries. Surgical bypass can be performed through either antegrade or retrograde reconstruction using either autogenous or prosthetic grafts. Single or multivessel reconstruction with outflow into the CA, SMA or rarely the IMA should be achieved. Isolated IMA revascularisation has been used for CMI in selected cases when it is not possible to revascularise either the CA or SMA.

Antegrade vs. retrograde inflow reconstruction

In antegrade reconstruction, the arterial inflow arises from the thoracic or supraceliac aorta, so the bypass is placed in the direction of normal blood flow to reduce anastomotic turbulence. This could be done through abdominal or thoracoabdominal incision.

In retrograde reconstruction (Fig. 2), inflow arises from the infrarenal aorta or the common iliac artery. A smooth C curvature of graft is maintained to avoid kinking of graft.

Apart from a slightly higher 30-day mortality with the antegrade approach, there is no statistically significant difference between the

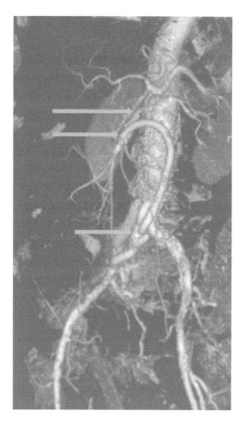

Figure 2.   Retrograde bypass. Top — superior mesenteric (SMA) stenosis. Middle — distal anastomosis to the proximal SMA. Bottom — proximal anastomosis from the right limb of the aorto-bi-iliac graft.

antegrade and retrograde approaches concerning symptom-free survival.

The drawbacks of retrograde revascularisation include kinking of the graft and progression of atherosclerosis to the origin of the retrograde bypass graft from the infrarenal aorta or the common iliac artery. Kinking of the vein grafts occurred immediately after surgery in the earlier series when short vein grafts were used. This problem has been avoided with the use of prosthetic grafts, especially when a long loop is constructed.

The retrograde approach is useful in high-risk patients requiring shorter surgical time, patients with previous abdominal surgery and those who have had a failed previous antegrade bypass [8].

Autogenous vs. prosthetic grafts

Both autogenous and prosthetic vascular reconstructions have been used with satisfactory results. Both the long saphenous vein and and superficial femoral vein have been used with equally good results although polytetrafluoroethane (PTFE) and Dacron have more long-term durability.

Outcome: Surgical reconstruction has been associated with morbidity and mortality (5–30%) in most series [8]. This could be expected in this group as many are elderly with significant weight loss, malnutrition, and low albumin levels, which are all predictors of increased morbidity and mortality after any major surgery. Postoperative multiorgan dysfunction as a sequel of ischaemia — reperfusion cascade is often encountered, especially manifesting as elevated transaminases.

Percutaneous transluminal angioplasty and stenting (PTA/stent)

In the last two decades, endovascular therapy has become a more acceptable approach for stenotic or occlusive lesions in the mesenteric arteries. This consists of percutaneous transluminal angioplasty and stenting (PTA/stent) of the mesenteric arteries. Short occlusive or stenotic lesions are ideal for this procedure (Figs. 3 and 4).

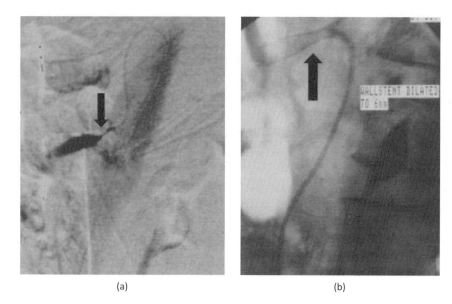

(a)   (b)

Figure 3.   (a) Tight stenosis at the origin of coeliac artery and (b) successful angioplasty and stent deployment.

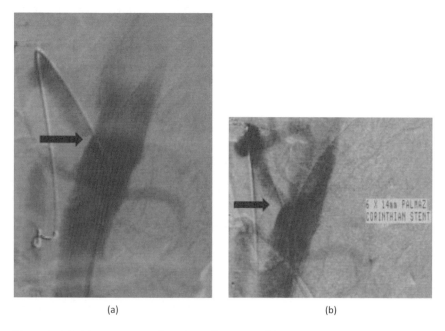

(a)   (b)

Figure 4. (a) Tight stenosis at the origin of SMA and (b) successful angioplasty and stent deployment.

An endovascular approach could also be used for graft angioplasty in the case of recurrent symptoms after surgical repair (Fig. 5).

In a systematic review of 12 studies comparing endovascular vs. surgical revascularisation for the management of CMI by Saedon *et al.*, there were no differences in mortality and morbidity in both the groups. Patency rates were better following Surgical revascularisation [10].

In a meta-analysis of contemporary clinical studies performed by Ansari *et al.*, a total of 13 studies (12 retrospective and one prospective) provided a total of 7446 patients, divided in two groups: 4281 (EVT — endovascular treatment group) and 3165 (OS — open surgery group). There was no difference in post-procedural mortality (EVT: 3.4% vs. OS: 11.3%, $p = 0.67$). Primary (59% vs. 85%) and secondary patency rates (73% vs. 92%) were better in the OS group ($p < 0.001$). There was no difference in long-term survival between EVT and OS (77% vs. 73%, $p = 0.52$). They concluded that endovascular therapy and open surgery have comparable post-procedural mortality and

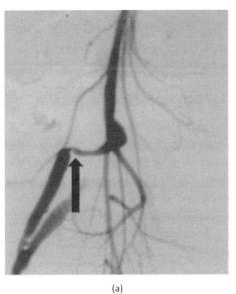
(a)

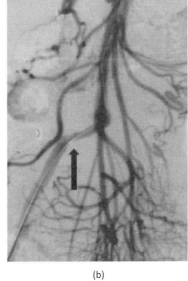
(b)

Figure 5.   (a) Tight stenosis in vein graft 18 months after surgery and (b) successful graft angioplasty.

Table 3.   A comparison of surgical and endovascular repairs.

	Surgical repair	Endovascular repair
Suitable lesions	Long flush occlusions	Stenotic/short lesions
Success rate	90–100%	80–100%
In-hospital complications	5–30%	5–15%
Peri-operative mortality	11.3%	3.4%
Primary patency	85%	59%
Secondary patency	92%	73%
Long-term survival	73%	77%
Reintervention	Lower	Higher

long-term survival, although surgery is associated with superior primary and secondary patency rates which is shown in Table 3 [11].

In another meta-analysis of eight studies by Cai *et al.*, they concluded that endovascular treatment offers a benefit of lower in-hospital complication rate, but a greater recurrence rate within 3 years after revascularisation compared with the open revascularisation, and both the groups have similar 30-day mortality and 3-year cumulative survival rate [12].

Retrograde Hybrid Revascularisation (retrograde open mesenteric revascularisation — ROMS)

Wyers and coauthors from Dartmouth reported a hybrid open-interventional approach for the treatment of acute on chronic atherosclerotic SMA thrombosis that involves an efficient, less invasive mesenteric revascularisation.

In this ROMS approach, the SMA is exposed at the base of the transverse mesocolon, and a local thromboendarterectomy/embolectomy of the SMA is performed. Placing a patch angioplasty then facilitates retrograde cannulation of the SMA with a sheath directed towards the aorta. Because of the superior pushability with sheath access so close to the obstruction, technical success was 100%. Long-term outcomes with this approach has not been established [13].

Conclusion

Although uncommon, CMI remains an important cause of abdominal pain that may lead to serious consequences if misdiagnosed. The clinician has to have a high degree of suspicion for its early detection. Diagnosis requires good history taking, physical examination and diagnostic testing. Non-invasive investigations, CTA or MRA are the standard investigations with high levels of accuracy. All patients with symptomatic CMI must have revascularisation.

Open revascularisation in either antegrade or retrograde bypass should be preferred in younger patients with less comorbidities. Endovascular therapy is beneficial to elderly high-risk patients with short, focal and stenotic disease.

References

1. Hansen KJ, Wilson DB, Craven TE, Pearce JD, English WP, Edwards MS *et al*. Mesenteric artery disease in the elderly. *J Vasc Surg* 2004;40:45–52.
2. Zwolak RM. Can duplex ultrasound replace arteriography in screening for mesenteric ischaemia? *Semin Vasc Surg* 1999;12:252–260.
3. Van Bockel JH, Geelkerken RH, Wasser MN. Chronic splanchnic ischaemia. *Best Pract Res Clin Gastroenterol* 2001;15(1):99–119.
4. Kirkpatrick ID, Kroeker MA, Greenberg HM. Biphasic CT with mesenteric CT angiography in the evaluation of acute mesenteric ischaemia: Initial experience. *Radiology* 2003;229:91–98.
5. Laissy JP, Trillaud H, Douek P. MR angiography: Noninvasive vascular imaging of the abdomen. *Abdom Imaging* 2002;27:488–506.
6. Lau H, Chew DK, Whittemore AD *et al*. Transaortic endarterectomy for primary mesenteric revascularization. *Vasc Endovasc Surg* 2002;36:335–341.
7. Kansal N, Logerfo F, Belfield A, Pomposelli F, Hamdan A, Angel N, Campbell D, Sridhar A, Freischlag J, Baldrich W. A comparison of antegrade and retrograde mesenteric bypass. *Ann Vasc Surg* 2002;16:591–596.
8. Cho JS, Carr JA, Jacobsen G, Shepard AD, Nypaver TJ, Reddy DJ. Long-term outcome after mesenteric artery reconstruction: A 37-year experience. *J Vasc Surg* 2002;35:453–460.
9. Kasirajan K, O'Hara PJ, Gray BH, Hertzer NR, Clair DG, Greenberg RK *et al*. Chronic mesenteric ischaemia: Open surgery versus percutaneous angioplasty and stenting. *J Vasc Surg* 2001;33:63–71.

10. Saedon M, Saratzis A, Karim A, Goodyear S. Endovascular versus surgical revascularization for the management of chronic mesenteric ischemia. *Vasc Endovasc Surg* 2015;49(1–2):37–44.
11. Ansari M, Garcia D, Cardoso R, Heaney C, Diaz- Sandoval L, Saab F, Mustapha J. Comparison of surgical repair and endovascular intervention for chronic mesenteric ischemia. *Catheteriz Cardiovasc Intervent* 2016; 87:S44–S45.
12. Cai W, Li, X, Shu C, Qiu J, Fang K, Li M, Chen Y, Liu D. Comparison of clinical outcomes of endovascular versus open revascularisation for chronic mesenteric ischemia: A meta-analysis. *Ann Vasc Sur* 2015;29(5):934–940.
13. Rutherford Textbook of Vascular Surgery 8th Edition- Mesenteric Vascular Disease-Chronic Ischemia- Gustavo S Oderich. Elsevier Saunders, Chapter 152, pp. 2393–2397.

Chapter 16

Acute Ischaemic Colitis

Vish Bhattacharya and Gerard Stansby

Key Points

- Acute ischaemic colitis can be due to occlusive or non-occlusive causes.
- A high index of suspicion should be present in elderly patients presenting with sudden abdominal pain and bloody diarrhea.
- Computed tomography (CT) scan may show a 'halo sign' and also rule out other abnormalities.
- D Lactate is more specific for intestinal ischaemia.
- Angiography and lysis may be considered in early cases with no sign of peritonitis.
- In the case of bowel resection, primary anastomosis is best avoided and a relook laparotomy recommended.
- Postaneurysm repair colitis can be prevented by selective reimplantation of the inferior mesenteric artery (IMA) in high risk cases.

Introduction

Ischaemic colitis is the result of an event that leads to a reduction in colonic blood flow sufficient to cause ischaemia or infarction of the colonic wall, but not sufficient to produce full thickness infarction and perforation.

The term *ischaemic colitis* was first introduced by Marston *et al.* [1] It is commonly due to acute thrombosis or embolism of the superior mesenteric artery (SMA) or IMA, causing compromise of the colonic blood supply or due to hypotension causing hypoperfusion and ischaemia.

The term is often used for cases where full thickness infarction is present acutely, but this usage is incorrect — not all ischaemic colons have ischaemic colitis, although the two may coexist if the involvement is patchy.

Pathophysiology

The following causes predispose the colon to ischaemia more readily than the small bowel:

1. The colon differs from the small bowel in having no villi and therefore no countercurrent mechanism.
2. The overall blood supplied per gram of tissue is lower in the colon compared to the small bowel.
3. The mucosa may be relatively hypoperfused in conditions of low cardiac output because it is at the end of the microvascular arcades supplying the colonic wall.
4. There is decreased capacity for autoregulation, especially when the perfusion pressure is lower than 50–60 mmHg [2].
5. In periods of physiological or surgical stress, blood is shunted away from the splanchnic circulation as part of the physiological responses to shock and vasoconstrictors.

The ischaemic colonic mucosa loses its barrier function rapidly allowing invasion by luminal bacteria and absorption of endotoxins. In less severe cases, inflammatory cytokine release may contribute to multiple organ failure with renal and respiratory impairment. The mucosa may also slough in a patchy fashion and this can result in increased peristalsis and diarrhoea mixed with blood. In the more severe forms of the condition, bacterial invasion leads to portal pyaemia and death.

The gut mucosa is rich in the enzyme xanthine dehydrogenase, which results in the production of reactive oxygen species and free radicals, such as superoxide. This causes oxidative tissue damage, which is actually most severe when reperfusion follows a period of ischaemia.

This reperfusion injury also results in the activation of polymorphonuclear leukocytes, which then result in systemic events, which may potentially lead to tissue injury and systemic inflammatory response syndrome (SIRS). In addition, endothelin 1 (ET-1), a potent vasoconstrictor, is released following ischaemia and reperfusion, and may lead to splanchnic vasoconstriction, thus further exacerbating the situation.

Aetiology

The following causes lead to ischaemic colitis:

1. occlusive vascular disease of the major vessels due to embolism, thrombosis, trauma or surgical ligation,
2. low perfusion states with low cardiac output, e.g., in cardiogenic or septic shock,
3. mesenteric venous occlusive disease, where increased venous resistance leads to impaired microcirculatory arterial perfusion, e.g., in portal hypertension, mesenteric venous thrombosis or sequestration of red cells in sickle cell disease,
4. drug-induced ischaemic colitis due to cocaine, catecholamines, oral contraceptives [3], phenobarbital and sumatriptan,
5. hypercoagulability states caused by dehydration and physiological shunting, e.g., in marathon runners [4], and
6. small, vessel disease, e.g., in acute pancreatitis, polyarteritis nodosa, systemic lupus erythematosus, Wegener's granulomatosis.

Anatomical Factors

The colon is normally supplied by the SMA and IMA, with some contributions from the internal iliac arteries via the superior haemorrhoidal vessels. This anatomical arrangement usually allows for free collateralisation between the coeliac, SMA and IMA territories, such that occlusion of individual vessels does not necessarily result in ischaemia.

Important in the collateral pathways between SMA and IMA territories is the marginal artery of Drummond, which runs along the splenic flexure and the Arc of Riolan forming a collateral between the left colic artery and the SMA (meandering mesenteric artery). These collaterals may not always be adequate, either because of congenital variations or previous surgery. In acute conditions, for example, after surgery or myocardial infarction, there may be no time for collaterals to form.

The internal iliac arteries provide an important collateral supply to the IMA territory of the rectum and descending colon via the middle and inferior haemorrhoidal vessels.

The watershed between the areas of the colon supplied by the SMA and IMA is usually described to be between the proximal two-thirds and distal third of the transverse colon, based on the embryological division between the mid- and hind-gut. This anatomical arrangement explains the vulnerability of the splenic flexure to ischaemia. However, in the arteriopath with an occluded inferior mesenteric artery (IMA), the watershed point will be shifted distally towards the rectum.

In up to 50% of people, the marginal artery of the colon may be poorly developed and this may result in right-sided ischaemic colitis. Right colonic involvement appears to be associated with severe forms of ischaemic colitis and occurs frequently in patients with chronic cardiac disease, such as aortic stenosis and in patients with chronic renal failure requiring haemodialysis.

Clinical Features

The typical presentation is of an elderly man with a history of vascular disease complaining of abdominal pain and tenderness with bloody diarrhoea.

Mild degrees of ischaemic colitis may in fact be subclinical and never diagnosed. Clinically evident ischaemic colitis appears to affect 1–2% of patients after aortic surgery, but it is found more frequently if colonoscopy or biopsy evidence is sought. In a study by Welch *et al.* [5] where colonoscopy and biopsies were performed post-aortic surgery a surprisingly high 30% were found to have features of ischaemic colitis on biopsy, although virtually all of these were asymptomatic. If only the submucosa and mucosa are involved, then the presentation is more likely to be mild. If the muscularis is involved, then symptoms are likely to be worse and the colitis may fail to resolve or cause subsequent stricture formation.

Full thickness infarction of the muscularis can lead to perforation and peritonitis. This situation should not be classified as true ischaemic colitis, but most series do include 10–20% of such cases, presumably reflecting the fact that full thickness infarcts and true ischaemic colitis can coexist in a patchy fashion.

Differential Diagnosis

This includes infective colitis, pseudomembranous colitis due to *Clostridium difficile* toxin, inflammatory bowel disease, an acute diverticulitis and radiation colitis.

Perhaps, the most common diagnostic dilemma is between *C. difficile* colitis and ischaemic colitis in the post-operative patient where *C. difficile* is probably more common.

The diagnosis can usually be made on a combination of microbiology for *C. difficile* and its toxin and histological features on biopsy. Hyalinization and haemorrhage in the lamina propria along and atrophic microcrypts and a diffuse microscopic distribution of pseudomembranes are more commonly seen in ischaemic colitis [6]. Full-thickness mucosal necrosis is also significantly more common in ischaemia than *C. difficile*.

Escherichia coli 0157 may cause a haemorrhagic colitis resembling ischaemic colitis. In addition, it may also be a cause of ischaemic colitis by causing thrombosis in the colonic vessels as a secondary event.

Investigations

The diagnosis of ischaemic colitis requires a high index of clinical suspicion and confirmation by further investigations.

Plain X-ray

Plain X-ray of the abdomen may show fluid levels in the colon, toxic colonic dilatation, intramural gas, or free gas if a perforation has occurred.

In severe cases, intraportal air may be seen, a finding that suggests an outcome with a high mortality. In the post-operative patient, it may help exclude mechanical obstruction or indicate the need for laparotomy.

Stool Culture

Stool samples should be sent for microscopy for ova cysts and parasites, culture and sensitivity and for analysis for *C. difficile* toxin.

Endoscopic Examination

Sigmoidoscopy may reveal blood in the lumen, but the mucosa may appear normal at this point if the 'watershed zone' is higher up. If the mucosa appears macroscopically normal but ischaemic colitis is suspected, mucosal biopsies should be taken.

Colonoscopy will determine the extent of ischaemia and may need to be undertaken in an unprepared bowel if the patient is unwell. Examination will determine the extent of the ischaemia. In mild disease, the mucosa has a pale appearance with petechiae. In more severe disease, the mucosa may be blue or black with slough and ulceration. Colonoscopy can help diagnose ischaemic colitis, but cannot separate transmural from mucosal ischaemia.

Barium

Enema

An instant enema may reveal thumb printing due to mucosal oedema. However, endoscopy with biopsy is preferable as a means of investigation, if available.

Computed tomography (CT)/magnetic resonance imaging (MRI) scanning

These may be normal in the early stages of ischaemic colitis or show non-specific thickening or oedema with a 'double halo' or 'target' appearance. CT can be used to confirm the clinical suspicion of ischaemic colitis and diagnose complications. In ischaemic colitis, CT typically demonstrates circumferential, symmetric wall thickening with fold enlargement. CT may also demonstrate a thrombus in the mesenteric vessel, toxic megacolon or gas in the colonic wall. Modern spiral CT may also allow assessment of patency of visceral vessels as may gadolinium-enhanced magnetic resonance angiography (MRA).

Blood gases

In severe intestinal infarction, the patient will develop a metabolic acidosis with a large base excess and low pH. However, these metabolic changes are usually signs of advanced full thickness infarction rather than ischaemic colitis.

L-lactate is produced by all cells as a product of glycolysis and is produced in excess during conditions of hypoxia. Raised levels of L-lactate are therefore related to inadequate tissue perfusion. However, since L-lactate from the intestine is mostly removed by the liver, it is not usually helpful in the diagnosis of ischaemic colitis, although it may be raised in colonic infarction. D-Lactate is produced by intestinal bacteria and may be more predictive of colonic ischaemia after aortic surgery than L-lactate, although there has been no prospective study.

Angiography/Duplex scanning

Angiography and duplex scanning of mesenteric vessels are rarely helpful or diagnostic for ischaemic colitis in the acute situation.

Management

Conservative

Conservative management is appropriate in most patients if they are clinically stable and there are no signs of full thickness involvement or peritonitis. Patients should be given intravenous fluids and antibiotics and be carefully monitored. If there are conditions predisposing to intestinal ischaemia, such as hypercoagulability, they should be treated.

Pharmacological

A number of pharmacological treatments have been shown experimentally to improve intestinal blood flow, such as glucagon and prostanoid infusions, but are not widely used clinically. Early colonoscopy should be carried out to confirm the diagnosis. The question of angiography and other investigations remains controversial. In the case of a patient who appears to be settling and who is systemically well, intervention is probably best avoided.

Surgical

In a patient who continues with significant bowel disturbance or systemic symptoms, angiography may be considered in order to assess the visceral circulation. If there is a significant stenosis or occlusion of visceral arteries, then thrombolysis followed by angioplasty may be considered. Thrombolytic therapy should be undertaken within 8 h of onset of symptoms and only if there is no sign of peritonitis or bowel necrosis. Angioplasty may be considered if there is any stenosis of the SMA. Heparin should be given concomitantly, provided there is no bowel necrosis.

In cases with embolic acute myocardial infarction (AMI), where lysis is not indicated, surgical embolectomy can be carried out. A transverse arteriotomy is made and the clot removed. If the embolectomy fails, an aorto bi-iliac graft can be inserted.

Patients who have peritonitis or who deteriorate should have a laparotomy with resection of the ischaemic segment and both ends of the bowel should be brought out as stomas. A primary anastomosis is probably always best avoided when the colon is involved. If attempted, then the anastomosis certainly should be covered by a defunctioning stoma. Relook laparotomy the following day should also be considered. Although there is a high-associated mortality, in patients who survive, it is often possible to reverse the stoma at a later date [7].

Mortality rates in patients requiring emergency surgery for peritonitis and resection of ischaemic bowel may be as high as 50%. This is due to the associated comorbid medical conditions including peripheral vascular disease, ischaemic heart disease and cerebrovascular disease. If the original surgery has involved aortic grafting, then there is also a high risk of subsequent graft infection.

Colonic stricture may develop as a late complication of ischaemic colitis, especially where the muscularis has been involved. Clinically, these patients will typically present with features of subacute obstruction. Bowel resection and anastomosis for these strictures may lead to anastomotic dehiscence in cases where there has been an occlusive aetiology.

As post aortic ischaemic colitis is commonly seen, this will be discussed in detail below.

Post Aortic Surgery Ischaemic Colitis

The single commonest cause of ischaemic colitis is post aortic surgery where a combination of inferior mesenteric occlusion, post-operative hypoxia or hypotension and a vulnerable, elderly patient are predisposing factors.

Incidence

Its clinical incidence is of the order of 1–2% in most series. In ruptured aortic aneurysm repair, however, the Incidence is much higher, up to 30%. Studies with colonoscopy or sigmoidoscopy have, however, shown an even higher incidence: 7–35% of elective cases and up to 60% of survivors of ruptured aneurysm repair.

Fanti *et al.* [8] reported a series of 105 patients who underwent rectosigmoidoscopy within 72 h of aortic surgery. Colonic ischaemia was found in 12 patients, but 7 were asymptomatic and all were managed conservatively.

Welch *et al.* studied a group of patients undergoing elective aortic surgery with pre- and post-operative colonoscopy with biopsy in order to assess the true incidence of the condition. They studied 28 patients each in two groups having aneurysm repair and reconstruction for occlusive aortoiliac disease, respectively. Post-operative colonoscopy and biopsy was carried out at 1 week. All patients had normal appearances and biopsies before surgery. Post-operatively, however, 30% had features of ischaemic colitis upon biopsy. Interestingly, there was no difference in the incidence of this finding between those with occlusive and those with aneurysmal disease.

It has also been described following aortic stent grafting.

Risk Factors in Aneurysm Surgery

Renal disease, emergency surgery, age, type of hospital, aortobifemoral graft, operating time, cross-clamping time and ligation of one or both internal iliac arteries are independent risk factors for developing ischaemic colitis. Duration of hypotension, temperature less than 35°C, pH <7.3, fluid requirement of >5 L and packed red cells >6 units have been found to be predictive of ischaemic colonic complications following ruptured aortic aneurysm repair.

Ischaemic colitis after aortic surgery may be due to interruption to colonic blood supply due to division of the IMA, hypotension and hypoxia in the peri-operative period and stenosis of other visceral vessels due to the underlying atherosclerotic disease process. IMA ligation is probably the most important factor in the majority of cases. Other possible factors include embolisation into the IMA territory during dissection of the aneurysm, injury to mesenteric vessels by retractors and mesenteric compression by haematoma.

Prevention

As post-operative ischaemic colitis occurs in an unpredictable fashion, there are no clear guidelines as to how surgeons may avoid its development. The normal IMA is not well demonstrated at routine angiography and pre-operative angiography may demonstrate only the occasional at-risk patient with enlarged collaterals. Routine angiography can therefore not be justified in all patients undergoing aortic surgery.

Various suggestions have been made to either reimplant the patent IMA routinely, or selectively based on stump pressure, Doppler and intra-operative inspection.

Seeger *et al.* [9] reimplanted all patent IMAs routinely in 151 aortic reconstructions. None of the patients developed colonic infarction compared with 2.7% of patients in the previous series of 186 patients where reimplantation was done based on stump pressure, Doppler and inspection.

Killen *et al.* [10] used IMA stump pressure of less than 50 mmHg as an indicator for implantation of the IMA. However, this did not improve the incidence of ischaemic colitis in his series.

Routine reimplantation of IMAs may increase the risk of bleeding from the anastomosis, is technically demanding and takes extra time. However, this is recommended in patients whose pre-operative angiography has shown occlusion or stenosis of the SMA, if neither of the internal iliac is reconstructed and the colon appears ischaemic post-operatively.

In summary, the following steps can prevent this complication after aneurysm repair:

1. At least one internal iliac artery should be revascularised whenever possible.
2. Blood pressure and oxygen levels should be maintained as any fall may be critical in patients with an already compromised colonic mucosal perfusion.
3. Inspection of the colon after surgery is important, although confounding factors such as hypovolemia, hypotension and the use of inotropes can make this unreliable.
4. Selective reimplantation of the IMA in high-risk patients as mentioned above.

Conclusions

Acute mesenteric ischaemia is a serious condition associated with a 60–80% mortality. The SMA is the main vessel usually involved in 85% of cases. Computer tomography angiography with 3D reconstruction is the diagnostic tool of choice. Conventional angiography is only useful if this is associated with thrombolysis and or stenting.

The elderly are most commonly affected due to their higher incidence of underlying systemic pathology, most notably atherosclerotic cardiovascular disease. A high index of suspicion should be present, especially in the elderly arteriopath presenting with abdominal pain. Early recognition and an aggressive therapeutic approach are essential if the usually poor outcome is to be improved. Blood pressure support typically involves careful, but often massive, fluid resuscitation and pharmacologic support. Thrombolysis and stenting have a limited role and only in the early hours of diagnosis. A second look laparoscopy or laparotomy is indicated in the case of bowel resection.

References

1. Marston A, Pheils MT, Thomas ML, Morson BC. Ischaemic colitis. *Gut* 1966;7:1–115.
2. Kvietys PR, Granger DN. Physiology, pharmacology and pathology of the colonic circulation. In: Shepherd AP, Granger DN (eds.), *Physiology of the Intestinal Circulation.* New York: Raven Press, 1984.
3. Mann DE Jr, Kessel ER, Mullins DL, Lottenberg R. Ischemic colitis and acquired resistance to activated protein C in a woman using oral contraceptives. *Am J Gastroenterol* 1998;93:1960–1962.
4. Lucas W, Schroy PC 3rd. Reversible ischaemic colitis in a high endurance athlete. *Am J Gastroenterol* 1998;93:2231–2234.
5. Welch M, Baguneid MS, McMahon RF, Dodd PDF, Fulford PE, Griffiths GD, Walker MG. Histological study of colonic ischaemia after aortic surgery. *Br J Surg* 1998;85:1095–1098.
6. Dignan CR, Greenson JK. Can ischaemic colitis be differentiated from *C difficile* colitis in biopsy specimens? *Am J Surg Pathol* 1997;21:706–710.
7. Longo WE, Ward D, Vernava AM 3rd, Kaminski DL. Outcome of patients with total colonic ischaemia. *Dis Colon Rectum* 1997;40:1448–1454.
8. Fanti L, Masci E, Mariani A, Chiesa R, Jannello A, Melissano G, Castellano R, Guerini S, Tittobello A. Is endoscopy useful for early diagnosis of ischaemic colitis after aortic surgery? Results of a prospective trial. *Ital J Gastroenterol Hepatol* 1997;29:357–360.
9. Seeger JM, Coe DA, Kaelin LD, Flynn TC. Routine reimplantation of patent inferior mesenteric arteries limits colon infarction after aortic reconstruction. *J Vasc Surg* 1992;15:635–641.
10. Killen DA, Reed WA, Gorton ME, Muehlebach GF, Borkon AM, Piehler JM, Wathanacharoen S. Is routine postaneurysmectomy hemodynamic assessment of the inferior mesenteric artery circulation helpful? *Ann Vasc Surg* 1999;13:533–538.

Chapter 17
Vascular Trauma

Paul Blair

Key Points

- Remember the whole patient, do not just focus on the vascular injury.
- Time is of the essence, avoid delay.
- Massive haemorrhage is the major preventable cause of death after major trauma.
- Do not attempt to mobilise large veins, use local pressure.
- Consider temporary intravascular shunts in complex limb injuries.
- Consider damage limitation surgery in patients developing hypothermia or acidosis.

Trauma is the fourth leading cause of mortality in western countries and the commonest cause of death in the first four decades of life. Vascular surgeons are often involved in the management of a multiply-injured patient who may have limb- and/or life-threatening vascular injuries. In addition, the extended range of procedures carried out by open and minimally invasive surgical and radiological techniques has created its own unique set of associated vascular injuries. It is beyond the scope of this short chapter to deal with specific vascular injuries in detail, however, general principles will be discussed with specific details given in the more common sites of injury.

General Considerations

Vascular trauma can occur as a result of a variety of mechanisms including penetrating, blunt, crush, irradiation and iatrogenic injuries. The majority of penetrating injuries in civilian life in the UK are caused by knives whilst in the USA, a higher proportion of vascular injury is due to gun-shot wounds. Penetrating injuries in military and terrorist theatres are more often associated with high-velocity weapons, bombs and missiles. The latter can cause extensive damage due to a combination of blast and shrapnel injuries. Blunt vascular trauma is usually seen following road traffic accidents, falls, building collapses, major disasters and the like.

Time is of the essence when dealing with vascular trauma and the need for early control of haemorrhage and the restoration of blood flow must be balanced with potential delay caused by over investigation. Patients should be managed along the principles of the Advanced Trauma Life Support (ATLS) system and it is important not to miss occult torso injuries. Rapid exsanguinating local haemorrhage is best controlled with local pressure to allow distal perfusion of tissues via collateral supply. The use of vascular clamps should be avoided in the emergency department. A small but significant number of trauma patients may benefit from immediate transfer to the operating room without further investigation (see Table 1).

The Role of Endovascular Techniques [1]

Endovascular techniques may be helpful in vascular trauma to arrest haemorrhage and maintain vital organ function, particularly in vessels that are difficult to access surgically. In patients with traumatic rupture of

Table 1.   Indications for immediate transfer to the operating room.

Cardiopulmonary resuscitation (CPR) in progress and penetrating torso injury
Systemic blood pressure <90 systolic after 2 L of fluid
Major amputation of hip/shoulder
Major complex wounds and hypotension

the thoracic aorta, [1] Thoracic endovascular aortic repair (TEVAR) is associated with a lower mortality, transfusion of fewer blood products and reduced incidence of procedure-related paraplegia than open repair and has now become the accepted form of treatment.

Axillo-subclavian injuries are associated with high morbidity and mortality and given the anatomy of the thoracic inlet with a large number of vital structures within a small area, endovascular management is potentially very attractive. In a review of 160 cases of subclavian and axillary injury, patency rates of 84.4% were reported at follow-up. Further favourable reports exist in the literature relating to endovascular treatment of arterial injuries to the carotid, vertebral, visceral, iliac and peripheral vessels, however, these are largely case reports with no robust trials.

The decision to employ endovascular therapies in the management of arterial trauma must also consider the potential for undue delay and long-term complications and local expertise.

Limb Trauma

Pathophysiology

Distal ischaemia can result from a wide range of arterial injury, including complete transection or laceration of vessels, contusions and haematomas, dissections, thromboses, occlusion by haematoma from adjacent injury false aneurysms and delayed presentation of arteriovenous fistula.

Arterial injury affects distal flow and results in ischaemia and tissue hypoxia. Striated muscle will likely undergo irreversible damage if warm ischaemia exceeds 6–8 h and may result in multi-organ dysfunction. Limb ischaemia is associated with oedema; tight fascial compartments can cause a further fall in perfusion pressure with worsening of ischaemia resulting in compartment syndrome. Revascularisation of ischaemic limbs can result in significant ischaemia reperfusion injury and rapidly destabilise an already unwell patient as toxic metabolites are washed out. Although the upper limb will tolerate a prolonged period of warm ischaemia, >6 h ischaemia is poorly tolerated in the lower limb. Revascularisation of a non-viable limb is futile and hazardous to the patient.

Table 2.   Clinical signs of vascular injury in a limb.

Hard signs	Soft sign
Absent pulses	Pulses present but decreased (compare with opposite limb and/or measure ABPI)
Arterial thrill or bruit over or near the artery	History of haemorrhage at the scene
Observed pulsatile bleeding	Unexplained hypotension
Signs of distal ischaemia	Peripheral nerve deficit
Haematoma (large or expanding)	

Initial assessment and management

Clinical signs of limb vascular injuries can be classified into hard and soft signs (see Table 2). The majority of patients with a single-level penetrating injury and one hard sign should be transferred immediately to the operating theatre, without further imaging, for immediate exploration. Exceptions to this rule include the following:

- Proximal upper limb injuries or multiple entry wounds;
- Extensive bone or soft tissue injury;
- Close range shotgun injuries or multiple entry wounds;
- Elderly patients with coexisting peripheral vascular disease (PVD).

Other issues to be considered are as follows:

- Assessment for neurological deficit.
- Duration since injury, i.e., warm ischaemia time.
- Any features of compartment syndrome — is the arm/calf soft.

Investigations [2]

It can be difficult to assess distal limb perfusion in a hypothermic, hypovolaemic, multiply-injured patient. Hand-held Doppler can be helpful but should be used with caution. Accuracy is improved significantly when formal ankle brachial pressure index (ABPI) measurements are performed. An ABPI <0.9 should raise the suspicion of upstream compromise. Stable patients with hard signs of vascular trauma, not falling into the urgent category (Table 1), or those patients with single-level penetrating injury and hard sign of vascular trauma, may be investigated in a more timely fashion.

Computer tomography (CT) is widely available and can provide superb contrast resolution with the additional visualisation of non-vascular structures, particularly useful in the investigation of a trauma patient. Multi-slice technology has further expanded the image quality of run-off vessels, although images can be suboptimal. Catheter-directed angiography remains the gold standard, particularly if therapeutic interventional procedures are required. The development of endovascular surgery has improved the quality of digital subtraction angiography (DSA) available in the operating theatre.

The investigation of patients with soft signs of vascular trauma is more controversial. The majority of publications concerning investigation of such patients are produced from high volume North American or South African trauma centres and are, therefore, not always applicable to the UK where the incidence of vascular trauma s relatively low. While it is not appropriate to over investigate patients, once the suspicion of a vascular injury is raised it should be excluded or confirmed by appropriate imaging. There is a high incidence of occult arterial injury with posterior knee dislocations and investigations should be utilised freely in this situation.

Over-investigation of penetrating proximity injury, with 'soft signs', should be balanced with the risk of late sequelae of missed injuries such as false aneurysms and arteriovenous fistulae.

The absence of any hard or soft sign in an injured limb effectively excludes a surgically significant vascular injury as reliably as any imaging modality. If all hard and soft signs are absent, no further vascular injury is necessary and the patient can proceed to management of skeletal and soft tissue injuries.

General principles of arterial repair

Prior to exploring any vascular injury, proximal and distal control must be attempted, with the use of additional axial incisions, if required. Major bleeds from the femoral vessels in the groin are best controlled by direct pressure until proximal control of the external iliac vessels is obtained via extraperitoneal approach in the iliac fossa. The contralateral limb should be prepped in case great saphenous vein (GSV) harvest is required and the abdomen should also be prepped in case iliac control is required. Axillary artery injuries may require proximal control of the subclavian artery in the supraclavicular space while the axillary artery itself is approached through an incision just below the clavicle with division/separation of pectoralis fibres. Axillary and subclavian artery injuries should be approached with care due to the close association of the brachial plexus. Embolectomy catheters may be employed to gain temporary proximal control.

In complex limb injury, or delayed management of a single arterial injury, the use of a temporary intravascular shunt should be considered [3, 4]. This allows early restoration of tissue perfusion prior to a planned arterial repair with appropriate soft tissue cover. It is important to have healthy vessel exposed proximally and distally, particularly in crush injury, and a gentle distal embolectomy should be performed to remove distal thrombus prior to shunt insertion. Temporary intraluminal shunts may also be employed in venous injury although this is rarely required. Once the shunt is in place, associated damage to bone, nerve, muscles and skin can be fully assessed and may require the presence of an orthopaedic and plastic surgeon. If there is an associated fracture, bony stability via internal or external fixation can be achieved with the shunt in place. This allows stability prior to definitive arterial and/or venous repair. Intravenous heparin may be employed although is best avoided in unstable hypovolemia trauma patients.

Arterial repair can be in the form of lateral suture, patch angioplasty or some form of arterial patch. Patch angioplasty can be difficult in a young patient, due to spasm, and if in doubt a short segment GSV graft is the operation of choice. It is the authors' opinion that resection of a damaged vessel with end-to-end anastomosis is rarely possible and an inter-position graft is preferable. In the majority of cases, GSV should be harvested from the contralateral limb in case of deep vein damage in the traumatised limb. The majority of venous injuries require lateral suturing or occasionally ligation. Venous repair is rarely required in the upper limb but may be required in the lower limb at the popliteal level. Complex venous repair employing panel or spiral grafts is best avoided in the majority of trauma patients.

Limb distal vessel injury

Isolated distal radial or ulnar artery injuries can be ligated if the collateral circulation as assessed by Allen's test (negative if colour fails to return following release of the ulnar artery) is adequate. However, they frequently need exploration because of the risk of associated nerve injury. Isolated lower limb crural vessel injury rarely requires repair and may be ligated in the majority of cases. If both anterior and posterior tibial vessels have been transected in a young patient, attempts should be made to repair at least one of them, preferably the posterior tibial artery. Achieving tissue cover for the vascular repair is critical to success. Use of soft tissue flaps and involvement of the plastic surgeons is very helpful. In extensive soft tissue loss extra-anatomic bypasses may be utilised.

Fasciotomies should be used liberally as compartmental hypertension from a combination of ischaemic damage, direct trauma, haematomas and third space losses associated with trauma can all compromise blood flow.

Strong indications for fasciotomy include an ischaemia time greater than 6 h, major artery and vein injury, significant soft tissue injury or evidence of muscle damage, proximal half of below-knee vascular tree injury or compartment pressures of greater than 40 mmHg.

Primary limb amputation should be considered in cases in which the salvage of a functional limb is unlikely and possibly harmful to the patient's recovery. Although there are a variety of scoring mechanisms, the decision to perform a primary amputation is difficult and should ideally involve a second consultant and if possible a Plastic Surgeon when the upper limb is involved.

Risk factors for amputation include the following:

- Gustilo III-C injuries (comminuted, open tibial-fibular fractures with vascular disruption);
- Large nerve transaction;
- Prolonged ischaemia (>6 h) or muscle necrosis;
- Crush injuries with destruction of soft tissue;
- Significant wound contamination;
- Multiple or severely comminuted fractures or segmental bone loss;

- Old age and presence of multiple or severe comorbidity;
- Lower vs. upper extremity;
- Failure of revascularisation.

Abdominal Vascular Trauma

Patients with significant abdominal vascular trauma are usually haemo-dynamically unstable with obvious signs of haemorrhage. A small group of patients, however, may present late with relatively subtle signs. Abdominal vascular trauma can present as hypovolemia, limb ischaemia, anuria or obvious intraperitoneal haemorrhage. Most patients, unless extremely unstable, will have a contrast CT of the abdomen and pelvis. Resuscitation and diagnosis usually take place simultaneously and unstable patients should proceed, without delay, to the operating room as stated in Table 1.

Stable patients, who have sustained blunt trauma and after CT evaluation, may proceed to attempted embolisation of arterial bleeding points as might be associated with pelvic fractures, distal renal artery and lumbar vessels. It is important, however, to exclude non-vascular injuries in these patients such as occult bowel perforation.

Operative management

A standard mid-line laparotomy is performed with the patient prepped for additional thoracotomy, if required. Initial assessment requires four quadrant packing and careful evaluation of injuries. If faced with uncontrollable haemorrhage, from multiple sites, control of the aorta at the diaphragmatic hiatus may be a useful manoeuvre. Mobilisation of the left lobe of the liver is required and care must be taken to avoid damaging the oesophagus (more easily identified if a nasogastric tube is inserted). Finger dissection of the diaphragmatic crus in a vertical plane is required before the aorta can be visualised and clamped in a vertical fashion. Formal vascular repair, in the abdomen, depends on the location of the injury and also the general condition of the patient. In the extremely unstable patient, principles of damage control surgery should be applied. The presence of metabolic acidosis, hypothermia and coagulopathy may preclude formal vascular repair. In such patients, packing the abdomen and pelvis, followed by a period of resuscitation in intensive care, may be entirely appropriate prior to second-look laparotomy.

Laparoscopy is now widely available and represents a feasible option for screening (confirmation of peritoneal penetration), diagnosis (involving a full inspection of all intraperitoneal and retroperitoneal structures and therapeutic intervention (active repair of injured structures). There is, however, a published missed injury rate with diagnostic laparotomy.

Management of retro-peritoneal haematomas

The decision to explore a retro-peritoneal haematoma depends on the mechanism of injury, stability of the patient and the appearance of the haematoma. Exploration of a retro-peritoneal haematoma can be challenging and it may be best to simply pack the area and wait for additional help to arrive. Retro-peritoneal haematomas, caused by penetrating trauma, usually require mandatory exploration, while a more selective policy may be employed for those caused by blunt trauma. They are classified into three zones — central, lateral and pelvic.

Ventral haematomas (zone 1) are always explored as the likely sources of bleed are the great vessels, pancreas or duodenum. For suprarenal haematomas, the proximal control of the aorta is obtained at the diaphragmatic hiatus. The lesser sac is then opened to isolate the injury. If that fails, left or right visceral rotation is carried out to expose the aorta and inferior vena cava (IVC), respectively. Infrarenal haematomas or those at the base of the mesentery are approached after infrarenal aortic control. Special care must be taken to avoid injury to the extremely delicate IVC, renal or iliac veins.

Lateral (zone 2) haematomas are likely of renal pedicle origin and should be explored if expanding or pulsatile or if there is radiological evidence of serious injury. Renal vessels should be controlled prior to opening the haematoma. Avulsed or lacerated renal arteries are best treated with saphenous graft although outcomes are often poor.

Pelvic fracture associated injuries (zone 3) can be due to torn pelvic veins or injury to the iliac vessels. In case of a pelvic fracture, fixation of the same is essential to reduce the pelvic volume and therefore blood loss. If the patient is reasonably stable following pelvic fracture fixation, investigation via catheter guided angiography may be particularly useful in achieving embolisation of arterial bleeders.

The retro-peritoneum often provides tamponade for zone 3 haematomas and if this is entered catastrophic blood loss may occur. When faced with incontrollable venous haemorrhage in this situation, damage limitation surgery and packing should be considered. If the haematoma is actively bleeding or expanding and pulsatile, especially with a missing pulse in the groin, it should be explored. Some of these injuries can be managed by endovascular means.

Resuscitative endovascular balloon occlusion of the aorta (REBOA) [5]

Haemorrhage within the torso is particularly challenging since control of bleeding cannot be achieved without a haemostatic intervention such as surgery or embolisation. REBOA involves accessing the aorta and deploying a balloon within the lumen with aim of achieving control of haemorrhage and return of cardiac afterload and coronary and cerebral perfusion.

REBOA has been used in the management of post-partum haemorrhage, upper gastrointestinal bleeding, pelvic haemorrhage during pelvic/sacral tumour surgery, traumatic abdominopelvic haemorrhage and haemorrhage due to ruptured abdominal aortic aneurysms. It is employed as a temporary haemorrhage control measure and resuscitation adjunct. The most common access sites are the femoral and brachial arteries with a combination of percutaneous and open-cut-down techniques described. Fluoroscopy is used to assist and confirm placement and deployment of the endovascular balloon.

Whilst the majority of studies have found a positive impact on systolic blood pressure as a result of using REBOA, the two largest controlled studies have found conflicting results regarding its impact on mortality. Norii and colleagues found that REBOA was associated with an increase in mortality whilst Moore and co-workers found the opposite. The establishment of the American Association for the Surgery of Trauma-sponsored observation study (AORTA) and the European registry (ABOTrauma Registry) should yield information regarding the indications, outcomes, morbidity and mortality associated with this intervention.

Mesenteric vessel injuries [6]

The superior mesenteric artery (SMA) proximal to the trunk of the middle colic should be repaired if at all possible or a saphenous graft taken off the aorta or iliac arteries. Segmental branches to the small bowel can be ligated and in between injuries should be repaired or ligated, dependent on the patient's condition.

- Coeliac artery injuries will tolerate ligation but should be repaired if possible.
- IVC injuries are best controlled by direct pressure and suture repair where possible. For major uncontrollable haemorrhage, IVC ligation is the best option and is well tolerated. Retrohepatic IVC injuries have over 80% mortality. Patient may need a median sternotomy and atrio-caval shunt or total occlusion of the portal system to achieve control and repair.
- Portal vein injuries are also associated with an extremely high mortality. Where possible, they should be repaired by direct suturing and interposition grafting. Failing that, ligation would be the best option.
- Renal vein injuries on the right side need repair as the right kidney does not tolerate ligation. On the left, the renal vein can be ligated providing adequate drainage via the gonadal and adrenal vein is preserved.
- Iliac vein injuries are treated by packing if associated with pelvic fractures. Where possible, common or external iliac vein injuries should be repaired but ligation is a feasible option as well.

Vascular Injuries of the Neck [7, 8]

Carotid artery injury accounts for approximately 10% of all vascular traumas with penetrating trauma responsible for 90% of cases. The carotid artery is most commonly involved in penetrating trauma with the vertebral artery more commonly damaged by blunt trauma. Mortality remains around 10–30% and in survivors permanent neurological sequelae are present in approximately 40%.

Diagnosis and assessment of penetrating neck vascular injuries: If a penetrating injury has breached the platysma, surgical exploration or arterial imaging is essential. Besides active bleeding, a cervical bruit or thrill or a rapidly expanding haematoma and an absent carotid pulse are diagnostic of carotid artery injury. It is essential to look for evidence of neurological deficits, which may be the result of vessel occlusion (contralateral deficits) or direct cranial nerve injuries (IX–XII). Associated head injuries, psychotropic substance or systemic hypotension and hypothermia may make neurological assessment difficult.

Investigations and management of penetrating carotid injuries: Carotid artery injuries are classified into three zones and management is dependent on the zone of injury.

Zone 1 — injuries from clavicle to cricoid cartilage.
Zone 2 — injuries from cricoid to angle of mandible.
Zone 3 — injuries above the angle of mandible.

Surgical access in zones 1 and 3 injuries is problematic and, therefore, imaging is essential. The gold standard imaging modality is catheter angiography although CTA and occasionally duplex may be employed. Catheter-directed angiography has the additional benefit of offering therapeutic endovascular interventions. Most patients, unless unstable, will need further investigation to rule out concomitant aero-digestive tract injury.

Injuries with active bleeding, expanding cervical haematomas or airway compromise should undergo immediate surgical exploration. In such patients, early control of the airway by intubation must be considered.

Management

Patients with minor angiography abnormalities, such as small pseudoaneurysms, small intimal defects and non-obstructive downstream intimal plaques may be managed non-operatively with close follow-up.

Patients with carotid artery occlusion on angiography and a dense neurological deficit due to brain infarct have a poor outcome, regardless of operative management.

Those with an occluded vessel but no neurological deficit should be managed with anticoagulation to prevent thrombus extension. High zone three injuries and those involving the vertebral artery may be best managed by endovascular methods, such as the use of embolisation and covered stents. Most other injuries seen on angiography are likely to need surgical intervention.

Operative management

The carotid artery is approached by an incision along the anterior border of the sternocleidomastoid with the chest being prepped for access if needed. If possible, proximal and distal control should be obtained prior to entering a haematoma although this may not always be possible. Digital pressure may be used prior to vessel control, but care should be taken to avoid damaging the vagus, hypoglossal and recurrent laryngeal nerves. Repair is undertaken by suture, patch or interposition or transposition grafting as required. Occasionally, a thrombosed occluded vessel may be ligated to reduce the risk of embolic stroke. Thorough exploration of the aerodigestive tract is essential to ensure that no other injuries are missed.

Blunt Carotid Artery Injury in the Neck

Blunt injury may cause dissection and thrombosis of the carotid or, more commonly, vertebral arteries. These injuries can be extremely difficult to diagnose and may be missed in up to two-thirds of patients. High risk criteria for associated blunt cerebrovascular injuries include severe hyperextension, rotation or flexion of the neck, a significant anterior triangle haematoma or soft tissue injury, transient ischaemic attack (TIA) or stroke, cervical spine fracture (vertebral artery), seat belt around the neck, bruit or thrill and a basilar fracture involving the petrous bone (carotid artery). Occasionally, patients develop transient neurological signs at the time of injury. There may be a classic history of a neurologically intact road traffic victim later developing hemiparesis or other lateralising neurological signs. Some patients may present with Horner's syndrome. Diagnosis is usually by CT or MRI.

The keystones of management are to optimise haemodynamics and anticoagulation. Hypotension must be avoided to prevent thromboses. Hypertension risks the development of an intimal flap and dissection. Systemic anticoagulation is the preferred treatment for most patients.

Endovascular placements of stents may have a role in the management of pseudoaneurysms but their role in the management of dissections remains unclear. These patients need to be followed-up with MRI to detect late onset of false aneurysm formation.

Vertebral Artery Injuries

The majority of vertebral artery injuries are silent due to the vertebral artery's capacity for collateral flow. However, in 2–3% of patients, the contralateral artery may be hypoplastic, precipitating the development of neurological signs. Injuries occur rarely in the setting of penetrating trauma and are more commonly associated with cervical spine injuries. Where possible, endovascular interventions are the treatments of choice, as surgical access can be very difficult.

Vascular Injuries in Intravenous Drug Users [9]

Intravenous drug use (IVDU) is a worldwide socioeconomic problem. The most common arterial injury is a femoral pseudoaneurysm. The septic technique of injection, substances injected, late presentation and potential for inadvertent arterial puncture increase the risk of complications. Limb ischaemia due to chemical arteritis can present with intense pain and is frequently associated with the presence of distal pulses. Infected pseudoaneurysms are common in this group, are diagnosed by duplex ultrasonography and managed by open surgical techniques of ligation, excision and debridment of surrounding tissues. Formal dissection and vessel exposure are usually very difficult due to intense fibrosis and scarring of the tissues, however, despite crude oversewing of the femoral vessels a surprising number of patients do not proceed to amputation

There is little evidence of successful conservative management of infected pseudoaneurysms. Routine revascularisation is not associated with reduced amputation rates. Deep vein thrombosis with or without superimposed infection and chronic venous insufficiency are also vascular complications of IVDU.

Iatrogenic Injuries

Injures of arterial and venous catheterisation and endovascular procedures

Arterial catheterisation and puncture may cause bleeding, stenosis or occlusion as a result of laceration, thromboembolism, dissection or foreign body occlusion. If recognised at the time of intervention, numerousendovascular interventions in the form of angioplasty and covered stents are available.

Major haemorrhage can occur especially if the back wall of an artery is perforated and a concealed bleed into the retroperitoneum occurs. If suspected after a groin puncture, and time allows, a CT scan can confirm the diagnosis. Most such injuries in the femoral artery can be explored and controlled from the groin.

Thromboembolic occlusion or dissection will require surgical exploration.

Pseudoaneurysms formed as a result of arterial catheterisation should proceed directly to surgical repair if there are any signs of active bleed or impending rupture. In stable patients, duplex sonography can confirm the diagnosis. Pseudoaneurysms <2 cm in maximum diameter will likely respond to thrombin injection and compression.

Central venous line insertion can inadvertently puncture the subclavian artery or carotid artery. If the catheter is withdrawn, especially after a dilator has been used, significant bleeding can occur. A bleed from the carotid artery can rapidly cause airway compromise. If the carotid artery is punctured and dilated, it will need formal exploration and repair and the dilator should remain in place until control of the vessel has been achieved. Surgical access to the subclavian artery can be especially difficult and endovascular solutions should be considered.

Endovascular procedures with catheters and balloons can also cause vascular trauma in the form of perforation and rupture of vessels distant from the site of puncture.

Immediate control can usually be achieved by balloon tamponade followed by surgical exploration.

Specific injuries relating to open surgery

Lumbar disc surgery, especially at L4/L5 level can cause vascular injury to the aorta, IVC or iliac vessels. Significant intra-operative bleeding may necessitate an immediate laparotomy and repair. Patients can also present with an arteriovenous fistulae, which are ordinarily best dealt with by endovascular means.

Hip and knee surgery and fracture fixation have all been associated with injury to major lower limb vascular structures. Vascular injuries after hip/knee arthroplasty/replacement are rare but have been known to result in amputations.

Varicose vein surgery has resulted in femoral vein injuries, ranging from laceration to stripping of the vein. Redoing groin surgery and attempts to pass a vein stripped from distal to proximal are significant causative factors. Blind attempts at applying haemostats can make a bad situation worse. Compression will control bleeding until help is available. Repair may be by a simple lateral suture, patch or interposition grafting.

Accidental injection of sclerosant into arteries can produce significant tissue damage. If that is suspected and the needle is still *in situ*, heparinised saline and an α-blocker should be injected through it.

Laparoscopic surgery and especially the creation of a pneumoperitoneum have been reported to cause major vascular trauma, which will require rapid recognition and treatment if a successful outcome is to be achieved.

Hepatic artery injury during cholecystectomy is often best dealt with by ligation, rather than attempts at repair. Significant hepatic damage is unlikely to occur given the dual vascular supply to the liver.

A variety of other vascular injuries have been reported to be associated with abdominal surgery, hernia repairs and gynaecological surgery amongst others. The application of the general principles and approaches to vessels should allow control and management of such injuries.

References

1. Nagarsheth K, Dubose J. Endovascular management of vascular trauma. *Trauma* 2015;17(2):93–101.
2. Fishman EK, Horton KM, Johnson PT. Multidetector CT and three-dimensional CT angiography for suspected vascular trauma of the extremities. *Radiographics* 2008;28(3):653–665; discussion 665–666.
3. Barros D'Sa AA, Harkin DW, Blair PH, Hood JM, McIlrath E. The Belfastapproach to managing complex lower limb vascular injuries. *Eur J Vasc Endovasc Surg* 2006;32(3):246–256.
4. Taller J, Kamdar JP, Greene JA *et al*. Temporary vascular shunts as initial treatment of proximal extremity vascular injuries during combat operations: The new standard of care at Echelon II facilities? *J Trauma* 2008;65(3):595–603.
5. Morrison JJ, Galgon RE, Jansen JO, Cannon JW, Rasmussen TE, Eliason JL. A systematic review of the use of resuscitative endovascular balloon occlusion of the aorta in the management of hemorrhagic shock. *J Trauma Acute Care Surg* 2016;80(2):324–334.
6. Asensio JA, Forno W, Roldan G *et al*. Visceral vascular injuries. *Surg Clin North Am* 2002;82:1–20.
7. Rathlev N, Medzon R, Bracken M. Current Concepts in the Management of the Trauma Patient. *Emerg Med Clin N Am* 2007;25:679–694.
8. Newton E, Love J. Acute complications of extremity trauma. *Emerg Med Clin N Am* 2007;25:751–661.
9. Fiddes R, Khattab M, Abu Dakka M, Al-Khaffaf H. Patterns and management of vascular injuries in intravenous drug users: A literature review. *Surgeon* 2010;8(6):353–361.

Chapter 18

Indications and Management of Lower Limb Amputation

Mark Kay and Colette Marshall

Key Points

- Peripheral vascular disease is the leading cause of amputation in the Western world.
- Diabetics are 8–12 times more likely to suffer amputation.
- Mortality and subsequent loss of the contralateral limb following amputation are high.
- The level of amputation requires careful consideration of the rehabilitative potential of the patient, level and pattern of vascular disease and likely healing.
- Careful pre-operative assessment and peri-operative care using the multidiscliplinary team is essential for successful outcomes.
- Epidural analgesia provides the best peri-operative analgesia, but does not prevent subsequent phantom pain.
- The general principles of amputation surgery apply to all sites of amputation.
- Rehabilitation of the patient should start immediately post-operatively.

- Post-amputation pain is the commonest post-operative complication, is multifactorial and requires thorough assessment and possible onwards referral to a multidisciplinary pain team for management.
- Phantom limb pain is common and effective treatments remain elusive.

History of Amputation [1, 2]

Amputation, derived from the latin *amputare*, 'to cut away', is one of the oldest surgical operations. The first recorded amputation appears in the book of the Vedas, written in Sanskrit in India, dated between 3500 and 1800 BC. It records that the leg of Queen Vishpla was amputated in battle, and after healing, an iron leg was fitted to enable the Queen to return to the battlefield.

The early descriptions of amputation by Hippocrates and Celsus focused on amputation for the treatment of gangrene. Hippocrates, in the latter half of the 5th century BC, recommended amputation for gangrene of the joint below the 'boundaries of blackening' as soon as it is 'fairly dead and lost its sensibility.' Celsus described the use of ligatures to control bleeding, although the use of cautery was more commonly used. By 100 AD, Archigenes and Heliodorus described amputation for the management of ulcer, tumour, injuries and deformity.

War served as the impetus for surgical developments in amputation. The mid-14th century saw the arrival of gunpowder into the wars of Europe, and with it came a new era of injury that required control of major haemorrhage and limb fracture.

Amboise Paré, surgeon to the Colonel General of the French infantry, is most famous for reintroducing the use of the ligature to control bleeding. Paré first employed the ligature in amputation of the leg at the siege of Danvier in 1552, and published his technique in 1564. Paré is also known for his work on prosthetics, having designed an artificial hand and above- knee prosthesis with a knee joint. The introduction of the tourniquet in 1674, by the French barber surgeon Morell, further advanced surgical practice of haemorrhage control during amputation.

During the Napoleonic wars, Dominique Larrey, Napoleon's chief of surgery, advocated the use of amputation 'on-site' rather than waiting for transfer to conventional hospital settings. This practice was continued in the American civil war with immediate transfer to adjacent field surgical sites, where some 50,000 amputations were carried out.

The introduction of ether anaesthetic by Morton and Warren in 1846 and the antiseptic technique by Lord Lister in 1867 reduced mortality from amputation and allowed better healing of wounds. Prior to antisepsis, mortality following limb amputation due to sepsis was approximately 60%. However, as medical advances have developed, so too have weapons of increasing destruction. World War I saw somewhere between 300,000 and 500,000 amputations carried out.

Epidemiology of Amputation

In the Western world, peripheral vascular disease is the dominant cause of lower limb amputation. Implicit to this is an increased prevalence of diabetes, currently over 1.7 million in the UK, obesity, together with an ageing population. Amputation carries with it a significant economic burden and a high mortality rate, approaching 50% in diabetics at 2 years. A 1.6% annual incidence of major limb amputation is reported in patients with intermittent claudication [3].

The incidence of amputation is reported to be 8–12 times higher in diabetics than non-diabetics [4]. The mortality rate in both groups increases with age and the level of amputation, and is twice as high in men compared to women. A half of all diabetics who have a major amputation will lose their contralateral leg within 5 years [5].

The National Vascular Registry annual report 2015 indicates that approximately 2300 below-knee amputations and 2500 above-knee amputations were performed in 2014 in the UK. The mean age was 70, with 77% being performed in males.

In the USA, an estimated 134,000 amputations occur annually, such that there are approximately 1.7 million amputees. Dysvascularity accounts for 82% of amputations, with the highest incidence among males.

Rates of trauma-related and cancer-related amputations have both declined by approximately half over the past 20 years. However, unlike in the UK, the risk of traumatic amputations in the USA has increased steadily with age, reaching its highest level among people aged 85 or older.

There is evidence that focused management can reduce the incidence of amputation. Regional UK studies have shown significant reduction of lower limb amputation rates in diabetics of 70–80%, following the introduction of diabetic foot care monitoring [6].

These improvements are unlikely to be due to any single factor. Dedicated diabetic foot care services with a multi-disciplinary approach, advances in radiology such as the use of subintimal angioplasty, and tighter control of risk factors with statins, antihypertensives and antiplatelet agents are all important developments.

Aetiology of Amputation

- Critical limb ischaemia
- Sepsis
- Trauma
- Neoplasm
- Congenital

Critical limb ischaemia warrants revascularisation by angioplasty or bypass, to relieve rest pain or for the management of tissue loss/gangrene, in order to avoid major amputation. Amputation may become necessary after unsuccessful attempts at revascularisation or it may be considered as a primary option to control symptoms. Some patients choose primary amputation over potentially complex and lengthy surgery, or it may be recommended if they have significant comorbidities. The aims of amputation are to improve patient function and quality of life.

Sepsis +/− gangrene is most commonly seen in the diabetic foot, but can result from systemic infections such as meningitis. The diabetic foot is subject to a combination of neuropathy, ischaemia and biomechanical changes that result in abnormal weight bear- ing. Pressure ulceration ensues and ischaemia impairs healing, allowing superimposed infection. Minor infection may be treated with antibiotic treatment, but diabetic foot sepsis can progress rapidly and have devastating consequences if not managed appropriately. The diabetic patient with foot sepsis and palpable pedal pulses has a good prognosis with early surgical intervention. Digital gangrene is treated by amputation of the digit and metatarsal head with the wound left open. However, the extent of underlying infection is often more extensive than is apparent externally, necessitating a higher and more major level of amputation. This should be borne in mind when consenting such patients. In diabetics with absent pulses, attempts at revascularisation should be made at the earliest opportunity, ideally prior to surgery, but this may not be practical until after.

Trauma was a common reason for amputation during wartime, but in the UK amputation is now more commonly performed following traumatic injury sustained in road traffic or machinery accidents. Thermal injury by severe burns or extreme cold exposure may also necessitate amputation.

Bone or soft tissue tumours (e.g., osteosarcoma, fibrosarcoma) may require limb amputation as their management. Finally, congenital deformities such as polydactyly may require amputation to improve patient function.

Pre-operative Assessment

Pre-operative assessment of the patient includes consideration of the level of amputation. Decision on the level of amputation should include the likely rehabilitative potential of the patient. Patients with peripheral vascular disease often have concomitant disease that will limit ambulation due to the energy expenditure required for more proximal amputations. A summary of the key considerations for major amputations are given in Table 1.

Pre-operative assessment should involve a multidisciplinary approach with input from physiotherapists, occupational therapists, prosthetists, rehabilitation medicine specialists, psychologists, nursing staff, and the surgical and anaesthetic teams. As well as the rehabilitative considerations, a decision on the level of amputation should also include an assessment of the likelihood of the flaps healing. This should take into account the degree of tissue loss and ulceration, pattern and severity of vascular occlusion and the viability of tissues in the area of the proposed flaps. Toe pressures measured by Doppler should be >40 mmHg for successful

Table 1.   Key considerations in decision making about the level of major lower limb amputation.

Level of amputation	Energy expenditure above normal (%)	Ambulation rate (%)	Advantages	Disadvantages
Below-knee amputation, long stump	10	>80	Best chance of restoring ambulation.	Flaps require well-perfused tissues, up to 10% conversion rate to above-knee amputation. Not suitable for bed-bound patients who are unlikely to ambulate due to stump contracture and pressure ulceration.
Below-knee amputation, short stump	40	80	May excise poorly perfused tissues.	If stump is too short a prosthesis cannot be successfully used.
Through-knee amputation	71.5	31	Useful if orthopaedic metalware present in femur.	Unpredictable healing of skin flaps.
			Provides long stump for balance in a wheelchair.	Poor cosmesis from prosthesis with leg appearing to dangle further than the normal side.
Above-knee amputation	63	38–50 (less in vascular patients)	Excellent healing rates.	Vascular or elderly patients unlikely to become ambulant, poor balance due to short stump.

healing of toe amputations. Several adjunctive tests exist to aid decision making, e.g., laser Doppler flowmetry, transcutaneous oxygen measurement or isotopic measurement of skin blood flow. However, the role of these tests is currently unclear and usually decision making is based on clinician judgement.

A checklist of the other pre-operative tests and assessments routinely required is given in Table 2. Additional, more detailed tests and referral on to the appropriate subspecialty may be required for individual patients based on clinical findings. Amputation patients are often very sick, frail and elderly. Careful attention to detail with delivery of optimal peri-operative care is essential for successful outcomes. It is recommended that surgery is performed on an elective list under direct consultant supervision. The Vascular Society's best practice care pathway sets out a framework for delivering high quality care to this group of patients [7].

Types of Amputation

Amputation may be divided into minor or major: minor amputation involves amputation of digits, major amputation is removal of most of the limb.

Principles of Amputation Surgery

The underlying general principles of amputation surgery apply to all surgical sites:

- Avoid undermining or devitalising skin flaps.
- Use a tourniquet to control haemorrhage — a recent randomised trial has shown that this reduces blood loss, but does not compromise healing [8].
- Ligate vessels as they are encountered.
- Divide nerves cleanly and away from bone ends to avoid neuroma formation.
- Presence of muscle that does not bleed or contract in response to diathermy stimulation indicates devitalisation and that a higher level should be selected for amputation.

Table 2.   Pre-operative checklist of tests and assessments required routinely prior to major lower limb amputation.

Test/assessment required	Reason	Action required
Full blood count	Patients often anaemic from chronic ulceration or other cause. Raised white cell count may indicate ongoing infection.	Consider transfusion. Pre-operative antibiotic treatment may be required if clinical supporting evidence of infection.
Urea and electrolytes	Vascular patients often have associated renal disease and often are on medications that may disturb electrolyte balance.	Peri-operative intravenous rehydration whilst patient is fasted. Treatment of individual disturbances. Involve renal team if necessary.
Clotting screen	Vascular patients may often be on a variety of anticoagulants or may have disturbed clotting function secondary to sepsis.	Stop anticoagulants peri-operatively to bring INR < 1.5. Patients at high risk of cardiac thromboembolism may need peri-operative intravenous heparin or treatment dose low molecular weight heparin — consult local protocols. Correct clotting disorders in discussion with a haematologist.
Crossmatch (usually two units)	Transfusion frequently required peri-operatively due to high blood losses. Concomitant disease such as ischaemic heart disease dictates maintaining relatively high haemoglobin levels.	Monitor haemoglobin post-operatively.

Blood glucose	Many amputation patients are diabetic. Good peri-operative diabetic control is associated with better outcomes.	Monitor BMs peri-operatively, prescribe insulin sliding scale or glucose/potassium/insulin infusion for insulin dependent diabetics depending on local protocols. Put diabetic patients first on the operating list. Refer to specialist team.
Electrocardiogram	Patients often have concomitant ishaemic heart disease.	Referral to cardiology if necessary based on clinical findings.
Chest X-ray	Only if clinically indicated for suspected acute or new chest problems tests and referral to a respiratory physician if indicated.	Delay surgery if possible until active problems treated. Consider pulmonary function.
Thromboprophylaxis risk assessment	Major amputation puts patients at high risk of thromboembolic disease.	Prescription of low molecular weight heparin. Avoid TED stocking in patients with known peripheral arterial disease.
MRSA screening/ microbiological screen	Guides use of peri-operative antibiotics. Allows isolation of MRSA-positive patients.	Routine prescription of intravenous broad spectrum antibiotics at induction of anaesthesia. Modify according to swab results.
Anaesthetic assessment	To assess and plan analgesic requirements. To plan safe anaesthesia. To plan level of critical care facilities required.	Instigate pre-operative epidural analgesia, if possible. Book bed at appropriate level of care (levels 1, 2 or 3). Consultant vascular anaesthetist presence (or senior trainee).

(Continued)

Table 2. (*Continued*)

Test/assessment required	Reason	Action required
Careful history and examination	To detect unexpected conditions that may impact on surgery, e.g., previous orthopaed c metalware or vascular prostheses.	Inform operating surgeon and other team members.
Consent	Some patients undergoing amputation may be unable to give consent. Life-changing procedure that requires careful counselling. Surgery high risk with associated high mortality and morbidity rates.	In-depth discussion with patient and family about procedure, its risks and impact on quality of life. Two doctor consent form may need to be signed if necessary. Supply written information.
Other assessments	The Vascular Society best practice pathway mandates a number of pre-operative assessments in order to ensure that amputation patients receive the best standard of care that meet all of their complex needs.	Nutrition assessment by dietitian; Pain team assessment; Falls assessment; Pressure area assessment; MDT assessment; Rehabilitation assessment; Discharge team/coordinator; Prosthetics assessment; Surgical counsellor/psychologist.

Notes: INR, international normalised ratio; BM; TED thromboembolic deterrent; MRSA, methicillin-resistant Staphylococcus aureus.

- Guilotine amputation of highly-infected tissue with later stage completion of amputation is indicated for severe sepsis and may reduce revision rates.
- Avoid unnecessary tension on the flaps and unnecessary bulk in the stump when closing.
- Use a suction drain/s for major amputation.
- Avoid stump bandaging, which can cause skin breakdown.

Lower Limb Amputation

Toe amputation

An evaluation of the vascular supply must be performed prior to toe amputation. Fishmouth or circular incisions are used to excise the affected toe. Amputation should not be performed through a joint as the avascular cartilage that is exposed prevents healing. Therefore, toe amputations are usually performed through the proximal phalanx (Fig. 1).

Ray amputation

This involves removal of a toe through the metatarsal bone. A tennis racquet-shaped incision is used to expose the distal part of the

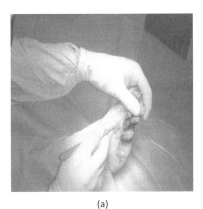
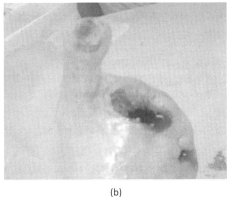

(a)   (b)

Figure 1.   Toe amputation: amputation of diabetic gangrenous toes.

metatarsal bone and amputation is performed through the neck. Dissection must be kept close to the bone to avoid damaging the blood supply to neighbouring toes. Tendon remnants need to be excised as far proximally as possible. Ray amputation usually involves subsequent near normal ambulation, but amputation of the hallux or fifth toe can sometimes cause ulceration of the plantar skin due to tendon imbalances and abnormal weight bearing.

Transmetatarsal amputation

This involves amputation of all the toes through the mid-metatarsal bones. A plantar flap is fashioned to cover the end of the foot. Excellent ambulation results from a well-healed amputation.

Mid-foot amputation

For more proximal foot disease, amputation can be carried out proximal to the metatarsal bones. Named amputations include the Chopart amputation — a disarticulation of the talonavicular and calcaneocuboid joints, or the Lisfranc amputation between the metatarsal and tarsal bones. Other unnamed amputations at this level can also be successful. Healing rates at this level may be unpredictable and ambulation limited by the development of equinus varus deformity due to sacrifice of tendons. Mid-foot amputation should only be considered in patients without or with corrected ischaemia.

Ankle-level amputation

The Syme and Pirogoff amputations at ankle level are seldom performed in vascular surgical practice. The Syme amputation occurs through the ankle joint with the distal tibia and fibula cut in line with the joint. The Pirogoff modification conserves a piece of posterior calcaneum, which is screwed onto the distal tibia. Problems associated with these amputations include difficulty fitting a prosthesis, posterior migration of the heel pad and sloughing of the skin. The failure rate in dysvascular patients is approximately 41%. Usually, below-knee amputation is preferable and allows a more reliable stump to be fashioned.

Below-knee amputation (BKA)

The most common technique for BKA is the long posterior flap technique, first described by Burgess and Romano in 1967. The preferred site for section of the tibia is 14 cm below the knee joint or 10–12 cm below the tibial tuberosity. The absolute minimum required for successful limb-fitting is a length of 7.5 cm below the joint line. The flaps are marked out accurately using the rule of thirds (Fig. 2). The tibia is divided 1 cm proximal to the skin wound and bevelled smoothly. The fibula is divided 2 cm proximally. The posterior flap is fashioned by excluding soleus from the wound to provide suitable coverage for the bone end that is not too bulky. An alternative technique uses skew flaps. This technique is useful when a long posterior flap is unsuitable due to tissue loss or non-viability extending onto the proposed site of the posterior flap. Evidence

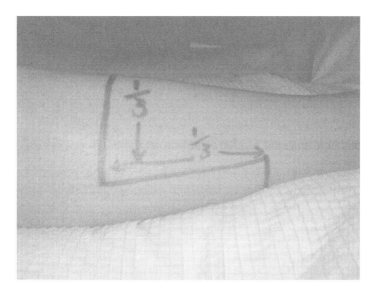

Figure 2.   Marking the amputation flaps of a below- knee amputation using the rule of thirds.

demonstrates equivalence of the two techniques with regard to healing and functional outcome.

Through-knee amputation

Through-knee amputation may be useful when a BKA is contraindicated due to tissue non-viability. The through-knee amputation provides a long lever and an end-bearing stump. The patella may be preserved and wired onto the end of the femur (Gritti–Stokes amputation) or may be sacrificed. Problems with through-knee amputation include unpredictable healing of tissues and a stump that cosmetically is bulbous with unequal levels of the knee when fitted with a prosthesis. However, when successful it can provide good ambulation with less energy demands than a more proximal amputation. For the non-ambulant patient, the long stump provides good leverage for transfer and good balance for sitting.

Above-knee amputation (AKA)

The preferred site of AKA is at the mid-femoral level, at least 15 cm above the tibial plateau. The aim is to achieve a stump long enough to act as a lever arm for locomotion whilst allowing adequate clearance at the knee for a jointed prosthesis. The shortest stump recommended is 8 cm below the inferior pubic ramus. The flaps are fashioned using fishmouth incisions to achieve equal anterior and posterior myoplastic flaps.

Hip disarticulation and hindquarter amputation

These may occasionally be required in cases of severe ischaemia extending proximally, usually due to occlusion of aorto-iliac inflow. Mortality is high and successful ambulation exceedingly low.

Upper Limb Amputation

Upper limb amputation is rare in vascular surgical practice and may result from trauma, failed or delayed revascularisation or infection. Amputations for congenital causes or malignancy may be undertaken by other specialities. The general principle considerations for amputations apply to amputations of the upper limb.

Post-operative Complications

Early complications

- Deep vein thrombosis
- Flap necrosis
- Wound infection
- Post-amputation pain
- Stump haematoma
- Flexion contractures
- Psychological problems

Late complications

- Excess bulbosity of the stump
- Bone erosion through the skin
- Neuroma formation
- Ischaemia
- Osteomyelitis
- Adherent scar tissue
- Ulceration

Post-amputation pain

Because post-amputation pain is so common and challenging to treat, it deserves special mention. Post-amputation occurs in about 80% of patients following amputation. There are several different causes, which are categorised in Table 3. A careful history and examination is the key to identifying the cause of the pain and a treatment plan can then be tailored to the underlying cause. Phantom limb pain occurs in about 70% of patients. Despite the wide variety of treatments described, none has been conclusively proven to be of benefit in preventing or treating phantom limb pain. Pre-emptive epidural analgesia does not prevent phantom

Table 3.   Causes of post-amputation pain.

Type of pain	Definition	Treatment strategies
Immediate post-operative pain	Pain occurring in the immediate post-operative period due to the trauma of surgery.	Opiate analgesia. Epidural analgesia.
Phantom limb sensation	Any sensory phenomenon (except pain) felt in the amputated limb.	Reassurance.
Phantom pain	Pain felt in the amputated limb or a portion of the absent limb.	Referral to a multidisciplinary pain team. Useful approaches may include: simple analgesia, opiates, amitriptyline, gabapentin or pregabalin, ketamine, biofeedback, transcutaneous nerve stimulation, psychological techniques, spinal cord stimulation, use of metallic stump liners and application of hot or cold to stump. No treatment has been conclusively proven in robust randomised trials to be elective.
Residual limb pain *Internal pain:*		
• Neuroma formation	Overgrowth of nerve-ending in stump — may cause spontaneous or mechanically induced pain.	Nerve injections, amitriptyline, gabapentin or pregabalin. Surgical excision/revision of nerve.

• Bony overgrowth	New bony formation may produce spurs that cause local pain.	Revision of stump.
• Ischaemic pain	Coldness, blueness and pain associated with elevation in the stump +/– ulceration.	Revascularisation using inflow procedure, amputation at higher level.
• Sympathetically mediated pain	Rare type of pain maintained by the sympathetic nervous system and similar to complex regional pain syndrome. Associated with coldness, blueness, increased sweating and allodynia (pain associated with a stimulus that is not usually painful).	Referral to multidisciplinary pain team.
• Neuropathic pain	Neuropathic pain usually associated with diabetes may affect a stump.	Amitriptyline, gabapentin, pregabalin.
External pain:		
• Mechanical causes from ill-fitting prosthesis	Ill-fitting prosthesis.	Adjustment of prosthesis.
Myofascial pain syndrome	Pain occurring at the supporting joint usually from an ill-fitting or heavy prosthesis.	Physiotherapy, adjustment of prosthesis.

pain in the long term, but does provide superior peri-operative analgesia [9]. For cases recalcitrant to treatment with first-line oral agents, referral to a multidisciplinary pain team is recommended. Mirror therapy is gaining in popularity with many cases of anecdotal success, but currently is not supported by well-evidenced research from large trials.

Rehabilitation and Prosthetics

Rehabilitation of the amputee should start as soon as possible post-operatively. Physiotherapy in the early period is important to prevent flexion contractures and to commence practice in transferring, sitting in bed, etc. Once the stump is healed, elasticated graduated compression stump socks are used to shrink the stump to an acceptable shape for fitting of a prosthesis. Early walking aids allow the patient to stand and start walking early. The Pneumatic Post Amputation Mobility Aid uses a maximal pressure of 40 mmHg to attach a pneumatic aid to the stump to achieve early walking in the physiotherapy gym.

Limb fitting is usually delayed until about 6 weeks post-operatively, when oedema in the stump has subsided and it has shrunk to an acceptable size. A prosthesis is a device that is designed to replace, as much as possible, the function or appearance of a missing limb or body part. Advances in prosthetic technology have developed very sophisticated artificial limbs that use microchip technology to anticipate and respond to movements. These can be useful for young athletic patients to maintain prior levels of activity. However, for elderly dysvascular patients simpler and lighter modular components are recommended. Modern materials such as silicone or thermoplastic materials are used for stump liners and sockets to achieve a good fit with the stump [10].

References

1. Ellis H. *The Cambridge Illustrated History of Surgery*. Cambridge: Cambridge University Press, 2009, pp. 127–128.
2. Stansbury LG, Branstetter JG, Lalliss SJ. Amputation in military surgery. *J Trauma Injury, Infect Crit Care* 2007;63:940–944.
3. Dormandy JA, Murray GD. The fate of the claudicant. *Euro J Vasc Surg* 1991;5:131–133.

4. Johannesson A, Larsson GU, Ramstrand N *et al.* Incidences of lower limb amputation in the diabetic and nondiabetic general population. *Diabetes Care* 2009;32:275–280.
5. Nathan DM. Long-term complications of diabetes mellitus. *New Eng J Med* 1993;328:1676–1685.
6. Canavan RJ, Unwin NC, Kelly WF, Connolly VM. Diabetes- and nondiabetes-related lower extremity amputation incidence before and after the introduction of better organized diabetes foot care: continuous longitudinal monitoring using a standard method. *Diabetes Care* 2008;31:459–463.
7. A best practice clinical care pathway for major amputation surgery. Vascular Society, April 2016.
8. Choksey PA, Chong PL, Smith C, Ireland M, Beard J. A randomized controlled trial of the use of a tourniquet to reduce blood loss during transtibial amputation for peripheral arterial disease. *Eur J Vasc Endovasc Surg* 2006; 31:646–650.
9. Halbert J, Crotty M, Cameron ID. Evidence for the optimal management of acute and chronic phantom pain: A systematic review. *Clin J Pain* 2002;18: 84–92.
10. Tang PCY, Ravji K, Key JJ, Mahler DB, Blume PA, Sumpio B. Let them walk! current prosthesis options for leg and foot amputees. *J Am Coll Surg* 2008;206:548–560.

Chapter 19

Leg Swelling and Lymphoedema

Ahmad Rafizi Hariz Bin Ramli and Tim Lees

Key Points

- Worldwide, the commonest cause of lymphoedema is filariasis.
- In the Western world, the commonest cause is malignancy and its treatment.
- Oedema is initially pitting, but becomes non-pitting due to fibrosis of subcutaneous tissues.
- Diagnosis is confirmed by isotope lymphangioscintigraphy.
- Satisfactory treatment can usually be achieved by conservative measures that include manual drainage, compression hosiery, complex decongestive therapy and prevention of infection.

    The two most common causes of leg swelling are chronic venous insufficiency and lymphoedema. Lymphoedema is a debilitating condition that has no cure. Several million people are affected worldwide and approximately 1.3/1000 population in the UK [1].

Definition

Lymphoedema can be defined as the accumulation of fluid rich in protein in the skin and subcutaneous tissues due to a defect in the lymphatic system resulting in swelling of the limb.

Classification

Lymphoedema can be primary or secondary.

Primary

Primary lymphoedema can be classified based on the age of onset (Table 1). Women are more likely to be affected than men. The lower limbs are more frequently affected than the upper limbs. The

Table 1. Causes of lymphoedema

Primary	Secondary
• Syndromic (Turner's, Noonan's, Prader Willi, oculo-dento-digital dysplasia)	• Malignant disease
• Systemic/visceral involvement (Hennekam)	• Surgery
• Disturbed growth and/or cutaneous/vascular anomalies (CLOVE, Klippel Trenaunay, Parkes-Weber, Lymphangiomatosis)	• Radical mastectomy
• Congenital (Milroy's)	• Radical groin dissection
• Late onset (distichiasis, Meige's)	• Radiotherapy
	• Infection
	• Parasitic (filariasis)
	• Pyogenic (β haemolytic streptococci, *Staphylococcus aureus*)
	• Tuberculosis
	• Arterial surgery
	• Venous disease and venous surgery

classification pathway of primary lymphoedema now includes increasingly well-described single gene disorders [2]:

- Syndromic — Lymphoedema is a recognised part of several syndromes, and these patients display a number of abnormal features alongside the oedema. Examples of such syndromes include Turner's (45XO), Noonan's (mutations in PTPN11 and others), Prader Willi (mainly 15q11 microdeletion) and oculo-dento-digital dysplasia (mutation in GJA1).
- Systemic/visceral involvement — These individuals show a widespread developmental abnormality of the lymphatic system, not confined to the peripheries. Disease may be segmental/multi-segmental or show a uniform and widespread pattern of oedema in all body segments (e.g., Hennekam Syndrome, caused by mutations in CCBE1 and FAT4).
- Disturbed growth and/or cutaneous/vascular anomalies — This group includes individuals with CLOVE syndrome due to increased signalling via the PIK3/AKT/mTOR signalling pathway, giving rise to the potential use of mTOR inhibitors (e.g., rapamycin) in treating these patients. Klippel Trenaunay, Parkes Weber and Lymphangiomatosis are also conditions within this classification.
- Congenital lymphoedema — This is present at birth (<1 year of age) and can be autosomally inherited (Milroy's disease). About 70% of cases are due to mutations of vascular endothelial growth factor receptor 3. Oedema is present at birth and two-thirds of affected patients have bilateral lymphoedema. It accounts for 25% of all cases.
- Late onset (>1 year) primary lymphoedema — This group includes patients with lymphoedema distichiasis (which is caused by mutations in FOXC2) and Meige's disease (genetic cause unknown). It was described classically as follows:
  o Lymphoedema praecox (1–35 years of age), which occurs usually during adolescence, is the commonest form of congenital lymphoedema. Most patients have unilateral limb involvement.
  o Lymphoedema tarda (>35 years of age) is the least common form and accounts for about 10% of cases.

All forms of primary lymphoedema are likely to arise from an abnormality present at birth that may manifest at birth or later in life. It is likely that these groups all represent different parts of the same spectrum of disease, which has been attributed to aplasia, hypoplasia or hyperplasia of the lymph vessels during development.

Secondary

Secondary lymphoedema occurs when the lymphatic vessels become occluded by an acquired pathology. The lymphatic channels distal to the obstruction become dilated and the valves secondarily incompetent. Worldwide, the commonest cause is an infection caused by the parasite Wuchereria bancrofti resulting in filariasis.

In the Western world, the commonest cause is neoplasia and its treatment, resulting in damage or removal of lymph nodes, for example, post-mastectomy lymphoedema of the upper limb. This is particularly common in patients who undergo radiotherapy following axillary lymph node removal.

The causes of secondary lymphoedema are listed in Table 1.

Pathophysiology

Interstitial fluid is composed of proteins, lipids and water. It is formed by the high hydro-static pressure in the capillaries that forces fluid into the interstitial space. This results in an increase in the oncotic pressure, which attracts more water. Normally functioning lymphatics return interstitial fluid to the intravascular space. High molecular weight proteins and associated water pass through the lymphatics and eventually into the venous system.

Disease causes obstruction of the lymphatics and the above transport system is overwhelmed. There is a stagnation of protein-rich fluid in the interstitial space. High concentrations of protein result in accumulation of more water. The lymphatic vessels dilate and this results in secondary valvular incompetence.

Limbs may swell due to other local or systemic conditions. Chronic venous insufficiency results in a rise in venous pressure. This pressure is transmitted to the capillary bed, resulting in structural changes in the endothelium, causing an increase in capillary permeability. This results in an increase in interstitial fluid volume, causing oedema. Systemic conditions such as congestive cardiac failure, hypoproteinemia and nephrotic syndrome result in a state of retention of salt and water, causing oedema. This may compound the situation in the presence of diseased lymphatics or overwhelm a normally functioning lymphatic system.

Initially, the oedema is pitting. The accumulation of protein and fluid in the interstitial space results in an inflammatory reaction. This, in time, leads to fibrosis of subcutaneous tissues and the oedema becomes non-pitting.

Presentation

Patients initially present with peripheral oedema. Lymphoedema can be differentiated from other causes of limb swelling by history and examination. A detailed history and examination of the patient may help differentiate primary from secondary lymphoedema.

History

The initial presentation is swelling of the limb of varying degrees. As the swelling progresses, the patient may have difficulty fitting into clothes and footwear. As the oedema progresses, skin complications develop. Bacterial and fungal infections are common. Patients may have discomfort related to the size of the limb, cosmetic concerns, difficulty mobilising and impairment of activities of daily living. Primary lymphoedema occurs predominantly in females in their early teens. Patients with secondary lymphoedema will commonly have a history of previous surgery, neoplastic disease or radiotherapy.

Examination

The patient may have unilateral or bilateral limb swelling. Initially, the oedema is pitting, but with time, the swelling becomes non-pitting due to fibrotic changes in the skin and subcutaneous tissues. The swelling is

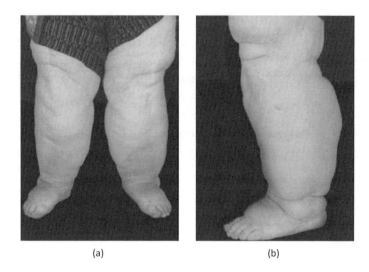

(a)   (b)

Figure 1.   (a) Chronic lymphoedema of the leg with tree-trunk appearance and (b) 'buffalo-hump' of the foot.

Source: Copyright: © Saunders Ltd. 2013.

uniform, and as it progresses, the leg appears like a tree trunk (Figs. 1(a) and 1(b)). The skin gradually thickens and becomes less elastic. The dorsum of the foot is usually involved, producing the characteristic "buffalo hump" appearance (Fig. 1(b)). The skin becomes thickened and has a typical peau d'orange appearance. There are thick deposits of keratin on the epidermis.

Investigation

The diagnosis of lymphoedema can usually be made clinically. Investigation is needed when the diagnosis is uncertain, to confirm diagnosis, when considering surgery, to plan treatment and to exclude pelvic masses as the cause for lower limb lymphoedema. Oedema associated with generalised disorders such as hypoproteinemia, congestive cardiac failure and nephrotic syndrome are excluded or diagnosed by examination, biochemical analysis and urinalysis. Genetic testing should be strongly considered once primary lymphoedema is suspected. Referral to a geneticist is recommended.

Duplex ultrasonography

This is useful to exclude chronic venous insufficiency. Chronic venous insufficiency is the commonest differential diagnosis for lymphoedema. Deep venous thrombosis may cause unilateral lower limb swelling.

Lymphoscintigraphy (isotope lymphography)

This is the most commonly performed investigation (Fig. 2). It defines anatomy, evaluates dynamics and determines the severity of obstruction [3]. A radiolabelled (usually technetium) colloid is injected into the inter-digital space and gamma-camera pictures are taken at 5-min intervals to assess transit through the lymph channels. If the time taken for the tracer to appear in the regional lymph node is greater than 60 min, then this

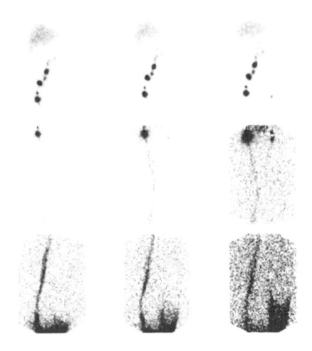

Figure 2.   Lymphangioscintigram confirming left-sided lymphoedema. On the right, the isotope is travelling up the lymphatics of the leg with concentration in the ilioinguinal nodes (normal). On the left, the isotope has remained in the foot (not seen).

Source: Copyright: © Saunders Ltd. 2013.

would suggest delayed lymphatic transport. A negative scintigram effectively excludes the diagnosis of lymphoedema. Primary and secondary lymphoedema are frequently associated with similar scintigraphic appearances, including delayed transit, the presence of collaterals, dermal backflow, and reduced uptake in one or more groups of lymph nodes. It can be used to distinguish between a venous and lymphatic cause of limb swelling [4]. The test cannot differentiate primary from secondary lymphoedema.

Computed tomography

The primary role of computed tomography is in the diagnosis of primary and secondary malignancy as a cause for lymphoedema. The common findings on computed tomography are skin thickening, thickening of subcutaneous fat and thickening of the perimuscular aponeurosis. It will also provide evidence of lymphoedema by the presence of a honey-comb appearance of fluid in the subcutaneous tissues [5] and has been used to monitor the response to compression therapy. Patients with a previous history of pelvic or abdominal malignancy should be scanned for recurrent disease in order to diagnose enlarged lymph nodes or pelvic masses that may be compressing the lymphatic channels.

Magnetic resonance (MR) imaging

The MR features of lymphoedema include circumferential oedema, increased volume of tissues, honeycomb pattern of subcutaneous tissues and thickening of the dermis. Nodal architecture can be demonstrated. It can distinguish between lymphatic and venous swelling, but is not good at separating primary and secondary causes of lymphoedema.

Contrast lymphangiography

Lymphangiography used to be the gold standard test for evaluating lymphatic disorders. It is an invasive test and can cause an inflammatory reaction in the lymphatics. This investigation is now rarely used in the diagnosis of lymphoedema and has been largely replaced by scintigraphy.

Treatment

The aim of treatment is to reduce limb swelling, reduce the risk of infection and improve function. Treatment can be surgical or non-surgical. If management begins early in the disease process, before irreversible fibrotic changes occur, then conservative measures should be successful. Once achieved, the improvement must be maintained. Surgery is indicated only in a small proportion of patients, is palliative and not curative.

General measures

There is no cure for lymphoedema. The nature of the condition and its management should be clearly explained to the patient. General measures are of benefit and should be followed religiously throughout life to obtain maximum benefit. These include the following:

- skin care is essential to maintain healthy skin and reduce risk of infection,
- elevation of the limb at rest,
- regular exercise to encourage flow of lymph,
- weight reduction,
- high protein and low sodium diet,
- avoiding pressure, tight footwear and constrictive clothing,
- simple lymphatic drainage, which involves gentle massage of the affected area by patients or their carers [6].

Manual lymphatic drainage

This is performed by specially trained therapists. Beginning with the proximal portion of the affected limb, the limb is massaged over short segments in a distal to proximal manner. Massage stimulates the flow of lymph via superficial lymphatics from an affected area to an adjacent normal area.

Compression therapy

Compression can be achieved by multi-layer bandaging during the intensive treatment phase. Multi-layer Lymphoedema Bandaging

(MLLB) involves the use of several layers of bandages to achieve compression [7]. The pressure is more uniformly distributed. Compression stockings need to exert a pressure of approximately 40–50 mmHg at the level of the ankle and are generally used during the maintenance phase. The compression should be graduated from distal to proximal. Support garments are essential to maintain limb size in the treatment of lymphoedema.

Intermittent sequential pneumatic compression therapy

Intermittent pneumatic compression is a means of reducing the size of a limb in lymphoedema. They can be used at home or in an outpatient setting. They work best if used before subcutaneous fibrosis sets in. The affected limb is placed in a sleeve or cuff that is alternately inflated and deflated, creating a pressure gradient that moves fluid out of the affected limb. These devices may have a single sleeve of uniform pressure or may consist of several chambers that can be inflated in sequence. The direction of inflation should be graduated from distal to proximal. Compression hosiery should be used between treatments.

Thermal treatment

Hyperthermia of the leg is produced by immersing the limb in hot water or by microwave heating. The reason behind its efficacy is not clear. It is presumed to mobilise fluid and soften tissues.

Complex decongestive therapy

Complex decongestive physiotherapy generally involves an intensive treatment programme over 4 weeks. The first phase (intensive therapy) involves skin care, exercise, multi-layer bandages and manual lymphatic drainage. Phase 2 (maintenance phase) aims to conserve and optimise the results obtained in Phase 1. It involves the regular use of support garments, continued exercise, skin care and massage therapy. Reduction in limb volume can be achieved and maintained. There is a reduction in the incidence of infection. Worldwide, people have achieved good results, but this process is resource intensive and compliance can be poor.

Prevention of infection

Macrophages and lymphocytes are activated by inflammatory processes and carried through the lymphatics to regional lymph nodes. Antigens are presented and an immune response is mounted. Stagnation of lymph prevents this and increases the risk and severity of infection. The common pathogens are β-haemolytic streptococci and Staphylococcus aureus. With each episode of infection, there is further destruction of the lymph channels, making the oedema worse. Well-fitting comfortable shoes prevent small cracks in the skin that may act as a portal of entry. The affected limb should be washed daily with a mild soap and the feet must be dry before putting on shoes. The patient must keep a very careful eye on the foot and any early signs of infection must be treated aggressively with antibiotics. Recurrent infection can be managed by long-term, prophylactic, low-dose antibiotics such as amoxicillin, flucloxacillin or a cephalosporin.

A Consensus Document on the Management of Cellulitis in Lymphoedema has been published by the British Lymphology Society and the Lymphoedema Support Network [8].

This document makes recommendations about the use of antibiotics for cellulitis in patients with lymphoedema, and advises when admission to hospital is indicated. Prompt treatment is essential to avoid further damage to the affected part, which in turn may predispose to repeated attacks.

Drugs

Drug therapy for lymphoedema is limited. Diuretics can be used in the early stages, but have no value in long-term treatment. Underlying filarial infection should be treated with diethylcarbamazine. Benzopyrenes have been advocated by some. They induce phagocytosis of proteins and proteolysis. The resulting fragments are more readily removed. New promising studies in primary lymphoedema evaluating the use of targeted therapy, e.g., rapamycin and adenoviral transfection of VEGFC, are still in progress.

Surgical treatment

Surgery is indicated only in a small proportion of patients as symptoms are usually controlled adequately by conservative measures. Surgery is indicated if conservative measures have failed and there is severe disability, gross deformity or lymphorrhagia. These can be divided into debulking operations and bypass procedures. Obliterative causes are best treated by debulking procedures, whereas in lymphatic obstruction surgical bypass is recommended.

Debulking operations

These procedures are indicated when there is gross oedema.

These procedures involve removal of variable amounts of the excess skin and subcutaneous tissue from the affected limb:

- Homan's operation involves making an incision along the length of the limb. Anterior and posterior skin flaps are fashioned and raised. Excess subcutaneous tissue is excised. Tissue is removed down to the level of the deep fascia. The skin flaps are then fashioned appropriately and closed primarily. The skin should be reasonably healthy to carry out this procedure.
- Charles' procedure involves excision of skin, subcutaneous tissues and deep fascia. The resulting defect is closed with a split skin graft. The cosmetic results of this procedure are poor and the procedure can be complicated by hyperkeratotic scars.
- Liposuction has been used to reduce the size of a lymphoedematous limb. It is generally more effective in patients with minimal pitting oedema. Post-procedure, patients are required to wear compression garments for life. The National Institute for Health and Clinical Excellence (NICE) has issued guidance regarding treating chronic lymphoedema by liposuction. NICE has said that if a doctor wants to use liposuction to treat chronic lymphoedema, they should make sure

that extra steps are taken to explain the uncertainty about how well it works in the long term, as well as the potential risks of the procedure. The patient should be told that they will need to wear compression garments indefinitely after the procedure. This should happen before the patient agrees (or does not agree) to the procedure. The patient should be given this leaflet (Treating chronic lymphoedema by liposuction, Interventional procedure guidance 251) and other written information as part of the discussion. There should also be special arrangements for monitoring what happens to the patient after the procedure [9].

Bypass procedures

Several procedures have been described (Table 2). Only a small number of patients show long-term improvement. Patients with proximal obstruction of lymphatics in the pelvis and patent distal lymphatics can have a bypass procedure. Of note are lymphovenous anastomosis and lympho-lymphatic anastomosis. They are physiological methods for correcting lymphoedema. Multiple lymphatics are anastomosed to subdermal venules using micro-surgical techniques to produce an improvement in signs and symptoms. Autologous lymphatic vessels harvested from the contralateral normal limb can be used to bypass obstruction by performing lympho-lymphatic anastomosis. For the procedures to succeed, the patients should have patent distal lymphatics and mild-to-moderate oedema. In patients with distal obliterative disease, reconstruction is not an option. The techniques of omental and enteromesenteric bridges have been described to help improve lymphatic drainage.

Table 2. Bypass procedures for lymphoedema.

- Skin and muscle flaps
- Omental bridges
- Enteromesenteric bridges
- Lymphatic–lymphatic anastomosis
- Lymphaticovenous anastomosis
- Silicone tube implant

Silicon tube insertion

Recently, a new technique of silicone tube implant has been described to facilitate distal lymphatic drainage in combination with compression therapy [10]. Three long multi-hole silicone tubes are implanted from the distal leg or forearm and tunnelled subcutaneously with the proximal end at the retroperitoneal or subscapular region. This technique shows promising mid-term outcome, but long-term data are still lacking.

Lipedema

This condition is often diagnosed as lymphoedema. It is characterised by symmetrical enlargement of the lower limbs, excluding the feet. The age of onset is early and the condition almost exclusively affects women. There is no cure for the condition. Treatment is multi-modal and mainly involves the use of exercise and compression hosiery. Liposuction has been used with some effect. Patients require adequate support.

References

1. Moffatt CJ, Franks PJ, Doherty DC, Williams AF, Badger C, Jeffs E, Bosanquet N, Mortimer PS. QJM Lymphoedema: An underestimated health problem. *QJM: Int J Med* 2003;96(10):731–738. DOI:10.1093/qjmed/hcg126.
2. Connell F, Brice G, Jeffery S, Keeley V, Mortimer P, Mansour S. A new classification system for primary lymphatic dysplasias based on phenotype. *Clinical Genetics* 2010;77: 438–452.
3. Mortimer PS. Evaluation of lymphatic function: Abnormal lymph drainage in venous disease. *Int Angiol* 1995;14:32–35.
4. Brautigam P, Vanscheidt W, Foldi E, Krause T, Moser E. The importance of the subfascial lymphatics in the diagnosis of lower limb edema: Investigations with semi quantitative lymphoscintigraphy. *Angiology* 1993;44:464–470.
5. Hadjis NS, Carr DH, Banks L, Pflug JJ. The role of CT in the diagnosis of primary lymphoedema of the lower limb. *AJR Am J Roentgenol* 1985;144: 361–364.
6. Lymphoedema Support Network. What is lymphoedema? 2004 www.lymphoedema.org.

7. Lymphoedema Support Network. What is lymphoedema? 2004 www. lymphoedema.org.
8. British Lymphology Society. Cellulitis Management Consensus 2007 www. thebls.com.
9. National Institute for Health and Clinical Excellence. Treating chronic lymph-oedema by liposuction 2008 www.nice.org.uk/IPG251 (accessed 13 June 2009).
10. Olszewski WL, Zaleska M. A novel method of edema fluid drainage in obstructive lymphedema of limbs by implantation of hydrophobic silicone tubes. *J Vasc Surg Venous Lymphat Disord* 2015;3(4):401–408.

Chapter 20

Varicose Veins and Chronic Venous Insufficiency

Ahmad Rafizi Hariz Bin Ramli and Tim Lees

Key Points

- Truncal varices are common with an age-adjusted prevalence of 40% in men and 32% in women.
- Varicosities may be primary, or secondary due to previous deep vein thrombosis (DVT), pelvic obstruction or deep venous reflux.
- Patients present with discomfort, aching, swelling, pain, pruritus, bleeding, thrombophlebitis and skin changes.
- Hand-held Doppler has replaced the tourniquet test as a 'bedside examination' for evaluating venous reflux. Patients having treatment will normally undergo duplex scanning.
- Surgery involves high tie and stripping and has a recurrence rate of 15–20%. It has been largely replaced by less invasive catheter ablation techniques.
- Foam sclerotherapy and catheter ablation techniques can be performed under local anaesthesia. Tumescent anaesthesia is used for laser and radiofrequency ablation. Tumescent anaesthesia is not required for mechanochemical ablation and cyanoacrylate ablation.

- Chronic venous insufficiency affects between 7% and 9% of the adult population and is due to venous reflux, outflow obstruction and calf pump failure.
- Clinical signs include swelling, venous eczema, pigmentation, lipodermatosclerosis and ulceration.
- Multilayered compression bandaging is the gold standard for healing venous ulceration compression.
- Venous reconstruction is rarely performed, but there remains a role for venous bypass surgery. The use of venous angioplasty and stenting is increasing.

Varicose veins

Epidemiology

Varicose veins have a prevalence of 20% with a range of 21.8–29.4% in the adult Western population. Of these 5% (range 3.6–8.6%) have venous oedema, skin changes or venous ulceration. Up to 0.5% have active ulceration and 0.6–1.4% have healed ulceration. [1].

Data from the Edinburgh Vein Study (EVS) suggest a slightly greater prevalence of varicose veins in males compared to females (4:3.2). The age-adjusted prevalence of truncal varices was found to be 40% in men and 32% in women. Mild varices (hyphenweb and reticular varices) were identified in 80% of the population aged 18–64 years.

Asymptomatic disease detected with Duplex scanning and defined as significant venous reflux greater than or equal to 0.5 seconds is estimated to occur in 35% of the population between the ages of 18 and 64 years. The prevalence of varicose veins increases with age and affects approximately 15% of the population aged between 25 and 34 years and 50–60% of the population aged 55–64 years [2].

Aetiology

Primary varicose veins

Primary varicose veins occur in the absence of any known underlying cause. Risk factors for developing primary varicose veins include age, parity, weight, posture and bowel habit.

- **Pregnancy:** Although not consistent, pregnancy is presumed to be a major contributory factor in the increased incidence of varicose veins in women [3]. Hormonal changes, such as an increase in relaxin and progesterone levels, weaken the blood vessel wall and have a vasodilator effect. In addition, fetal growth and weight gain increase intra-abdominal pressure and impair venous return. There is a significant increase in blood volume, which is primarily caused by plasma volume expansion. This increases the pressure on the venous valves in the lower limbs. Interestingly most varices appear in the first trimester when uterine size is unlikely to cause obstruction to venous return. Multiparity is also a risk factor for venous disease with a 20–30% increased risk associated with two or more pregnancies.

- **Weight:** Increased weight is a risk factor for varicose veins and the evidence for this is stronger in women. The association with elevated body mass index (BMI) has been shown in numerous studies. In the EVS, being overweight (BMI 25.0–29.9 kg/m^2) was a risk factor for venous reflux, but not obesity (BMI $>$ 30 kg/m^2) [4]. Currently it is not clear at what BMI level the risk is greatest.

- **Posture:** It has been suggested that prolonged standing may exacerbate varicose veins. Prolonged sitting has also been linked in some studies. The mechanism may be related to prolonged, increased hydrostatic pressure making the veins more susceptible to other factors.

- **Diet:** The effect of diet is suggested by the geographical variation in venous disease. Varicose veins are more common in Western societies with low fibre diets. Western diets result in straining during defaecation associated with raised intra-abdominal pressures. This pressure may be applied hydrostatically to leg veins.

- **Genetics:** Patients frequently describe the occurrence of varicose veins in other family members suggesting an inherited component to the occurrence. Although this is plausible, the evidence for genetic factors is limited. The prevalence of venous disease is so high that it is of no surprise that other family members are afflicted.

Secondary varicose veins

Secondary varicose veins occur as a consequence of another condition (post deep venous thrombosis, pelvic tumours, congenital malformations, deep venous reflux and outflow obstruction). In these situations the superficial veins act as a collateral venous return.

Clinical features (Table 1)

Asymptomatic varicose veins

The majority of patients with varicose veins are asymptomatic. Many seek medical attention for cosmetic reasons. This may have psychological implications altering a patient's confidence. Such concerns should be identified and discussed prior to any intervention to ensure that the expectations of any treatment are realistic. Some patients have concerns about the risk of future complications. Many have a fear of developing ulceration and some are concerned about the risk of deep venous thrombosis.

Other patients are concerned about the risk of developing a DVT during flying. These patients should be offered reassurance as not all patients develop skin changes. If a patient is likely to be travelling on a long-haul flight they should take the same precautions as a person without varicose veins. Many of the available treatments have an underlying risk of DVT and hence treatment of varicose veins should not be offered as a form of DVT prophylaxis.

Table 1.   Clinical features of varicose veins.

Symptoms	Types of varices	Chronic skin changes	Acute complications
Pain	Corona phlebectatica	Eczema Lipodermatosclerosis	Haemorrhage
Swelling Heaviness	Hyphenweb varices	Pigmentation	Superficial thrombophlebitis
Pruritus	Reticular varices	Ulceration	
Burning Restlessness	Truncal varices	Atrophie blanche	
Cramps			

Symptomatic varicose veins

Symptoms can be variable and may include pain, swelling, heaviness, pruritus, burning, restlessness and cramps. These symptoms may be exacerbated by ambulation and alleviated by lower limb elevation. Consequently symptoms may be more troublesome during the day or in the evening after prolonged standing or sitting and less problematic in the morning after the legs have been elevated overnight.

Presentation with acute complications of varicose veins is not uncommon. The acute complications are those of haemorrhage and thrombophlebitis (Fig. 1).

Haemorrhage can be torrential, occasionally life threatening and frequently associated with trauma (frequently trivial). Bleeding is initially managed with compression and elevation. Thereafter patients frequently seek definitive treatment in order to avoid further haemorrhage. Such bleeding can be very distressing for the patient and treatment of the affected veins is indicated to prevent further bleeding.

Superficial thrombophlebitis is a consequence of thrombosis and subsequent inflammation of the vein. The clinical presentation is that of

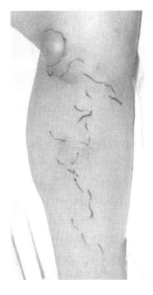

Figure 1.   Superficial thrombophlebitis.

an inflamed swollen tender vein. The early phase is managed with anal-gesics and anti-inflammatory agents. It is not uncommon for patients to receive a course of antibiotics in the community, although these are unnecessary as the process is that of a sterile inflammation. Subsequent fibrosis can result in a thickened nodule with subsequent skin pigmenta-tion, but many affected veins will recanalise. As recurrent phlebitis is common many surgeons regard this as an indication for surgery if the vein recanalises, once the acute phase has settled down.

Chronic complications (pigmentation, eczema, lipodermatosclerosis and ulceration) are more commonly seen with chronic venous insufficiency (CVI) although they can occur with isolated superficial venous reflux.

Clinical signs

Varicose veins show features of tortuosity, elongation and dilatation. They are described as hyphenweb varices, reticular or truncal varicosities.

- Hyphenweb varices are also referred to as telangiectasia, thread veins, spider veins and venous flare. They are intradermal dilated venules occurring in isolation or in association with truncal or reticu-lar varices.
- Reticular varices are subcuticular varices that do not belong to the main trunk or its tributaries. They frequently appear as a bluish reticu-lar pattern of veins beneath the skin and can occur physiologically.
- Truncal varices arise from the long or short saphenous veins or their major tributaries (first- and second-order tributaries). Chronic venous skin changes include eczema, lipodermatosclerosis and ulceration.
- Eczema results in dry, scaly, itchy skin. Scratching can result in bleed-ing, infection and subsequent ulceration.
- Lipodermatosclerosis is the term given to the pigmented skin associ-ated with thickened/inflamed subcuticular and cutaneous tissue. The mechanism is unclear but it is believed that elevated venous pressure facilitates extravasation of cells and fluid, leading to inflammation.
- Pigmentation/skin staining is a consequence of haemosiderin deposits.
- Chronic venous ulceration is most commonly (albeit not exclusively) seen in the gaiter area above the medial malleolus. It commonly

occurs in an area of pre-existing lipodermatosclerosis following trauma. Long-standing ulcers are at risk of malignant conversion to squamous cell carcinoma (Marjolin's ulcer) and this should be considered in long-standing ulceration and those that fail to heal.

- Other skin changes seen include malleolar flare/corona phlebectatica (intradermal or subdermal collection of dilated veins at the medial malleolus) and atrophie blanche (scar tissue at a site of previous ulceration).

Many studies have advocated the use of a classification to stratify the severity of disease as a guide for its management. Such classifications that are widely used are CEAP (clinical, aetiological, anatomical and pathophysiological) classification and Venous Clinical Severity Score (VCSS) (Tables 2 and 3). These can be beneficial when used in research to compare the treatment outcome of different modalities. These classifications should only be used as supportive assessment tools, however and decisions about treatment should be tailored to a patient's specific condition and personal preference. Some classifications are difficult to use routinely due to their complexity.

In 2013, the National Institute for Health and Care Excellence (NICE) issued guidelines for referral of a patient with varicose veins to a vascular service [5]:

- Refer people with bleeding varicose veins to a vascular service immediately.

Table 2.   CEAP classification.

C0	No visible or palpable signs of venous disease
C1	Telangiectasia or reticular veins
C2	Varicose veins >3 mm diameter
C3	Oedema
C4	Skin changes, lipodermatosclerosis, eczema, atrophie blanche
C5	Healed venous ulcer
C6	Active ulcer

Table 3.   Venous clinical severity score (VCSS).

Attribute	Absent = 0	Mild = 1	Moderate = 2	Severe = 3
Pain	None	Occasional	Daily	Limit activities
Varicose veins	None	Few, scattered	Multiple (LSV)	Extensive (LSV, SSV)
Venous oedema	None	Evening, ankle	Afternoon, leg	Morning, leg
Pigmentation	None	Limited area	Wide (lower 1/3)	Wider, above 1/3
Inflammation	None	Cellulitis	Cellulitis	Cellulitis
Induration	None	Focal (< 5 cm)	< lower 1/3	Entire lower 1/3
Number of AC	0	1	2	3
Duration of AC	None	< 3 months	3 months – 1 year	> 1 year
Size of AC	None	< 2 cm diameter	2–6 cm diameter	> 6 cm diameter
Comp therapy	Not used	Intermittent use	Most days	Continually

Notes: LSV, long saphenous vein; SSV, short saphenous vein; AC, active ulceration; lower 1/3, lower 1/3 of the leg.

- Refer people to a vascular service if they have any of the following.
  o Symptomatic primary or symptomatic recurrent varicose veins.
  o Lower-limb skin changes, such as pigmentation or eczema, thought to be caused by chronic venous insufficiency.
  o Superficial vein thrombosis (characterised by the appearance of hard, painful veins) and suspected venous incompetence.
  o A venous leg ulcer (a break in the skin below the knee that has not healed within 2 weeks).
  o A healed venous leg ulcer.

Investigations for venous disease

Hand held doppler

Hand held Doppler has replaced the tourniquet test in assessing the source of incompetence. It is now the initial choice of investigation at the bedside. The test is performed with the patient standing. The probe is placed at the junction suspected of being incompetent and the calf muscle compressed. This produces a characteristic venous signal. On releasing the muscle the presence of an audible signal suggests reflux. The long saphenous vein, saphenofemoral junction and saphenopopliteal junction can all be assessed although false positives are more commonly seen at the saphenopopliteal junction due to the variability of its location. Hence reflux at this site should always be confirmed with a Duplex scan.

Duplex

Duplex combines B-mode ultrasound and Doppler. This allows identification of individual vessels and can generate information on the direction of flow in a vessel. It therefore provides both anatomical and functional information. It is used to define the communication points between the deep and superficial venous systems (perforators, saphenofemoral and saphenopopliteal junctions) and the presence or absence of venous reflux. Duplex is non-invasive, quick and cheap. It is the first-line imaging technique for venous disease and frequently the only imaging ever required.

Whilst some surgeons rely on hand held Doppler for the diagnosis of straightforward long saphenous incompetence there is increasing evidence to support the use of Duplex scanning for all patients presenting with varicose veins who require treatment. Reliance on clinical examination alone can result in inappropriate surgical procedures being performed [6, 7]. The increasing availability of affordable portable scanners allows quick and convenient scanning in the outpatient environment, reduces diagnostic error and avoids the need for multiple clinic attendances.

Venography

Duplex scanning has almost abolished the need for this investigation for uncomplicated venous disease. Occasionally more detailed imaging is required (e.g., for the investigation of venous outflow obstruction). This can be done using magnetic resonance venography (MRV) and computed tomography venography (CTV). Some patients with complex venous disease will still require catheter contrast venography, particularly those in whom angioplasty or stenting is contemplated.

Magnetic resonance venography (MRV)

Magnetic resonance venography is useful for imaging the venous system, especially within the main body cavities (thorax, abdomen and pelvis) where Duplex imaging may be limited (especially in the obese). It can be used to diagnose deep venous occlusions, stenosis, thrombosis and mal-formations. Various techniques exist including non-contrast imaging, which utilises time of flight techniques and contrast enhanced MRV. The contrast-enhanced techniques have the advantage of being quicker and less susceptible to flow artefact in parallel vessels. It is also able to dif-ferentiate between acute and chronic deep venous thrombosis and is less invasive than conventional venography. The main limitation of MRV is its cost compared to other forms of venography and Duplex, and its availa-bility. In recent years increasing numbers of MRVs are performed for surveillance of patients with venous stents in place for treatment of venous outflow obstruction such as in May Thurner's syndrome. MRV has the advantage over CTV of avoiding radiation in this cohort of patients who are often young fertile females.

Computed tomography venograpy (CTV)

Computed tomography venography, like MRV, may provide better imag-ing of the iliac and caval venous systems than Duplex scanning. Extrinsic compression of the iliac veins or vena cava (inferior and superior) can also be identified and pelvic/abdominal masses can be visualised. CT pulmonary angiography has become the investigation of choice for pul-monary embolism.

Contrast venography

Venography requires the injection of the contrast into a vein followed by X-ray imaging. Historically it was used to investigate varicose veins but the main indications now are in those patients in whom endovascular inter-vention is being considered. This includes patients with suspected ovar-ian vein reflux, those with proximal (e.g., iliac) venous outflow obstruction, and patients with venous malformations. In addition there is increasing use of thrombolysis for patients with iliofemoral deep vein thrombosis and this is performed via a catheter inserted into the popliteal or femoral vein. Such patients may require iliac stenting for residual stenosis following lysis.

Functional calf measurements

Plethysmography

Overall lower limb venous function is influenced by valvular function, venous outflow and calf muscle activity. All of these will affect venous filling, which subsequently influences calf volume. The change in calf volume can be quantified using plethysmography. Photoplethysmography utilises infrared light absorption to quantify the change in blood flow within cutaneous veins. This is correlated with ambulatory venous pressure refilling time.

Air plethysmography involves enclosing the leg in a bag and measuring changes in the pressure within the bag following ankle exercise. From these measurements, changes in calf volume can be measured. A similar principle is used in foot volumetry where patients stand in water filled steel boots. Changes in foot volume are detected by measuring the volume of water expelled.

Ambulatory venous pressure (AVP)

This is an invasive technique requiring the cannulation of a dorsal foot vein and direct measurement of the superficial venous pressure by connection to a pressure transducer, amplifier and a computer. It remains the gold standard method for measuring venous pressure. Patients are asked to tip-toe ten times and the pressure changes are recorded. Although AVP can provide detailed information its use is now largely confined to research of venous disease.

Treatment

Reassurance

Many patients require no treatment other than reassurance. Patients with asymptomatic varicose veins who have no cosmetic concerns can be discharged after the benign nature of the disease has been explained. Patients who are due to fly on long-haul flights should be advised to wear anti-embolism stockings and to exercise their calves as for patients without varicose veins. The risk of developing DVT with varicose veins is not significant enough to justify intervention and patients should be reassured of this, especially as intervention itself is associated with a risk of DVT.

Compression stockings

These can provide symptomatic relief in patients with varicose veins and should be offered to those who do not want any form of invasive intervention. They have an important role in the management of chronic venous insufficiency and reduce ulcer recurrence after healing with compression dressings. They enhance the efficacy of surgery in venous ulceration by reducing the ulcer recurrent rate compared to compression alone [8]. They create a graduated pressure on the leg, aiding the action of the venous calf pump and improving deep venous blood flow, which in turn reduces reflux into the superficial system.

Compression stockings are classified (and should be described) according to the pressure applied at the ankle. These stockings may be described as class I to IV but this should be avoided due to the significant differences between the British and European pressure classification (Table 4). The most commonly used stockings are those that produce a pressure ranging between 25 and 35 mmHg at the ankle. Before prescribing compression stockings it is vital to exclude coexisting occlusive arterial disease. They should be used with caution in diabetic patients. Stockings can result in ulceration in these groups of patients and hence close monitoring is required.

Foam sclerotherapy

Foam sclerotherapy is a modification of a technique used for many years to treat varicose veins. The original use of sclerosing agents for varicosities became less popular after the recurrence rate was shown to be significantly higher compared to surgery. The efficacy of sclerosing agents was found to be improved however, by mixing with air and administering

Table 4.   Classification of compression stockings.

Indication	Support	European standard class pressure	British standard class pressure
Mild varices, deep vein thrombosis, prophylaxis	Light	I 18–21 mmHg	I 14–17 mmHg
Marked varices, oedema, chronic venous insufficiency	Medium	II 23–32 mmHg	II 18–24 mmHg
Chronic venous insufficiency, lymphoedema, prevention of venous ulcers	Strong	III 34–46 mmHg	III 25–35 mmHg
Severe lymphoedema, chronic venous insufficiency	Heavy	IV 49–70 mmHg	
	Super	IV 60–90 mmHg	

the agent as foam. This facilitated the displacement of blood from the vein and improved contact with the vein wall. Sclerosing agents react with the endothelium causing endosclerosis and endofibrosis.

Foam sclerotherapy injection is performed under ultrasound guidance. The most common agents used are sodium tetradecyl sulphate (1–3%) and polidocanol (0.5–3%). These agents are converted to foam by mixing with air using two syringes and a 3-way tap. Using ultrasound the long saphenous or short saphenous vein is cannulated with a venflon and the foam administered in 1 mL aliquots. Smaller tributaries are cannulated with butterfly needles and treated with lower concentrations of foam. Whilst the foam is administered, the leg is elevated and the patient encouraged to dorsiflex the ankle. This latter manoeuvre encourages blood flow in the deep veins, reducing the risk of deep venous thrombosis.

After treatment, compression bandaging is applied for one or two weeks. The more common complications include thrombophlebitis, haemosiderin skin staining and ulceration from extravasation of sclerosant (Table 5). Less common complications include deep venous thrombosis, transient visual disturbance and stroke (only a handful of cases have been reported worldwide). Foam sclerotherapy can be offered as an outpatient treatment and is also suitable for recurrent varicosities. It is the first-line treatment for patients unfit for general anaesthetic. A well-performed foam sclerotherapy treatment can achieve excellent results in patients with venous ulcers. Long-term studies are required to compare recurrence rates of foam with conventional surgery.

Catheter ablation

Catheter ablation is a technique used to induce transmural injury to the vein wall and cause it to thrombose. It is now divided into treatment categories of thermal and tumescence (TT) and non-thermal and non-tumescence (NTNT).

There are two techniques for TT based catheter ablation that are in common use: radiofrequency ablation (RFA) and endovenous laser treatment (EVLT). One trial comparing RFA with surgery has shown that RFA is associated with less postoperative pain and faster recovery compared to surgery [9]. Early results have shown that both are effective in eliminating reflux. Endovenous laser treatment has been shown to produce less postoperative bruising and swelling compared to surgery [10]. One trial has shown RFA to be superior to EVLT in postoperative pain and quality of life parameters [11]. Large randomised controlled trials are lacking.

For NTNT based ablation therapy, there are currently two devices on the market. The first device uses a mechanochemical ablation (MOCA) technique. When compared to RFA, one study demonstrated that patients who had MOCA had a lower average pain score on visual analogue score (VAS) [12]. This is otherwise no significant difference in term of occlusion rates, quality of life and complication rates between MOCA and RFA.

The second NTNT device uses a slightly different technique than MOCA. It is a new technique using medical grade super glue, cyanoacrylate (CA) to ablate the vein. Several recent studies have shown that endovenous CA embolisation (CAE) has the advantage of causing less bruising with similar occlusion rates, periprocedural pain and quality of life compared to RFA [13]. CAE may negate the need for compression stockings since the technique does not cause perforation of the vein wall.

Radiofrequency ablation (RFA)

Radiofrequency energy is used to cause a thermal injury to the inside of the truncal vein being treated. Using a Seldinger technique the vein (e.g., long saphenous vein) is cannulated under ultrasound guidance and the RFA catheter inserted and guided to a position just distal to the saphenofemoral junction. Radiofrequency energy is applied to the vein wall and this heats the vein wall to 120°C, causing denaturation of the collagen and contraction of the vessel such that no blood can flow through it. Complications include nerve injury (resulting in paraesthesia) and skin burns (Table 5). The risk is reduced or prevented by using tumescence anaesthesia (ultrasound guided injection of anaesthetic solution into the facial envelope surrounding the vein). The solution injected usually consists of a vasoconstrictor such as adrenalin and local anaesthetic diluted in a 0.9% saline solution. This type of anaesthesia protects the surrounding tissue from thermal insult, anaesthetises and vasoconstricts the vein compressing it against the catheter/electrode within the lumen. This latter effect drains blood from within the vein and facilitates contact of the catheter with the wall of the vein. This is aided further by manual compression. Successful long saphenous vein ablation is seen in approximately 85% of patients at 2 years [14].

Endovenous laser treatment (EVLT)

The main difference between EVLT and RFA is with the use of a laser diode to generate the thermal insult required for ablation of the vein. The technique of vein cannulation (ultrasound guidance, Seldinger technique) and tumescent anaesthesia is comparable to that of RFA. The catheter contains a laser diode that generates a laser beam (usually of 810 nm wavelength). This heats blood around the laser tip, generating steam, which heats the vein wall. The risks are similar to RFA, although the temperatures generated are higher, and the results are comparable. Both RFA and EVLT avoid the complications associated with groin incisions and thigh haematomas, and have improved postoperative recovery with less postoperative pain. Both techniques are dependent on causing cell death in the vein wall whilst avoiding perforation. Although there are no large randomised controlled trials to compare recurrence after EVLT

Table 5. Complications of treatment.

Catheter ablation (RFA/EVLT)	Surgery	Foam sclerotherapy	Mechanochemical ablation (MOCA)	Cyanoacrylate embolisation (CAE)
Bruising	Bleeding/bruising	Hyperpigmentation	Bruising	Bruising
Thrombophlebitis	Groin infection/abscess	Visual disturbance	Erythema	Erythema
Skin burns	Nerve injury	Skin necrosis	Deep vein thrombosis	Deep vein thrombosis
Nerve injury	Sensory loss	Deep vein thrombosis	Recurrence	Recurrence
Sensory loss	Motor loss	Thrombophlebitis	Hyperpigmentation	Hyperpigmentation
Neuralgia	Neuralgia	Stroke	Thrombophlebitis	Thrombophlebitis
Perforation of deep veins	Deep vein thrombosis	Recurrence	Stroke	Stroke
Erythema	Venous flare		Visual disturbance	Visual disturbance
Deep vein thrombosis	Residual varicosities			Multiorgan infarction
Recurrence	Arterial/venous injury			
	Recurrence			

with surgery, published case series indicate successful early ablation rates of 80–90% with EVLT [15, 16].

Mechanochemical ablation (MOCA)

MOCA has been introduced as an alternative treatment for varicose vein to avoid the use of heat and tumescent infiltration. It combines an endovenous mechanical method using a rotating wire with simultaneous injection of liquid sclerosant. The wire is shaped like a hockey stick with a ball tip. It rotates at 3500 rotations per minute with the tip causing damage to the venous intima while the sclerosant is infused (1–2 mm/s) through an opening close to the catheter tip. This mechanism allows deeper sclerotherapy penetration thus enhancing endothelial destruction. This explains why the results of MOCA appear to be superior to foam sclerotherapy with respect to medium-term occlusion.

The general principle of performing a MOCA procedure follows that of the other catheter-based endovenous ablation techniques. MOCA uses a smaller size sheath (4F) and catheter, hence, can be easily negotiated through a more tortuous vein with less risk of perforation. It only requires local anaesthetic at the skin puncture site and no tumescence is needed.

Some reported complications are minor bruising (ecchymosis) and haematoma. Recent multicenter studies have shown similar occlusion rates, improved post-operative pain and lower incidence of nerve injury [17].

Cyanoacrylate embolization

The second generation of NTNT devices uses cyanoacrylate embolisation (CAE) a super glue, to ablate the truncal vein. CA is an adhesive liquid monomeric agent, which quickly polymerises and becomes solid when it comes into contact with a solution containing anions (e.g., with the hydroxyl groups in blood). This leads to venous occlusion, a marked inflammatory endothelial response, and ultimately fibrosis. Similar glues have also been used intravascularly for the treatment of type I and II endoleaks following abdominal aortic aneurysm repair procedure, for the treatment of varicoceles, pelvic congestion syndrome and vascular malformations.

The delivery technique is similar to other catheter-based devices on the market. It is recommended that the catheter tip distance from the saphenofemoral junction is 5 cm in order to allow some propagation of the glue without the risk of extension into the common femoral vein. The most commonly reported complications of CA used for the treatment of varicose veins include ecchymosis and phlebitis. These are reported to be mild and resolve with over the counter non-steroidal anti-inflammatory agents. Other potential risks of CAE include systemic embolisation such as pulmonary embolism, stroke and multi-organ infarction via a patent foramen ovale. To date, however these have not been reported.

Surgery

Saphenofemoral junction ligation and long saphenous vein stripping

Surgical treatment of varicosities arising from an incompetent saphenofemoral junction and/or its tributaries is historically one of the most common procedures performed by the vascular surgeon. Flush ligation of the saphenofemoral junction, division of its tributaries and stripping of the long saphenous vein (ideally to a level of approximately one hand breadth below the knee) has been the gold standard surgical procedure. Stripping of the long saphenous vein to this level reduces the risk of recurrence, disconnects the vein from the more proximal calf perforator (Boyd's perforator) and minimises the risk of damage to the saphenous nerve. Saphenous neuralgia and chronic pain was a complication more commonly seen with full length long saphenous vein stripping. Conventional surgery of this nature has reduced considerably with the arrival of the catheter based ablation techniques.

Saphenopopliteal junction ligation

Varicosities associated with reflux of the saphenopopliteal junction are treated by ligation of the saphenopopliteal junction. Preoperative diagnosis of saphenopopliteal reflux requires Duplex confirmation, and prior to surgery all patients should have the saphenopopliteal junction marked with the aid of Duplex ultrasonography. This is to account for the great anatomical variation in saphenopopliteal junction location. Significant variation exists in the techniques for short saphenous vein surgery. Approximately 15% of UK surgeons strip the proximal third and there is evidence to suggest this reduces the risk of reoccurrence [18, 19]. Stripping of the short saphenous vein is not carried out routinely by all surgeons due to the risk of sural nerve damage, although the sural nerve normally joins the vein in the distal two thirds of the calf.

Multiple stab avulsions (phlebectomies)

The cosmetic part of the procedure takes the form of phlebectomies performed through tiny stab incisions and aided with a special vein hook. These should be sufficiently small enough to be closed with small steri-strip adhesive dressings. These can also be combined with the catheter based ablation techniques and can be performed under local anaesthetic.

Perforator surgery

Opinion remains divided regarding the relevance of perforator vein incompetence. Open surgical ligation of venous perforators may be complicated by poor wound healing and recurrence, particularly in the distal calf. A number of perforators identified as being incompetent on Duplex scan later become competent after treatment of truncal reflux. Ulceration may respond to treatment of truncal incompetence alone and hence many surgeons reserve perforator surgery for resistant venous ulceration not responding to treatment of either the long or short systems. In addition to open ligation, perforator ablation may also be performed using a small radiofrequency ablation probe designed specifically for perforator treatment.

Recurrent varicose veins

Recurrent varicose veins may develop for a number of reasons. Neovascularisation is the development of a new connection between the deep and superficial vein at the site of a previously ligated junction. The mechanism is not fully understood but is believed to be either the consequence of new vessel growth or the dilatation of pre-existing tributaries. This is the commonest cause of recurrence at the saphenofemoral junction. Other causes of recurrence include the development of incompetent perforators and the development of varicosities in a second saphenous system.

Approximately one in five patients treated for varicose veins are likely to develop recurrent varicosities. Surgery for recurrent varicose veins can be hazardous with a greater risk of injuring the deep veins, wound complications such as bleeding, infections, lymphatic leakage and seromas. In addition there is a greater risk of nerve injury especially at the saphenopopliteal junction. The need for re-exploration of the groin or saphenopopliteal junction has diminished with the expansion of techniques available to treat varicose veins. Foam sclerotherpy, RFA and EVLT can all be used and hence reduce the need for complicated groin and popliteal re-explorations and hence the risk of treatment.

Complications of treatment (Table 5)

When consenting patients for surgery, potential complications need to be discussed. General complications include bleeding, infection (more common with groin surgery), recurrence, nerve injury (parasthesia, chronic pain), deep venous thrombosis, residual varicosities, venous 'flare', haematoma, arterial and deep venous injury (common femoral vein, popliteal vein). Long saphenous vein stripping is associated with significant bruising to the thigh and patients should be warned of this. Saphenopopliteal ligation may be associated with injury to the common peroneal nerve and the risk of foot drop should be mentioned. The nerve can be affected by local anaethesia and foot drop that persists beyond the duration of the local anaesthetic should be referred for immediate investigation and treatment (nerve conduction studies, possible exploration, nerve repair/grafting or tendon transfer). Other nerve injuries can occur as a consequence of the phlebectomies. These can result in numbness or chronic neuralgia. Nerves at risk include the common peroneal, saphenous, sural and tibial nerves. The latter two are especially at risk when avulsing behind the malleoli. Neuropraxia has also been seen following application of compression dressings and staff should be advised to release dressings should the patient complain of significant pain and numbness in the post-operative recovery room. Any concern about perfusion to the foot following the application of dressings should be treated in the same way.

Chronic venous Insufficiency

Epidemiology

As with varicose veins, the prevalence of chronic venous insufficiency (CVI) is marginally greater in men (9% of the population aged between 18–64 years) compared to women (7% of the female population aged between 18–64 years) [2]. The prevalence increases with age. It is a major cause of ulceration and has significant economic implications both in lost working days and cost to the NHS.

Aetiology

This condition results from impaired venous return and causes elevated ambulatory venous pressure within the lower limbs. As a consequence of this elevated venous pressure, skin changes occur in the form of eczema, pigmentation, lipodermatosclerosis and ulceration. It is associated with lower limb oedema, varicose veins and chronic pain. There are a number of causes including venous reflux, venous obstruction and 'pump' failure of the calf muscle (Table 6).

The combination of normal venous anatomy and calf muscle contraction during exercise is responsible for reducing venous pressure in the

Table 6.   Aetiology of chronic venous insufficiency.

Aetiology	Example
Superficial venous reflux	Long saphenous/short saphenous varicosities
Deep venous insufficiency	Valvular damage e.g., post DVT
Venous outflow obstruction	Stenosis/occlusion e.g., post DVT, venous cannulation
Calf muscle pump failure	Immobility, obesity, prolonged sitting

lower leg and encouraging venous return. These mechanisms are impaired by venous reflux (affecting either the superficial, deep or perforating venous systems), venous occlusions (e.g., DVT) or abnormal calf pump action. Numerous causes exist for impaired calf muscle function and these range from neurological conditions to reduced mobility associated with morbid obesity. The relevance of perforator reflux remains a topic of debate and primary surgical treatment should be directed at the superficial system, with separate treatment of perforator reflux being reserved for resistant cases.

The mechanism by which raised ambulatory venous pressure generates skin changes is not fully understood. Numerous mechanisms have been suggested including the fibrin cuff hypothesis and white cell trapping hypothesis. The fibrin cuff hypothesis suggests that elevated pressure associated with chronic venous insufficiency results in capillary damage leading to the deposition of fibrinogen. This subsequently forms fibrin and is allowed to accumulate due to an impaired fibrinolytic system. Subsequently oxygen transfer is impaired and the resulting local ischaemia results in ulceration. The white cell trapping hypothesis suggests that the elevated venous pressure slows and halts the passage of large white cells through the capillaries. These become 'plugged' with white cells. These cells are activated and release proteolytic enzymes and free radicals causing local tissue damage. A series of events results in the release of factors, which favour increased vascular permeability facilitating the formation of the fibrin cuff. The latter and the trapped white cells cause local ischaemia and facilitate the formation of ulcers.

Clinical features

Patients complain of a variety of symptoms including swelling, itching, aching and heaviness. The symptoms tend to be exacerbated by prolonged standing and relieved by elevation. Initially, oedema is pitting but with chronicity becomes non-pitting. The venous eczema causes pruritus, which stimulates scratching and subsequent skin trauma. This can be the precipitating event leading to ulceration. The most common site of ulceration is the distal medial calf. Pigmentation results from haemosiderin deposition and when accompanied by fibrosis results in lipodermatosclerosis. Varicose veins may be present and superficial reflux should always be excluded. A previous history of deep venous thrombosis is not uncommon and symptoms of venous claudication (pain and swelling exacerbated with exercise, requiring rest and elevation for relief of symptoms) suggest significant venous occlusion (iliofemoral veins).

Management

Non-operative treatment

Certain comorbidities are known to be associated with the development of chronic venous insufficiency and these should be treated. Obesity and immobility should be improved. Leg elevation can reduce ankle venous pressure to 15 mmHg and should be encouraged. Bed rest and elevation above the level of the heart may be required for patients with ulceration resistant to other forms of treatment.

Most patients with chronic venous insufficiency are treated with either compression stockings or dressings. These apply a graduated compression that decreases proximally. The compression improves venous blood flow in the deep venous system. Multilayered compression is the gold standard used to heal venous ulceration. Stockings are used to prevent recurrence. Below-knee compression stockings of 25–35 mmHg are sufficient for most patients, but stronger stockings are available.

Operative treatment

Superficial venous surgery

The role of superficial surgery (e.g., ligation of saphenopopliteal junction, ligation of saphenofemoral junction and long saphenous vein stripping) in ulcer healing has been previously studied. The ESCHAR trial was a randomised trial involving 500 leg ulcers associated with isolated superficial incompetence and showed the one year recurrence rate of leg ulceration to be reduced with combined superficial venous surgery and elastic compression (9% recurrence) compared to compression alone (38% recurrence) [20]. The initial healing rate was not affected. Superficial surgery is recommended in patients with isolated superficial reflux and a history of ulceration.

Perforator surgery

The role of perforator surgery has already been discussed. There remains a debate regarding its benefits, as correction of superficial reflux is frequently associated with improvement in perforator reflux. The use of minimally invasive perforator surgery (SEPS) is associated with less morbidity but usually reserved for resistant ulceration.

Venous reconstruction

Venous reconstruction is reserved for patients with severe ulceration, and venous claudication and limb swelling that has not responded to compression and superficial/perforator surgery. In reality it is rarely done. The reconstruction may be either in the form of a venous bypass or, less commonly, valvular reconstruction. A variety of valvular reconstructive procedures have been described and include valvuloplasty, valve transplant, valve transposition, vein wall plication and external banding with a Dacron or polytetrafluoroethane (PTFE) cuff.

If the deep venous system is obstructed then deep venous bypass surgery or endovascular revascularization may be of benefit. Venous bypass is usually reserved for patients who are severely symptomatic despite allowing sufficient time (at least 12 months) for superficial collaterals to develop. Causes of deep venous obstruction include previous DVT, malignant disease, retro-peritoneal fibrosis and May–Thurner syndrome. Iliac vein obstruction can be treated with a Palma operation. Using the contra-lateral long saphenous vein a bypass is completed by anastomosing the distal end to the common femoral or profunda veins in the affected limb. In the absence of a suitable long saphenous vein a prosthetic conduit may be considered. Deep thigh vein occlusion can be treated with a saphenopopliteal vein bypass (May–Husni operation). Again the long saphenous vein is the conduit of choice. This procedure is very rarely performed. Reconstructive surgery is contra-indicated in early deep vein thrombosis, arterial disease and thrombophilias.

Endovascular treatment

The techniques of endovenous catheter ablation (RFA, EVLT, MOCA and CAE) and foam sclerotherapy described to treat the superficial system in varicose veins can also be used for treatment of the superficial venous system in chronic venous insufficiency. These are an alternative to surgery.

Recent advancements in endovascular techniques have led to deep venous balloon angioplasty and stenting becoming more widely used for deep venous outflow obstruction. This treatment has been shown to be efficient in reduction of venous hypertension and the prevention of post-thrombotic syndrome (PTS) and ulcer occurrence/recurrence [21]. The procedure should be done in a high volume vascular centre and care should be taken in patient selection, the use of an inferior vena cava filter and perioperative anticoagulation. Dedicated venous stents with high radial force should be used to ensure long-term patency and prevent stent related complications such as stent fracture and migration. This promising treatment has been shown to have a good mid term outcome with an 88% 5-year patency. Clinical relief of pain ranged from 86% to 94% and relief from swelling ranged from 66% to 89%; 58% to 89% of venous ulcers healed [22]. Long-term patency results are not known, however and have not been compared directly with surgery.

Management of Leg Ulcers

Venous ulceration accounts for approximately 80% of chronic leg ulceration. A significant number of ulcers are of mixed arterial and venous aetiology. Significant arterial disease should be treated especially if compression is to be considered. Neoplastic disease can be a cause of chronic ulceration and may occur in long standing ulcers (squamous cell carcinoma, Marjolin's ulcers). In ulcers resistant to healing biopsy needs to be considered.

In addition to management of the underlying venous disease, consideration should be given to appropriate skin dressings, emollients and nutritional supplements (vitamins and trace elements). Adjunctive surgical techniques that may facilitate wound healing should be considered e.g., wound debridement and skin grafts. Various techniques to facilitate debridement exist and range from topical applications to surgical debridement. Skin grafting may be considered to accelerate the healing. The graft is usually a split skin graft or pinch grafts.

Post-phlebitic Syndrome

After a deep venous thrombosis a number of patients will develop chronic venous insufficiency. This is frequently referred to as post-phlebitic or post-thrombotic syndrome. Mild disease is seen in up to one third of patients whilst severe disease may affect one in ten patients. The risk is increased with more proximal venous thrombosis. The underlying mechanism is of elevated ambulatory venous pressure. As a consequence of valvular destruction, out flow obstruction and calf muscle dysfunction ambulatory venous pressure fails to undergo the normal physiological reduction seen during walking. A normal pressure drop of 50% can be seen during ambulation compared to standing. In chronic venous insufficiency these pressures may actually rise and can result in venous claudication. The early management of DVT is aimed at preventing propagation of the thrombosis by anti-coagulation. Elevation and compression stockings are encouraged to minimise swelling. If detected early, preferably within 14 days, proximal/iliofemoral DVTs may be treated with thrombolysis with the aim of restoring venous patency and minimising the loss of venous function. Long-term treatment includes compression stockings and all patients are encouraged to preserve calf muscle function with regular exercise.

References

1. Rabe E, Pannier F. Epidemiology of chronic venous disorders. In: Gloviczki P, editor. Handbook of venous disorders: Guidelines of the American Venous Forum, 3rd edn. London: Hodder Arnold; 2009; pp. 105–110.
2. Evans CJ, Fowkes FG, Ruckley CV, Lee AJ. Prevalence of varicose veins and chronic venous insufficiency in men and women in the general population: Edinburgh vein study. *J Epidemiol Community Health* 1999;53:149–153.
3. Stansby G. Women, pregnancy, and varicose veins. *Lancet* 2000;355:1117e8.

4. LA Robertson, CJ Evans, AJ Lee, PL Allan, CV Ruckley, FGR Fowkes. Incidence and risk factors for venous reflux in the general population: edinburgh vein study. *Euro J Vascu Endovascu Surg* 2014;48(2):208–214.

5. NICE varicose veins management guideline 2013 (updated 2016).

6. London NJM. Duplex ultrasonograpy and varicose veins. *Br J Surgery* 2007;94:521–522.

7. Makris SA, Karkos CD, Awad S, London NJM. An 'all comers' venous duplex scan policy for patients with lower limb varicose veins attending a one stop vascular clinic: is it justified? *Eur J Vasc Endovasc Surg* 2002;32:718–724.

8. Comparison of surgery and compression with compression alone in chronic venous ulceration (ESCHAR study): randomised controlled trial Barwell, Jamie R *et al*. *Lancet* 1854;363(9424):1859.

9. Rautio T Ohinmaa A, Perälä J, Ohtonen P, Heikkinen T, Wiik H, Karjalainen P, Haukipuro K, Juvonen T. Endovenous obliteration versus conventional stripping operation in the treatment of primary varicose veins: A randomized controlled trial with comparison of the costs. *J Vasc Surg* 2002;35: 958–965.

10. de Medeiros CA, Luccas GC. Comparison of endovenous treatment with an 810 nm laser versus conventional stripping of the great saphenous vein in patients with primary varicose veins. *Dermatol Surg* 2005;31:1685–1694.

11. Almeida JI, Kaufman J, Göckeritz O, Chopra P, Evans MT, Hoheim DF, Makhoul RG, Richards T, Wenzel C, Raines JK. Radiofrequency endovenous ClosureFAST versus laser ablation for the treatment of great saphenous reflux: a multicenter, single-blinded, randomized study (RECOVERY study). *J Vasc Interv Radiol* 2009;20:752–759.

12. Bootun R, Lane T, Dharmarajah B *et al*. Intra-procedural pain score in a randomised controlled trial comparing mechanochemical ablation to radiofrequency ablation: The Multicentre Venefit versus ClariVein® for varicose veins trial. *Phlebology* 2016;31(1):61–65.

13. Morrison N, Gibson K, McEnroe S *et al*. Randomized trial comparing cyanoacrylate embolization and radiofrequency ablation for incompetent great saphenous veins (VeClose). *J Vasc Surg* 2015;61:985–994.

14. Suramonia S, Lees TA, Wyatt MG, Oates C. Radiofrequency ablation in the treatment of varicose veins. In Wyatt WA (ed.), *Endovascular Interventions*. Shrewsbury: TMF Publishing Ltd, 2004, pp. 271–276.

15. Disselhoff BC, der Kinderen DJ, Moll FL. Is there recanalization of the great saphenous vein 2 years after endovenous laser treatment? *J Endovasc er* 2005;12:731–738.

16. Sharif MA, Soong CV, Lau LL, Corvan R, Lee B, Hannon RJ. Endovenous laser treatment for long saphenous vein incompetence. *Br J Surg* 2006;93:831–835.

17. Bishawi M, Bernstein R, Boter M, *et al.* Mechanochemical ablation in patients with chronic venous disease: A prospective multicenter report. *Phlebology* 2013;29:397–400.

18. Winterborn RJ, Campbell WB, Heather BP, Earnshaw JJ. E management of short saphenous varicose veins: A survey of the members of the vascular surgical society of Great Britain and Ireland. *Eur J Vasc Endovasc Surg* 2004;28:400–403.

19. O'Hare JL, Vandenbroeck CP, Whitman B, Campbell B, Heather BP, Earnshaw JJ, Joint Vascular Research Group. A prospective evaluation of the outcome after small saphenous varicose vein surgery with one-year follow-up. *J Vasc Surg* 2008;48:669–673.

20. Gohel MS, Barwell JR, Taylor M, Chant T, Foy C, Earnshaw JJ, Heather BP, Mitchell DC, Whyman MR, Poskitt KR. Long term results of compression therapy alone versus compression plus surgery in chronic venous ulceration (ESCHAR): Randomised controlled trial. *BMJ* 2007;335:83.

21. Raju S, Darcey R, Neglén P. Unexpected major role for venous stenting in deep reflux disease. *J Vasc Surg* 2010;51(2):401–408, ISSN 0741–5214.

22. Raju, Seshadri, Treatment of iliac-caval outflow obstruction. *Sem Vasc Surg* 2015;28(1):47–53.

Chapter 21

Chronic Venous Insufficiency and Leg Ulceration

Tim Lees and Gerard Stansby

Key Points

- Clinical signs of chronic venous insufficiency (CVI) include swelling, venous eczema, pigmentation, lipodermatosclerosis and ulceration.
- The main area for venous change and ulceration is the medial calf "gaiter" area.
- The mechanisms involved are venous reflux, outflow obstruction and calf pump failure or a combination of these.
- Many cases (c. 50%) follow DVT when they are termed the post-thrombotic syndrome.
- Multi-layered compression bandaging is the gold standard for healing venous ulceration.
- Graduated compression stockings are used to maintain healing.
- All venous ulcer patients should be referred for a duplex scan.
- Those with superficial venous incompetence should be offered surgical intervention.
- Graduated compression is contraindicated in the presence of significant peripheral arterial disease.
- Venous reconstruction is rarely performed, but there remains a role for venous bypass surgery for deep venous obstruction.

- The use of deep venous angioplasty and stenting is increasing and has good results in selected patients.

Chronic Venous Insufficiency

Epidemiology

As with varicose veins, the prevalence of chronic venous insufficiency (CVI) is marginally greater in men (9% of the population aged between 18 and 64 years) compared to women (7% of the female population aged between 18 and 64 years) [1]. The prevalence increases with age. It is a major cause of leg ulcers and has significant economic implications both in lost working days and cost to the NHS.

Aetiology

The condition results from impaired venous return and causes elevated ambulatory venous pressure within the lower limbs. As a consequence of this elevated venous pressure, skin changes occur in the form of eczema, pigmentation, lipodermatosclerosis and ulceration. It is associated with lower limb oedema, varicose veins and chronic pain. There are a number of causes including venous reflux, venous obstruction and 'pump' failure of the calf muscle (Table 1).

The combination of normal venous anatomy, functional valves and calf muscle contraction during exercise is responsible for reducing venous pressure in the lower leg and encouraging venous return. These mechanisms are impaired by venous reflux (affecting either the superficial,

Table 1.   Aetiology of CVI.

Aetiology	Example
Superficial venous reflux	Long saphenous/short saphenous varicosities
Deep venous insufficiency	Valvular damage, e.g., post-DVT, congenital valve weakness
Venous outflow obstruction	Stenosis/occlusion, e.g., post-DVT, venous cannulation and external pressure (e.g., pelvic tumour)
Calf muscle pump failure	Immobility, obesity, prolonged sitting

deep or perforating venous systems), venous occlusions (e.g., DVT) or abnormal calf pump action. In practice, the cause of CVI is often multi-factorial due to a combination of venous valve failure and reflux, failure of the calf muscle pump, or deep venous outflow obstruction. Numerous causes exist for impaired calf muscle function and these range from neurological conditions to reduced mobility associated with morbid obesity. The relevance of perforator reflux remains a topic of debate and primary surgical treatment should be directed at the superficial system, with separate treatment of perforator reflux being reserved for resistant cases.

The mechanisms by which raised ambulatory venous pressure generates venous skin changes are not fully understood. The fibrin cuff hypothesis suggests that elevated pressure results in capillary damage leading to the deposition of fibrinogen which subsequently forms a fibrin cuff. This results in impaired oxygen transfer and the subsequent local ischaemia results in ulceration. The white cell trapping hypothesis suggests that the elevated venous pressure slows and halts the passage of large white cells through the capillaries. These become 'plugged' with white cells. These cells are activated and release proteolytic enzymes and free radicals causing local tissue damage and eventually ulcers. Both mechanisms probably coexist.

Clinical features

Patients with CVI complain of a variety of symptoms including swelling, itching, aching and heaviness. The symptoms tend to be exacerbated by prolonged standing and relieved by elevation. Initially, oedema is pitting, but with chronicity becomes non-pitting. The venous eczema causes pruritus, which stimulates scratching and subsequent skin trauma. This can be the precipitating event leading to ulceration. The most common site of ulceration is the distal medial calf. Pigmentation results from hemosiderin deposition and when accompanied by fibrosis results in lipodermatosclerosis. Varicose veins may be present and superficial reflux should always be excluded. A previous history of deep venous thrombosis is not uncommon and symptoms of venous claudication (pain and swelling exacerbated with exercise, requiring rest and elevation for relief of symptoms) suggest significant venous occlusion (iliofemoral veins).

Table 2.   The CEAP clinical classification.

C0	No visible or palpable signs of venous disease
C1	Telangiectasia or reticular veins
C2	Varicose veins
C3	Oedema
C4a	Pigmentation or eczema
C4b	Lipodermatosclerosis or atrophie blanche
C5	Healed venous ulcer
C6	Active venous ulcer

Classification

The most common classification system used for CVI is the CEAP classification. CEAP stands for Clinical, Etiological, Anatomical and Pathophysiological. The clinical part of CEAP is shown in Table 2.

Management of chronic venous insufficiency

In order to develop a management plan, a venous Duplex scan is usually the initial test carried out. This can identify sites of reflux in the superficial and deep systems and in cases of leg ulceration approximately one-third are due to deep reflux, one-third superficial reflux and one-third a mixture of deep and superficial. The presence of deep venous reflux in the popliteal vein is a marker for a high risk of ulcer recurrence. For more proximal disease such as lilac vein obstruction, MR or CT venography may be helpful and very occasionally direct venography or intravascular ultrasound (IVUS). Other tests, mostly for research purposes, include ambulatory venous pressure measurements where pressure in the long saphenous vein is measured directly and plethysmography tests such as air and strain-gauge plethysmography where leg volume on ankle movements is measured as a surrogate for venous function.

Non-operative management

Certain comorbidities known to be associated with the development of CVI such as obesity and immobility should ideally be improved. Leg elevation can reduce ankle venous pressure to 15 mmHg and should be encouraged. Bed rest and elevation above the level of the heart may be required for patients with ulceration resistant to other forms of treatment.

Most patients with CVI are treated with either compression stockings or dressings. These apply a graduated compression that decreases proximally. The compression improves venous blood flow in the deep venous system, reduces superficial venous pressures and may restore valve function. Multi-layered compression bandaging is the gold standard used to heal venous ulceration. Stockings are used to prevent recurrence. Below-knee compression stockings of 25–35 mmHg (Class 3) are sufficient for most patients with CVI, but stronger stockings are available for severe cases or lymphoedema as well as full leg stockings or tights (Table 3).

To be effective, graduated compression stockings need to be measured and fitted properly and patient compliance may also be a problem. Although usually safe, several adverse effects and complications, including allergic reaction and skin damage, have been reported. They are contraindicated in the presence of significant peripheral arterial disease (PAD). As about 10% of leg ulcers are mixed venous and arterial in origin, the ABI should be checked before graduated compression is used. If the ABPI is low investigations for occlusive arterial disease should be performed.

Operative treatment

Superficial venous surgery

The ESCHAR trial was a randomised trial involving 500 leg ulcers associated with isolated superficial incompetence and showed the 1-year

Table 3.   Classes of graduated compression stockings.

Class	Description	mmHg compression at ankle
Class 1	Light support	14–17 mmHg
Class 2	Medium support	18–24 mmHg
Class 3	Strong support	25–35 mmHg
Class 4	Severe CVI/lymphoedema	>35 mmHg

recurrence rate of leg ulceration to be reduced with combined superficial venous surgery and elastic compression (9% recurrence) compared to compression alone (38% recurrence) [2]. The initial healing rate was not affected. Superficial surgery is therefore recommended in patients with isolated superficial reflux and a history of ulceration.

Perforator surgery

Isolated perforator reflux is a rare cause of CVI and it is found usually in combination with other reflux either deep or superficial. There remains a debate regarding its benefits, as correction of other sites of superficial reflux is frequently associated with improvement in perforator reflux. In many cases, the incompetent perforators are simply acting as a re-entry site for refluxing blood back into the deep system. The use of minimally invasive superficial endoscopic perforator surgery (SEPS) is associated with less morbidity than direct surgery on the perforators, but is usually reserved for resistant ulceration.

Venous reconstruction

Venous reconstruction is usually reserved for patients with severe ulceration, and venous claudication and limb swelling that has not responded to compression and superficial/perforator surgery. In reality, it is rarely done. Reconstruction may be either in the form of a venous bypass or, less commonly, valvular reconstruction.

A variety of valvular reconstructive procedures have been described and include valvuloplasty (directly repairing the valve), valve transposition (for example, axillary vein valve to popliteal vein), vein wall plication (which brings the valve cusps together) and external banding with a Dacron or polytetrafluoroethane (PTFE) cuff (to produce a valve-like effect). These are technically difficult procedures, and no technique has yet become sufficiently reliable to be in routine use [3,4].

If the deep venous system is obstructed, then deep venous bypass surgery or endovascular recanalization may be of benefit. Venous bypass is usually reserved for patients who are severely symptomatic despite allowing sufficient time (at least 12 months) for superficial collaterals to develop. Causes of deep venous obstruction include previous DVT, malignant disease, retroperitoneal fibrosis and May–Thurner syndrome (compression of the left iliac vein behind the right iliac artery). Iliac vein obstruction that cannot be treated endovascularly can be treated with a Palma cross-over operation. Using the contralateral long saphenous vein, a bypass is completed by anastomosing the distal end to the common femoral or profunda veins in the affected limb. In the absence of a suitable long saphenous vein, a prosthetic conduit may be considered, but patency rates are poor. Deep thigh vein occlusion can be treated with a sapheno-popliteal vein bypass (May–Husni operation). Again, the long saphenous vein is the conduit of choice. Reconstructive surgery is contraindicated in early deep vein thrombosis, arterial disease and thrombophilias. In order to improve patency rates, venous bypass is often combined with the fashioning of a temporary arteriovenous fistula to maintain high flow and use of anticoagulants or antiplatelets. Prosthetic venous bypass has extremely poor long-term patency.

Endovascular treatment of CVI

The techniques of endovenous catheter ablation (RFA, EVLT, MOCA and CAE) and foam sclerotherapy (see Chapter 15) can also be used for treatment of the superficial venous system in CVI.

Recent advancements in endovascular techniques have led to deep venous balloon angioplasty and stenting becoming more widely used for deep venous outflow obstruction. This treatment has been shown to be efficient in the reduction of venous hypertension and the prevention of post-thrombotic syndrome (PTS) and ulcer occurrence/recurrence [5]. Dedicated venous stents with high radial force should be used to ensure long-term patency and prevent stent-related complications such as stent fracture and migration. This promising treatment has been shown to have a good mid-term outcome with an 88% 5-year patency. Clinical relief of pain ranged from 86% to 94% and relief from swelling ranged from 66% to 89%, 58% to 89% of venous ulcers healed [6]. Long-term patency results are not known however and have not been compared directly with surgery.

Venous Leg Ulcers

Pure venous ulceration accounts for approximately 70% of chronic leg ulceration (Table 4). However, a significant number of ulcers (c. 10%) are of mixed arterial and venous aetiology. The ABI should be measured before using compression and significant arterial disease should be treated. Neoplastic disease can be a cause of chronic ulceration and may occur in long-standing ulcers (squamous cell carcinoma, Marjolin's ulcers). Other important causes are vasculitis and rheumatoid arthritis. In ulcers resistant to healing, biopsy needs to be considered and a blood and clinical screen for vasculitis carried out. Most venous ulcers occur in the medial 'gaiter' area of the leg (i.e., the area extending from just above the ankle to the mid-calf) which is thought to be due to the presence of medial calf perforators transmitting deeper raised venous pressure to the surface.

In addition to the management of the underlying venous disease, consideration should be given to appropriate skin dressings,

Table 4.   Causes of chronic leg ulcers.

Aetiology	%	Characteristics
Venous	70	Medial lower calf, shallow, irregular margins, granulating base. Oedema and exudate, eczema, pigmentation, lipodermatosclerosis, varicose veins.
Arterial	5–10	Painful, below ankle distal, especially toes, small, dry base. Associated intermittent claudication/rest pain.
Mixed arterial and venous	10–15	Combined features of venous and arterial disease.
Vasculitis	1–2	Associated with rheumatoid arthritis or other vasculitis syndromes. Purpuric or other rashes. Vasculitis signs away from legs, e.g., nail-fold infarcts or splinter haemorrhages. Vasculitic leg ulcers will usually be multiple, necrotic, deep and have an atypical distribution.
Malignancy	<1	Raised lesion. Basal cell carcinoma, squamous cell carcinoma, melanoma (pigmented).
Neuropathic	1–2	Common in diabetes, wet, deep, sharp borders on pressure points. Often on sole of foot. Associated neuropathy. In diabetics, necrobiosis lipoidica may be present and can also ulcerate.

emollients and nutritional supplements (vitamins and trace elements). Adjunctive surgical techniques that may facilitate wound healing should be considered, e.g., wound debridement and skin grafts. Various techniques to facilitate debridement exist and range from topical applications including larval therapy to surgical debridement and negative-pressure wound therapy. Skin grafting may be occasionally considered to accelerate healing. The graft is usually a split skin graft or pinch grafts.

The mainstay of treatment of venous leg ulcers is multi-layer graduated compression bandaging. Various systems are available and for venous ulcers, a compression kit should be chosen that gives 35–40 mmHg at the ankle, graduating to 17–20 mmHg under the knee. Appropriately trained nurses should apply compression. Venous ulcers often recur if the underlying CVI is not corrected and most patients should be referred for venous Duplex assessment to look for correctable reflux. The majority should also be fitted for below knee compression hosiery to wear on a permanent basis. There is increasing interest in using foam sclerotherapy of the subulcer venous plexus to aid healing despite the fact that the ESCHAR trial of superficial venous surgery showed no effect on ulcer healing rates although recurrence was reduced.

Post-thrombotic Syndrome

After a deep venous thrombosis, a number of patients will develop CVI. This is frequently referred to as the post-thrombotic syndrome (PTS). In patients with symptomatic DVT, the reported incidence of PTS is 20–50%, with the onset of symptoms typically occurring within the first 2 years of the initial thrombotic episode. Mild disease is seen in up to one-third of patients whilst severe disease may affect one in 10 patients. The risk is increased with more proximal venous thrombosis.

The underlying mechanism is of elevated ambulatory venous pressure. As a consequence of valvular reflux, outflow obstruction and calf muscle dysfunction ambulatory venous pressure fails to undergo the normal physiological reduction seen during walking. A normal pressure drop of 50% can be seen during ambulation compared to standing. In CVI, these pressures may actually rise and can result in venous claudication.

The early management of DVT is aimed at preventing propagation of the thrombosis by anticoagulation.

If detected early, preferably within 14 days, proximal/iliofemoral DVTs may be treated with thrombolysis with the aim of restoring venous patency and minimising the damage to venous valves (7). Long-term treatment includes compression stockings and all patients are encouraged to preserve calf muscle function with regular exercise.

Examination of the affected limb in PTS may reveal limb swelling and pigmentation secondary to hemosiderin deposition, telangiectasia, venous eczema and lipodermatosclerosis as well as varicose veins and ulcers or scarring from healed ulcers.

PTS can be assessed using the Villalta scale, which is specific for PTS. It combines five subjective symptoms and six objective clinical signs (Table 5). Points are assigned to each category according to severity, ranging from 0 for not present to 3 for severe. A Villalta score of 5 or more, or the existence of a venous ulcer supports the diagnosis of PTS. A score of 5–9 represents mild disease, 10–14 moderate disease, and greater than 15 indicates severe disease. The presence of a venous ulcer

Table 5.   Villalta scale for PTS

Subjective symptoms

    Pain

    Cramps

    Heaviness

    Paraesthesia

    Pruritus

Objective clinical signs

    Pre-tibial oedema

    Hyperpigmentation

    Venous ectasia/varicose veins

    Skin induration

    Redness

    Pain during calf compression

Venous ulceration

automatically classifies the condition as severe, regardless of the contribution from other symptoms and signs (8).

References

1. Evans CJ, Fowkes FG, Ruckley CV, Lee AJ. Prevalence of varicose veins and chronic venous insufficiency in men and women in the general population: Edinburgh Vein Study. *J Epidemiol Community Health* 1999;53:149–153.
2. Gohel MS, Barwell JR, Taylor M, Chant T, Foy C, Earnshaw JJ, Heather BP, Mitchell DC, Whyman MR, Poskitt KR. Long term results of compression therapy alone versus compression plus surgery in chronic venous ulceration (ESCHAR): Randomised controlled trial. *BMJ* 2007;335:83.
3. Gloviczki P, Kalra M, Duncan AA, Oderich GS, Vrtiska TJ, Bower TC. Open and hybrid deep vein reconstructions: To do or not to do? *Phlebology* 2012; 27:103–106.
4. Caggiati A, Caggiati L. Surgery of venous valve. *Rev Vasc Med* 2013;1:15–23.
5. Raju S. Treatment of iliac-caval outflow obstruction. *Seminars in Vascular Surgery* 28;1:47–53.
6. Raju S, Darcey R, Neglén P. Unexpected major role for venous stenting in deep reflux disease. *J Vasc Surg* 2010;51(2):401–408, ISSN 0741-5214.
7. Watson L, Broderick C, Armon MP. Thrombolysis for acute deep vein thrombosis. *Cochrane Database Syst Rev* 2014;1:CD002783.
8. Soosainathan A, Moore HM, Gohel MS, Davies AH. Scoring systems for the post-thrombotic syndrome. *J Vasc Surg* 2013;57:254–261.

Chapter 22

Management and Prevention of Venous Thromboembolism

Omar Ashour and Vish Bhattacharya

Key Points

- Deep vein thrombosis (DVT) and pulmonary embolism (PE) are the leading causes of preventable in-patient mortality following surgery.
- Many DVTs are asymptomatic, but are still a risk for PE.
- Validated clinical prediction rules should be used to estimate the pre-test probability of venous thromboembolism (VTE), e.g., Wells score.
- D-dimer level measurements are useful screening tests.
- Ultrasonography is the current first-line imaging investigation for DVT.
- Newer anticoagulants such as rivaroxaban and dabigatran are now being used for prophylaxis and treatment of VTE.
- Inferior vena caval filters (IVCFs) should be used when anticoagulation is contraindicated or further VTE occurs despite adequate anticoagulation.
- DVT can lead to post-thrombotic syndrome (PTS) in the longer term.
- Thrombolysis should be considered in younger, fitter patients with ileofemoral DVT to reduce PTS risk.

Background

Deep vein thrombosis (DVT) and pulmonary embolism (PE), are manifestations of a single disease process known as venous thromboembolism (VTE) — and together represent the leading causes of preventable mortality after hospital admission and surgery. Hospital acquired VTE is defined as VTE happening within 90 days of a hospital admission.

Epidemiology

Many DVTs are asymptomatic and almost half of all fatal cases of PE are associated with asymptomatic DVTs [1]. It has an annual incidence of 1 in 1000 people and has an annual mortality of 14.6%.

DVT is one of the most prevalent medical problems today. Early recognition and appropriate treatment of DVT and its complications is vital. The inconsistent use of prophylactic measures for VTE in hospital patients has been widely reported. A UK survey suggested that 71% of patients assessed to be at medium or high risk of developing DVT did not receive any form of mechanical or pharmacological VTE prophylaxis. In the NHS, risk assessment for VTE and appropriate prophylaxis have now become the norm.

Pathophysiology

DVT formation and risk is multifactorial with interaction between hereditary and acquired risk factors. The Virchow triad (i.e., venous stasis, hypercoagulable state, vessel wall injury) continues to serve as the unifying concept in the pathogenesis of DVT. However, the significance of interplay between the elements of Virchow's triad and environmental or acquired risk factors is also important. The formation, propagation and dissolution of venous thrombi represent a balance between thrombogenesis and the body's protective mechanisms, specifically the circulating inhibitors of coagulating and fibrinolytic systems. Several risk factors in combination are usually needed for thrombosis to develop and the risk is cumulative.

Inherent hypercoagulable states include thrombophilias, which can be primary or secondary. They probably account for 5–10% of VTE events, but screening for them is not done routinely as initial management will not be affected. Three naturally occurring anticoagulant mechanisms exist to prevent inadvertent activation of the clotting process. These include antithrombin III (AT III), protein C and thrombomodulin protein S, and the tissue factor inhibition pathways.

Congenital thrombophilias include conditions such as AT III deficiency, protein C and protein S deficiency. Antiphospholipid syndrome is the most common cause of acquired thrombophilia and is considered a disorder of the immune system. It is characterised by the combination of antiphospholipid antibodies, such as lupus anticoagulant, anticardiolipin antibodies or β2-glycoprotein I. This syndrome is usually secondary to cancer or an autoimmune condition such as systemic lupus erythematosis. More recently, the factor V Leiden mutation and the prothrombin G20210 mutation have been shown to carry an increased risk of venous thrombosis. Factor V Leiden is a mutation that results in a form of factor Va that resists degradation by activated protein C, leading to a hypercoagulable state. It is found in 3–5% of healthy individuals in the western world and in about 20–30% of patients with venous thrombosis. In the setting of venous stasis, these factors are allowed to accumulate in thrombosis-prone sites, where mechanical vessel injury has occurred, stimulating the endothelium to become prothrombotic [1,2].

Clinical Features of DVT

Traditional clinical features such as swollen tender calf and venous distension are unreliable and are present in less than 50% of patients. No single physical finding or combination of symptoms and signs is sufficiently accurate to establish the diagnosis of DVT, but you should know about them. Homan's sign, which is pain on dorsiflexion of the affected foot, is specific but insensitive and is rare. Phlegmasia alba dolens (phlegmasia = inflammation, alba = white, dolens = painful) was originally used to describe massive iliofemoral venous thrombosis and associated arterial spasm. The affected extremity is often pale with poor or even absent distal pulses. The physical findings may suggest acute arterial occlusion, but the presence of swelling, petechiae and distended superficial veins point to a DVT.

In rare cases, the leg is cyanotic from extensive DVT where thrombosis extends into the collateral circulation, resulting in severe venous congestion. This ischaemic form of venous occlusion was originally described as phlegmasia cerulean dolens or painful blue inflammation. The leg is usually markedly oedematous, painful and cyanotic. Petechiae are often present and the viability of the limb maybe threatened.

Calf vein thrombi are usually benign unless there is propagation into the proximal veins which occurs untreated in about 1 in 6 cases. Thrombi in the proximal veins can result in PE in 40–50% of cases, and isolated calf vein DVTs cause PE in about 15% of cases. When symptomatic DVT is diagnosed, approximately 40% of patients have had a silent PE and 4% of individuals treated for DVT develop symptomatic PE. Almost 1% of postoperative hospitalised patients develop PE. These statistics highlight the importance of prevention of this complication.

Post-thrombotic syndrome (PTS) can appear up to several years after an episode of DVT, manifesting as chronic leg swelling, pain, varicose veins, venous eczema, pigmentation and venous ulcers. It is graded using the Vilalta score. It occurs because of damage to deep venous valves, resulting in chronic venous hypertension. It affects up to 40% of patients after DVT and is more common after extensive iliofemoral DVT. Traditionally, it has been believed that long-term use of graduated compression stockings after DVT can reduce the incidence of PTS although that has not been clearly shown in randomised trials. Graduated compression is however the mainstay for treatment of established PTS (Table 1).

VTE Risk Assessment

Risk assessment, ideally both for VTE risk and bleeding risk, allows identification of cases at risk and institution of appropriate prophylactic measures. In the UK NHS in line with NICE guidance the Department of Health risk assessment tool is usually used (Ref to online DOH tool). An

Table 1.   Villalta PTS score [2].

Clinical feature	None	Mild	Moderate	Severe
Syndrome				
Pain	0	1	2	3
Cramps	0	1	2	3
Heaviness	0	1	2	3
Paresthesia	0	1	2	3
Pruritus	0	1	2	3
Signs				
Pretibial oedema	0	1	2	3
Indurated skin	0	1	2	3
Hyperpigmentation	0	1	2	3
Erythema	0	1	2	3
Venous ectasia	0	1	2	3
Pain on calf compression	0	1	2	3
Venous ulcer	Absent or present			

Notes: Mild PTS: 5–9 points; moderate PTS: 10–14 points; severe PTS: $\geq$ 15 points or the presence of venous ulceration.

alternative is the Caprini score developed in the USA, which is a points-based score allowing categorisation into low, moderate, high and very high risk groups.

Surgical patients are at increased risk of VTE if they meet one of the following criteria in the Department of Health risk assessment score (NICE guidelines January 2010, last updated June 2015) [4,5].

- Surgical procedure with a total anaesthetic and surgical time of more than 90 min or 60 min if the surgery involves the pelvis or lower limb.
- Acute surgical admission with inflammatory or intra-abdominal condition.
- Expected significant reduction in mobility.
- One or more of the risk factors noted in Table 2.

Table 2.   Patient-related risk factors for VTE.

Active cancer or cancer treatment (known or undiagnosed)

Age over 60

Male sex

Heart failure

Severe infection

Critical care admission

Dehydration

Known thrombophilia (acquired or familial)

Obesity with a BMI over 30 kg m^{-1}

Personal history or first-degree relative with a history of VTE

Smoking

Chronic low-grade injury to the vascular wall (for example from vasculitis)

Significant trauma or direct trauma to a vein, e.g., IV cannulation

Use of hormone replacement therapy

Varicose veins +/− phlebitis

Pregnancy and the postpartum period

Diagnosis of VTE

VTE is under-diagnosed and most cases of fatal PE are only diagnosed at autopsy. Diagnosis depends on a high level of clinical suspicion and the presence of risk factors that prompt diagnostic study. As the presentation is often non-specific, coupled with the serious consequences of missing the diagnosis, VTE must be excluded whenever it is a feasible differential diagnosis. Since the prevalence of the disease is 15–30% in the population at clinical risk, a widely applicable (inexpensive and simple) screening/diagnostic test is required. The clinical history, physical examination and assessment of risk factors should be used to determine who requires further objective diagnostic testing.

Diagnostic testing for acute DVT has changed considerably over the past two decades and has been the subject of numerous modes of research, resulting in dynamically changing national guidelines. Invasive tests such as conventional venous angiography or fibrinogen uptake test have now been replaced by duplex/compression ultrasonography and

D-dimer assay in an algorithm that starts with a clinical probability score. Duplex is 100% sensitive in detecting proximal thrombus, but is less so for calf vein thrombi [2,3].

Clinical probability score for assessing DVT likelihood

The two-level DVT Wells score incorporates risk factors, clinical signs, and the presence or absence of alternative diagnoses (as shown in Table 3) to estimate the clinical probability of DVT. The model enables physicians to reliably stratify their patients into *likely* or *unlikely* risk categories. Combining this with the results of objective testing greatly simplifies the clinical work-up of patients with suspected DVT. There is a similar clinical probability score for suspected PE.

D-dimers in DVT

Thrombus formation is normally followed by an immediate fibrinolytic response. The resultant generation of plasmin causes the release of fibrin

Table 3.   Wells clinical score for DVT.

Clinical parameter score	Score
Active cancer (treatment ongoing, or within 6 months or palliative)	+1
Paralysis or recent plaster immobilisation of the lower extremities	+1
Recently bedridden for >3 days or major surgery <4 weeks	+1
Localised tenderness along the distribution of the deep venous system	+1
Entire leg swelling	+1
Calf swelling >3 cm compared to the asymptomatic leg	+1
Pitting oedema (greater in the symptomatic leg)	+1
Previous DVT documented	+1
Collateral superficial veins (non-varicose)	+1
Alternative diagnosis (as likely or greater than that of DVT)	−2
Clinical probability simplified score	
DVT likely	2 points or more
DVT unlikely	1 point or less

degradation products (predominantly containing D-dimer) into the circulation [3]. A negative D-dimer test effectively rules out VTE and the request for unnecessary ultrasound scans is therefore reduced. It should be noted that whilst a positive result can indicate thrombosis, there may be other causes of a raised D-dimer including liver disease, inflammation, malignancy, pregnancy, trauma and recent surgery.

The sequential use of a clinical score, rapid quantitative D-dimer test, and compression/duplex ultrasonography appears to be a safe and cost-effective diagnostic work-up for DVT. More recently, a NICE guidance update advocated using D-dimer tests with reference to the use of *age-adjusted D-dimer intervals* to reduce the need for further imaging tests and prevent the continuation of treatment. An algorithm combining the use of a clinical prediction score and a D-dimer assay is shown in Fig. 1 [2,3,6,7]. Similar algorithms exist for the diagnosis of PE based on clinical risk prediction and D-dimer but using CT-pulmonary angiography as the imaging modality of choice.

Ultrasonography in DVT

Ultrasonography has the advantage over venography of being non-invasive and has been shown to have a high sensitivity and specificity for proximal DVT. Figure 2 shows a clot in the common femoral vein.

Calf vein DVTs which do not extend proximally, rarely lead to clinically significant emboli, but in those that do, the risk of PE is significant. This has led to two different ultrasound strategies for DVT diagnosis. Many clinicians deliberately restrict ultrasound to only look at the proximal veins and then perform a repeat test 1 week later in selected patients. The first test will detect any proximal thrombosis, a calf vein thrombus will remain undetected, but a repeat scan 1 week later will pick up the clinically important ones that have extended. A second strategy is to scan the whole leg (proximal and calf veins). This means that no repeat ultrasound is required although it does subject more patients to anticoagulation. Both strategies are acceptable and safe. Recent NICE guidance update (2014) suggest that there may be an indication for whole-leg ultrasound scan in circumstances where a serial

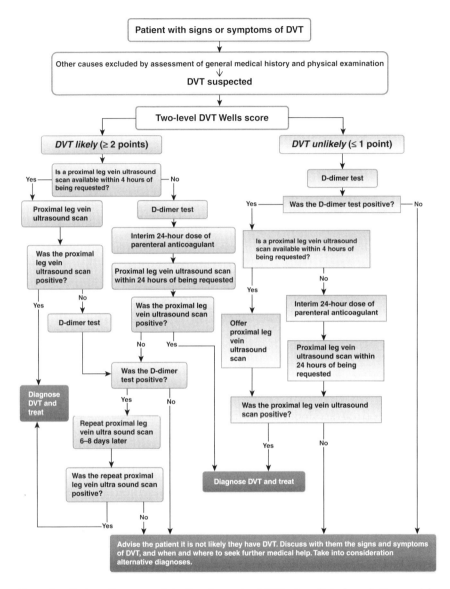

Figure 1.   Systematic approach to the diagnosis of DVT using clinical prediction models, D-dimer assays, and ultrasound [5].

ultrasound is not available, when a repeat scan would be very difficult to arrange or in patients receiving an anticoagulant prior to a D-dimer test [2,5].

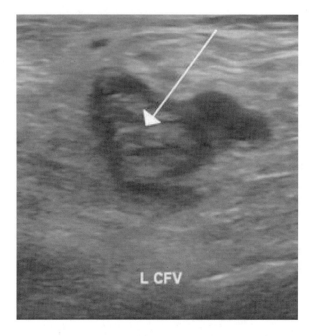

Figure 2.   Ultrasound showing blood clot in left common femoral vein.

Compression and duplex ultrasonography

Compression ultrasound consists of using gentle probe pressure to try and compress the venous lumen. If no residual lumen is observed the vein is considered to be fully compressible, which indicates the absence of DVT. Duplex ultrasonography is similar, but in addition a Doppler signal is used to determine blood flow characteristics. When the phasic (with respiration) pattern of venous blood flow is absent venous outflow obstruction is diagnosed. Colour-flow detail duplex imaging can augment the images further [5].

Thrombophilia testing

These are tests to look for heritable thrombophilias as described earlier in this chapter, especially the crucial antiphospholipid antibodies, which can be performed at specialist centres through a panel of diag-nostic blood tests. Thrombophilia testing should be considered for antiphospholipid antibodies in patients who have had unprovoked VTE +/− have a first-degree relative who has had VTE *and* if anticoagulation treatment is planned to stop. Testing might be useful in the finding of a thrombophilia that increases the risk of VTE recurrence, dictating long-term rather than short-term anticoagulation, and action can be taken to reduce the risk of VTE in a family member. Otherwise, routine testing is not recommended and in addition testing while the patient is already on anticoagulants is usually unhelpful [5].

Investigations for cancer in VTE patients

Tumours produce several proteins, such as tissue factor, which enable the tumour cells to invade and metastasize. Tissue factor simultaneously activates the coagulation cascade leading to VTE.

Investigating patients presenting with a VTE for cancer in unprovoked cases, or "cancer screening", is a concept that is controversial. NICE guidance states that patients diagnosed with unprovoked VTE who are *not* already known to have cancer should be initially investigated with a chest X-ray, full blood count, serum calcium, liver function tests and urinalysis. In addition, any patients >40 years of age should go on receive computed tomography (CT) scans (and mammograms in females) to look for cancer. This advice was based on series suggesting an incidence of about 10% of occult cancer, however, more recent studies suggest a lower incidence of about 3% which may not make such screening cost-effective [5].

Information and assessment

- All surgical patients should be assessed to identify their risk factors for VTE (Table 1), ideally prior to admission.
- They should be given verbal and written information, before surgery, about VTE, its risks, treatment, and the effectiveness of prophylaxis. In line with NICE guidance, this should include information on:
  - o how to use anticoagulants,
  - o duration of anticoagulant treatment,
  - o possible side effects of anticoagulant treatment and how to act on them,

- the effects of other medications, foods and alcohol on oral antico-agulation treatment ,
- monitoring their treatment,
- how anticoagulants may affect their dental treatment,
- taking anticoagulants in family planning,
- how anticoagulants may affect activities such as sports and travel,
- when and how to seek medical help.
- They should be informed that the immobility associated with pro-longed travel in the weeks before or after surgery may increase the risk of DVT.
- Oestrogen containing oral contraceptive should be stopped 4 weeks before elective surgery although there is no added risk with proges-terone only pills, implants or injections.
- Patients should be given verbal and written information on the signs and symptoms of DVT and PE, and the correct use of prophylaxis at home as part of their discharge plan if extended prophylaxis is required.
- Patients should be provided with an "anticoagulant information book-let", an "anticoagulant alert card" and be advised to carry the alert card with them at all times.
- Patients should be advised about the correct application and use of below-knee graduated compression stockings, how long they should be worn and when they should be replaced.
- Heparins of animal origin may be of concern to some patients — so they must be advised about that and alternatives provided if applica-ble [4,5].

Prophylaxis Against DVT [4,5]

NICE guidelines 2010 (updated 2015) made recommendations on assessing and reducing the risk of VTE in hospital inpatients. It offers guidance on the most clinically and cost-effective measures for VTE prophylaxis. The recommendations take into account the potential risks/side effects of the various options for prophylaxis as well as patient preferences. Several options for prophylaxis are summarised in Table 4.

Table 4.   Methods of VTE prophylaxis [4,5].

• General measures
Early mobilisation
Leg exercises
Hydration
• Mechanical methods
Antiemobolism stockings (thigh or knee length)
Foot impulse devices
Intermittent pneumatic compression devices (thigh or knee)
• Pharmacological methods
Heparin
(i) unfractionated
(ii) low molecular weight
Direct thrombin inhibitors
(i) dabigatran
(ii) rivaroxaban
Synthetic pentasaccharides (SP)
(i) fondaparinux
Anticoagulants, e.g., warfarin
Antiplatelet agents, e.g., aspirin, clopidogrel (not usually used alone for VTE prophylaxis)
• Vena caval fllters

- VTE prophylaxis for patients undergoing gastrointestinal, gynaecological, urological, vascular or thoracic surgery and who are assessed to be at risk of VTE should be started on mechanical prophylaxis at admission with antiembolism stockings (AES), foot impulse devices or intermittent pneumatic compression devices (if not contraindicated).
- Regional anaesthesia should always be considered as it carries a lower risk of VTE than general anaesthesia.
- Clinicians should use caution and clinical judgement when applying AES over venous ulcers or wounds. Contraindications to AES include the following:
  - suspected or proven peripheral arterial disease (PAD),
  - peripheral arterial bypass grafting,

- o peripheral neuropathy,
- o any local conditions in which stockings may cause damage, for example fragile "tissue paper" skin, dermatitis, gangrene or recent skin graft,
- o known allergy to material of manufacture,
- o cardiac failure,
- o severe leg oedema or pulmonary oedema from congestive heart failure,
- o unusual leg size or shape,
- o major limb deformity preventing correct fit.
- The stocking compression profile should be equivalent to the Sigel profile; approximately 18 mmHg at the ankle, 14 mmHg at the mid-calf and 8 mmHg at the upper thigh — in line with current British standards. These figures are based on Sigels work in 1975 when he showed that optimal compression for elastic stockings to be used by hospitalised patients confined to bed should be 18 to 8 mmHg (ankle to mid-thigh). At this compression, average femoral vein blood flow velocity is increased significantly. Graduated compression produced a greater femoral vein flow velocity than uniform compression of the lower limb.
- Pharmacological VTE prophylaxis for patients who have low risk of major bleeding should include fondaparinux sodium, LMWH or UFH (for patients with severe renal impairment or established renal failure). This should be continued until the patient no longer has significantly reduced mobility, generally for 5–7 days.
- Similar principles are applied in day surgery cases.
- NICE guidelines stipulate that in elective hip/knee replacement surgery and hip fractures, in addition to mechanical prophylaxis as stated above, VTE prophylaxis can be achieved with newer anticoagulants, such as:
  - o dabigatran etexilate, starting 1–4 h after surgery,
  - o fondaparinux sodium, starting 6 h after surgical closure,
  - o LMWH, starting 6–12 h after surgery,
  - o rivaroxaban, starting 6–10 h after surgery,
  - o UFH (for patients with severe renal impairment), starting 6–12 h after surgery.

- Pharmacological VTE prophylaxis for orthopaedic patients should be continued for 10–14 days in elective joint replacement surgery (knee replacement) and 28–35 days in traumatic orthopaedic surgery (e.g., hip fractures).
- Patients who are already on antiplatelet agents and who are at increased risk of VTE should have pharmacological prophylaxis if the risk of VTE outweighs the risk of bleeding. Conversely, if the risk of bleeding is higher, then mechanical prophylaxis should be used.
- If patients are on vitamin K antagonists (VKAs) and are within therapeutic range, no prophylaxis is required provided anticoagulant therapy is continued.
- When preparing patients for discharge, patients and their families/carers should be offered verbal and written information regarding their VTE prophylaxis as described previously in this chapter with specific advice and guidance to those patients who are discharged with AES and/or pharmacological prophylaxis. For example, this includes instructions for use, establishing appropriate support at home and leaving a point of contact if there is any concern. GPs must be made aware that their patients have been discharged with VTE prophylaxis.

Treatment of DVT

General principles

The primary objectives in DVT treatment are to prevent PE, reduce morbidity and prevent or minimise the risk of developing post-phlebitic syndrome. Because of the risk of proximal propagation with the potential risk of PE or PTS most authors believe that all DVTs should be treated. Anticoagulation remains the mainstay of treatment for DVT since the introduction of heparin in the 1930s. This section looks at the pharmacological management of VTE, strategies for continuing anticoagulation and the optimal length of time for treatment. The same classes of agents and doses are used for the treatment of PE and DVT.

In the initial treatment of acute DVT, it is important that a therapeutic level of anticoagulation is achieved quickly. Current guidelines stipulate that UFH, LMWH and fondaparinux are the only products with marketing authorisation in the UK for the *initial* treatment of VTE. All are injectable products, which achieve anticoagulation rapidly compared to VKAs, e.g., warfarin, which may take days to become effective [2].

The management of VTE has, in recent years, seen a paradigm shift from the use of traditional anticoagulants (LMWH overlapping with and followed by a VKA) to non-VKA oral anticoagulants (NOACs)/direct oral anticoagulants (DOACs). These terms are interchangeable. These classes of agents, encompassing direct factor Xa inhibitors and direct thrombin inhibitors have shown non-inferior efficacy and better safety to standard of care in randomised controlled trials (RCTs) [8].

Anticoagulation options for VTE include UFH, LMWH, fondaparinux and NOACs. Thrombolytic therapy is reserved for massive PE or extensive DVT.

One of the most recognised treatment regimens for the treatment of DVT is anticoagulation with heparin or LMWH followed by full anticoagulation with oral warfarin for 3–6 months. Warfarin therapy is overlapped with heparin for 4–5 days until the international normalised ratio (INR) is therapeutically elevated to 2–3.

The choice of anticoagulants, initial approach and duration of treatment are topics that have all been the subject of much speculation in recent years and there have been several important breakthroughs. One of the most significant were the results of the EINSTEIN [9] program which consisted of three randomised trials of rivaroxaban: one for the treatment of acute DVT, one for the treatment of acute PE and one for continued treatment in patients who have received treatment for acute VTE. There have been several pooled analyses of the EINSTEIN randomised studies which have advocated the use of rivaroxaban. As a result of that, the use of rivaroxaban has been approved for treatment of acute VTE and secondary prevention of recurrent VTE [9–11].

A single-drug approach with rivaroxaban resulted in similar efficacy to standard therapy and was associated with a *significantly* lower rate of major bleeding. It was found to be a safe and effective alternative to standard anticoagulation therapy in a broad range of patients, including high-risk groups (e.g., fragile patients, cancer patients, and patients with a large clot) [8–11]. Moreover, extended prophylaxis with single therapy reduced the incidence of symptomatic recurrent VTE to a greater extent than placebo in the EINSTEIN-Extension trial. Other studies have even shown favourable outcomes for rivaroxaban in terms of comparative hospital length of stay and efficacy in prophylaxis/treating VTE in patients with active cancer [12].

Duration of anticoagulation

Risk of recurrence determines the duration of anticoagulation following an episode of DVT/PE. These include the presence of reversible risk factors, non-reversible risk factors and no risk factors (idiopathic or unprovoked DVT). It is also influenced by the risk of bleeding and by patient preference. For the first episode of provoked DVT, patients should be treated for 3–6 months (e.g., proximal DVT due to reversible risk factors). Long-term anticoagulation is definitely indicated for patients with recurrent venous thrombosis and/or persistent or irreversible risk factors. Patients with non-reversible risk factors, such as malignancy and certain inherited thrombophilias with a strong family history of VTE will also require lifelong anticoagulation. The use of serial D-dimer measurements in clinical practice for the identification of VTE patients in whom anticoagulation can be safely discontinued has been evaluated, but is not yet recommended in routine practice [13].

Unfractionated heparin (UFH) and low molecular weight heparin (LMWH)

Heparin products used in the treatment of DVT include UFH and LMWH. UFH was the standard of care until the introduction of LMWH. Heparin prevents extension of the thrombus and has been shown to significantly reduce, but not eliminate, PE and recurrent thrombosis. The primary reason for this is that heparin has no effect on pre-existing non-adherent thrombus. It does not affect the size of existing thrombus and has no intrinsic thrombolytic activity. Heparin is a heterogeneous mixture of polysaccharide fragments with varying molecular weights. The key unit is a pentasaccharide sequence that is responsible for binding to AT III to inhibit thrombin. Heparin also activates the plasma protein heparin cofactor II, which inactivates thrombin. At higher concentrations it also binds to factor IXa, resulting in the modulation of factor Xa generation [2,4,5].

When IV UFH is initiated for DVT, the goal is to achieve and maintain an elevated activated partial thromboplastin time (aPTT) of at least 1.5 times control. After an initial bolus of 80 U kg^{-1}, a constant maintenance infusion of 18 U kg^{-1} is initiated. The aPTT is checked 6 h after the bolus and adjusted accordingly. The aPTT is checked every 6 h until two successive aPTTs are therapeutic. Thereafter, the aPTT, the haematocrit level and platelet count are monitored every 24 h. Heparin has a relatively short half-life of about 60–90 min and, therefore, the anticoagulant effect of therapeutic doses of heparin will mostly be eliminated at 3–4 h after termination of continuous intravenous administration. Protamine sulfate can be administered for a more immediate neutralisation of heparin. One of the complications of UFH use is heparin induced thrombocytopenia (HIT).

Overall, there is evidence to suggest that LMWH has more favourable outcomes than UFH, in both benefits and harms from treatment. There were fewer deaths and recurrent VTE with LMWH compared to UFH, and also less major bleeding and it is associated with a lower incidence of HIT. UFH is still preferred in patients with renal impairment. LMWH is prepared by selectively treating UFH to isolate the low-molecular-weight (<9000 Da) fragments. Its activity is measured in units of factor X inactivation, and monitoring of the aPTT is not required. The dose is weight adjusted. LMWH is administrated subcutaneously (SC), and its half-life permits single- or twice-daily dosing.

Acute DVT may be treated in an outpatient setting with LMWH. Patients with low-risk PE may be safely discharged early from hospital or receive only outpatient treatment with LMWH, followed by VKAs, although single-agent therapy with DOACs may be preferred (as discussed earlier in this chapter) [4,5,7].

Indirect factor Xa inhibitors (fondaparinux)

A recent further refinement of the heparin molecule is fondaparinux, a synthetic form of the pentasaccharide sequence of heparin that binds to antithrombin. It acts as a selective potent, indirect antithrombin-dependent inhibitor of factor Xa. It is administered once a day via SC injection and does not require laboratory monitoring. In recent years, fondaparinux has been shown to demonstrate good anticoagulative effect in clinical trials. Three types of fondaparinux are available: short-acting fonda-parinux, long-acting idraparinux and idrabiotaparinux (latter two not licensed for use in DVT). Pentasaccharides are not associated with HIT (like the other heparins) and are better tolerated than UFH, LMWH and warfarin. Low to moderate quality evidence shows that fondaparinux is more effective for short-term VTE, prevention when compared with LMWH. It can reduce total VTE, but does not demonstrate a reduction in deaths when compared with LMWH. A recent Cochrane review (2016) [14] showed that fondaparinux is effective for short-term prevention of VTE when compared with placebo. However, at the same time, moderate to high quality evidence shows that fondaparinux increases major bleeding when compared with placebo and LMWH. Despite its advantages, it is not recommended for patients with renal failure and has limited use due to its parenteral route of administration and lack of an antidote [4,5].

Direct factor Xa inhibitors

Factor Xa inhibitors include rivaroxaban and apixaban. Rivaroxaban is well tolerated, has high bioavailability and predictable pharmacokinetics and is orally available. It does not require dose adjustments and laboratory monitoring. The RECORD trials (four multi-centre double blind trials compared the efficacy of rivaroxaban compared to enoxaparin for the prevention of VTE following hip and knee replacements) showed significant reduction in primary efficacy end points (DVT, PE or death from all causes). As discussed previously, data from pooled analyses of the EINSTEIN studies showed that a dose of 15 mg twice daily for the first 3 weeks, followed by 20 mg once daily thereafter, without the need for laboratory monitoring, may provide an effective, safe, single-drug approach to the initial and continued treatment of venous thrombosis [4,5,15].

The AMPLIFY trial demonstrated that apixaban significantly reduced all-cause hospitalisations vs. enoxaparin/warfarin, and shortened the length of hospital stay in patients with acute VTE. It was also deemed a convenient option for cancer patients with VTE. Until recently, there were no approved drug-specific reversal agents for the DOACs. A number of drugs are currently being evaluated [16,17].

Direct thrombin inhibitors

Dabigatran and ximelagatran are a new class of drugs that act by binding directly to thrombin. There is no need for routine monitoring and drug interaction is rare. It was first approved to reduce the risk of stroke and systemic embolism in patients with non-valvular atrial fibrillation in 2008 and 2010, respectively. Dabigatran has since been approved for the treatment and prevention of recurrent VTE. Dabigatran is a specific, competitive and reversible direct thrombin inhibitor. Thrombin enables the conversion of fibrinogen into fibrin during the coagulation cascade. Clinical trials with dabigatran in patients undergoing hip and knee replacement surgery showed significantly less VTEs as compared to enoxaparin although bleeding risks were higher. Dabigatran remains an alternative to warfarin for the treatment of VTE. Selection of this therapy may be appropriate for those patients unable to comply with warfarin management requirements [4,5,18].

Complications of anticoagulant therapy

Hemorrhagic complications are the most common adverse effects of anticoagulant therapy. Initial management of bleeding patients on warfarin is withholding the drug and administering vitamin K if reversal is required. Severe life-threatening hemorrhage is managed with fresh frozen plasma in addition to vitamin K. In the case of serious and life-threatening bleeding, immediate correction of the INR can also be achieved by the administration of prothrombin complex concentrates. HIT is a serious but uncommon side effect. Type I HIT occurs in 10% and Type II in 5% of patients on heparin. Type I is due to a mild lowering of the platelet count as a result of platelet clumping and occurs in the first 24 h of therapy. Type II HIT results from the binding of heparin to platelets and subsequent generation of immune complexes consisting of immunoglobulin G and heparin platelet factor IV. This occurs 5 or more days after starting therapy and can cause thrombosis. Unfortunately, the subset of patients who develop thrombosis is unpredictable. Heparin can rarely cause hyperlipidaemia, hyperkalemia, osteoporosis, skin necrosis and hypersensitivity reactions [2,4,5].

Other Strategies

Inferior vena cava filters (IVCFs)

IVCFs should be considered for surgical inpatients with acute/recent (within 1 month) or existing DVT/PE and in whom anticoagulation is. They have also been advocated in trauma patients or those requiring abdominal surgery when anticoagulation is contraindicated or has to be discontinued. Other indications include recurrent PE while being adequately anticoagulated or if there is a complication with the anticoagulation therapy requiring its termination. Active bleeding complications requiring termination of anticoagulation therapy is another indication. Designs of filters have improved since Greenfield first described his filter in 1973. Temporary and retrievable filters are also available. Most of these can now be placed via 6–12 French sheaths using a percutaneous route under fluoroscopic or ultrasound guidance. They are usually inserted via the jugular vein route [19,20]. Complications include thrombosis of the filter and migration of the filter through the walls of the inferior vena cava. The evidence regarding their short-term and long-term efficacy is equivocal [21]. In the current era, most filters if used should be temporary and removed when the indication has passed.

Thrombolysis

The indications for thrombolysis in acute DVT remain controversial. Thrombolysis can be performed for acute (<10 days) ileofemoral DVT when there is no contraindication to use of anticoagulants or recent bleeding episodes, trauma or recent surgery. It is usually reserved for younger patients with major ileofemoral thrombosis with significant acute swelling and symptoms. Techniques vary considerably and are rapidly evolving [22]. Venous catheterisation can be performed via the internal jugular, femoral or popliteal vein, depending on the site of thrombus and treatment aims. Infusion of thrombolytic agents such as r-tPA is performed via a multiple side hole catheter embedded into the thrombus. A Cochrane review (third update of its series) in 2016 has shown that complete clot lysis and improved patency is more often seen with thrombolysis than conservative treatment with anticoagulation. Venous function is significantly improved and the incidence of PTS is reduced by a third following a proximal DVT. Strict eligibility criteria appear to improve safety in recent studies and may be necessary to reduce the risk of complications, e.g., bleeding. This may limit the applicability of this treatment [23].

Acute venous thrombectomy is now rarely performed. Mechanical devices for thrombus removal as adjuncts to thrombolysis have been developed. Some of them have a jet, suction or a brush tip to allow disruption and aspiration of the clot and one system utilises ultrasound to do the same thing [24].

Summary

It is essential to define the pre-operative risk of DVT and use best practice advice to reduce the risk in inpatients undergoing surgery. Treatment and care should take into account patients' needs and preferences. UFH, LMWH, fondaparinux and newer agents such as rivaroxaban and dabigatran are the main pharmacological agents currently used in the prophylaxis and treatment of DVT. In patients with contraindications to pharmacological prophylaxis, mechanical methods can be used. In the past decade, tremendous advances have been made with respect to the diagnosis and treatment of DVT. Current research in anticoagulants involves investigations into new agents that act on various phases of the coagulation cascade. The therapy of DVT is undergoing exciting changes with the development of targeted antithrombotics with greater therapeutic efficacy and safety, as well as considerably greater ease of use and clot removal with thrombolysis.

References

1. Rosendaal FR. Venous thrombosis: A multicasual disease. *Lancet* 1999;353:1167–1173.
2. Patel K, Brenner B, Chang JS *et al*. Deep venous thrombosis. *eMedicine Medscape*. Available at: http://emedicine.medscape.com/article/1911303-overview#a2 (Accessed 10 November 2016).
3. Bates SM, Kearon C, Crowther M *et al*. A diagnostic strategy involving a quantitative latex D-dimer assay reliably excludes deep venous thrombosis. *Ann Intern Med* 2003;138:787–794.
4. National Institute for Health and Clinical Excellence. Venous thromboembolism: Reducing the risk for patients in hospital. NICE Clinical Guideline CG92. January 2010. Updated June 2015. http://www.nice.org.uk.
5. National Institute for Health and Clinical Excellence. Venous thromboembolic diseases: Diagnosis, management and thrombophilia testing. NICE Clinical Guideline CG144. June 2012. Updated November 2015. http://www.nice.org.uk.
6. Michiels JJ, Gadisseur A, van der Planken M *et al*. Diagnosis of deep vein thrombosis: How many tests do we need? *Acta Chir Belg.* 2005;105 (1):16–25.
7. Michiels JJ, Gadisseur A, van der Planken M *et al*. Different accuracies of rapid enzyme-linked immunosorbent, turbidimetric, and agglutination D-dimer assays for thrombosis exclusion: Impact on diagnostic work-ups of outpatients with suspected deep vein thrombosis and pulmonary embolism. *Semin Thromb Hemost* 2006;32(7):678–693.
8. Streiff MB, Agnelli G, Connors JM *et al*. Guidance for the treatment of deep vein thrombosis and pulmonary embolism. *J Thromb Thrombolysis* 2016; 41(1):32–67.
9. The EINSTEIN Investigators. Oral rivaroxaban for symptomatic venous thromboembolism. *N Engl J Med* 2010;363:2499–2510.
10. Ageno W, Turpie AG. Spotlight on real-world evidence for the treatment of DVT: XALIA. *Thromb Haemost* 2016;116:S41–S49.
11. Burness CB, Perry CM. Rivaroxaban: A review of its use in the treatment of deep vein thrombosis or pulmonary embolism and the prevention of recurrent venous thromboembolism. *Drugs* 2014;74 (2):243–262.
12. Bookhart BK, Haskell L Bamber L *et al*. Length of stay and economic consequences with rivaroxaban vs. enoxaparin/vitamin K antagonist in patients with DVT and PE: findings from the North American EINSTEIN clinical trial program. *J Med Econ* 2014;17(10):691–695.

13. Agnelli G, Becattini C. Treatment of DVT: How long is enough and How do you predict recurrence. *J Thromb Thrombolysis* 2008;25(1): 37–44.
14. Dong K, Song Y, Li X *et al.* Pentasaccharides for the prevention of venous thromboembolism. *Cochrane Database Syst Rev* 2016;10:CD005134.
15. Robertson L, Kesteven P, McCaslin JE. Oral direct thrombin inhibitors or oral factor Xa inhibitors for the treatment of pulmonary embolism. *Cochrane Database Syst Rev* 2015;12:CD010957.
16. Liu X, Johnson M, Mardekian J *et al.* Apixaban reduces hospitalizations in patients With venous thromboembolism: An analysis of the apixaban for the initial management of pulmonary embolism and deep-vein thrombosis as first-line therapy (AMPLIFY) trial. *J Am Heart Assoc* 2015;4(12).
17. Agnelli G, Buller HR, Cohen A *et al.* Oral apixaban for the treatment of venous thromboembolism in cancer patients: Results from the AMPLIFY trial. *J Thromb Haemost* 2015;13(12):2187–2191.
18. Ogbonna KC, Dixon DL. Critical appraisal of dabigatran in the treatment of deep vein thrombosis and pulmonary embolism. *J Blood Med* 2015;6: 177–184.
19. Young T, Tang H, Hughes R. Vena caval filters for the prevention of pulmonary embolism. *Cochrane Database Syst Rev* 2010;2:CD006212.
20. Duffett L, Carrier M. Inferior vena cava filters. *J Thromb Haemost* 2016. DOI: 10.1111.
21. Wang SL, Siddiqui A, Rosenthal E. Long-term complications of inferior vena cava filters. *J Vasc Surg Venous Lymphat Disord* 2017;5(1):33–41.
22. Comerota AJ, Gravett MH. Iliefemoral vein thrombosis. *J Vasc Surg* 2007;46:1065–1076.
23. Prins MH, Lensing AW, Bauersachs R *et al.* Oral rivaroxaban versus standard therapy for the treatment of symptomatic venous thromboembolism: A pooled analysis of the EINSTEIN-DVT and PE randomized studies. *Thromb J* 2013;11(1):21.
24. Ageno W, Mantovani LG, Haas S *et al.* Safety and effectiveness of oral rivaroxaban versus standard anticoagulation for the treatment of symptomatic deep-vein thrombosis (XALIA): An international, prospective, non-interventional study. *Lancet Haematol* 2016;3(1):e12–21.
25. Watson L, Broderick C, Armon MP. Thrombolysis for acute deep vein thrombosis. *Cochrane Database Syst Rev* 2016;11:CD002783.
26. Robertson L, McBride O, Burdess A. Pharmacomechanical thrombectomy for iliofemoral deep vein thrombosis. *Cochrane Database Syst Rev* 2016; 11:CD011536.

Chapter 23

Infection in Vascular Surgery

Mike Clarke

Key Points

- Infection of prosthetic vascular grafts is associated with high mortality, morbidity and limb loss.
- Prosthetic grafts should be avoided if the risk of infection is high.
- Early diagnosis requires a low index of suspicion.
- The greatest chance of long-term success lies in complete removal of the infected prosthesis and revascularisation with autologous material.
- A groin abscess in an intravenous drug abuser should be considered to be an infected false aneurysm of the femoral artery until positively excluded.

Introduction

Managing the infective complications of arterial surgery represents one of the most complex challenges facing the vascular surgeon. Medical management alone seldom produces a satisfactory outcome, but the removal of an infected prosthesis in a debilitated patient, possibly in the face of life-threatening haemorrhage, is rarely straightforward. The problem of then restoring distal perfusion may require innovative approaches whilst minimising the risk to the patient's life and reducing the likelihood of recurrent infection.

Epidemiology

Conventional surgical teaching is that 'clean' operative procedures should carry a post-operative wound infection rate of less than 1% (Table 1). Data from the Health Protection Agency (HPA) surveillance of surgical site infection rates however suggest that this is rarely achieved and approaches the sort of rates generally seen with clean-contaminated or contaminated procedures [1].

Causative Organisms

Almost half of the organisms seen in early post-operative infections following vascular procedures are staphylococcal, two-thirds of these being methicillin-resistant *Staphylococcus aureus* (MRSA). Coagulase negative staphylococci are an unusual cause of early infection, but may be more important in the development of late-presenting graft infections. *Enterococcus* and *Enterobacter* species are responsible for around 30% of early post-operative infections with the remainder consisting of *Streptococci*, *Pseudomonas*, anaerobes, fungi and other bacterial species. Although MRSA is the commonest infecting organism, most studies suggest that outcomes are no worse with MRSA infection compared with other staphylococcal infections.

Table 1.   Incidence of infection following surgical procedures in England 1997–2005.

Category	No. of operations	Infected (%)
Knee prosthesis	62,031	1.0
Total hip prosthesis	74,677	1.8
Coronary artery bypass graft	27,447	4.1
Vascular surgery	8,959	6.0
Large bowel surgery	14,296	9.2
Limb amputation	2,670	13.1

The HPA data refer specifically to infection rates during the original hospital stay, and of these the vast majority relate to superficial wound infections. Nevertheless, the data are in keeping with some historical series that have suggested that the rate of vascular prosthesis implant infection may be as high as 7%.

Infection in following arterial reconstruction varies from simple superficial wound infection to deep infection involving the arterial conduit itself. The classification system proposed by Szilagyi in the 1970s remains relevant to vascular surgical practice today [2].

Grade 1 — dermis only
Grade II — involvement of subcutaneous tissues
Grade III — vascular graft involvement.

An alternative sometimes used is the Samson classification:

Group 1   Infection extends no deeper than the dermis.
Group 2   Infection involves subcutaneous tissues, but does not come into grossly observable direct contact with the graft.
Group 3   Infection involves the body of the graft, but not at an anastomotic site.
Group 4   Infection surrounds an exposed anastomosis, but bacteraemia or anastomotic bleeding has not occurred.
Group 5   Infection involves a graft-to-artery anastomosis and is associated with septicaemia and/or bleeding at the time of presentation.

Although it is grade Szilagyi III infections that are of the greatest concern, it is recognised that early grade I and II infections are associated with the later development of grade III infections and so should always be taken seriously. Table 2 shows how rates of grade III infection vary by the nature of the conduit and the site of arterial surgery. As can be seen, prosthetic grafts are more at risk than autologous forms of reconstruction, and risk is also increased by surgery involving the groin.

Aortic graft infection is defined as 'early' (<4 months) or 'late' (4 months) with respect to the time of clinical infection after graft implantation [8].

Table 2.   Rates of Szilagyi grade III infection following arterial reconstruction by nature of graft and anatomical location.

Graft type	Rate of grade III infection
Synthetic graft	1.9
Autogenous vein	0.4
Endarterectomies	0.2
Arterial allografts	0.4
Site of surgery	
Aortoiliac	0.7
Aortofemoral	1.6
Femoropopliteal	3.0
Femorofemoral	0.9
Other (intrathoracic, carotid, visceral)	1.0

Prevention

Although not always possible, there is correctly a keen focus on reducing infection rates in surgical patients. Some factors cannot be easily altered. Patient age and pre-operative health status (including the presence of diabetes) have both been shown to be associated with higher instances of post-operative infection. Other risk factors include prolonged pre-operative hospital stay, the presence of non-healing ulcers or other tissue loss, admission from a long-term care facility and excessive antibiotic usage.

Conduct of the operation

Surgical technique can go a long way to preventing infection following surgery. Simple measures include pre-operative washing of patients, reducing theatre traffic to a minimum, careful attention to the handling of tissues, avoidance of excessive retraction with self-retaining retractors, pre-operative marking of the long saphenous vein (LSV) to avoid undermining skin flaps, careful skin closure without undue tension and with suture techniques that avoid devascularising the skin edges. Other factors that may help reduce peri-operative surgical site infection include maintenance of normothermia during surgery and careful glycaemic control in patients with diabetes. Approximately 5% of patients undergoing arterial surgery will be colonised with MRSA prior to surgery. Pre-operative screening for MRSA allows attempts at eradication therapy prior to admission and patients known to be colonised with MRSA should not be nursed alongside patients who are free from MRSA.

Antibiotic prophylaxis

It is important to develop a local antibiotic prophylaxis policy in conjunction with your microbiologists. Consideration should be given to observed patterns of infection in vascular patients as well as sensitivity and resistance patterns amongst organisms encountered. As well as routine prophylaxis, it is well worth the policy including an alternative regime for patients with known sensitivities or renal/liver impairment that precludes them from receiving the standard regime as well as an option for second-line prophylaxis for those patients requiring early re-exploration.

Diagnosis

Clinical presentation

Graft infections may present in a multitude of ways and it is important to maintain a high index of suspicion. For superficial grafts, the diagnosis may be relatively straightforward with, for example, an obviously infected false aneurysm within the groin or a discharging sinus overlying a graft. Any signs of bleeding should raise the possibility of anastomotic disruption, and all too often a small herald bleed will be followed soon afterwards by major haemorrhage. The diagnosis of infection related to intracavity grafts can be somewhat more complicated. Patients presenting with upper gastrointestinal haemorrhage following previous aortic surgery should be considered to have an aorto-enteric fistula until proven otherwise. In many cases however, the presentation is more subtle and may include pyrexia of unknown origin, general malaise and weight loss, vertebral osteomyelitis and hydronephrosis.

Laboratory investigations

Routine laboratory investigations can provide evidence in support of the diagnosis of graft infection, but most are non-specific. They should, in the first instance, include full blood count, erythrocyte sedimentation rate, C-reactive protein, urea and electrolytes, serum albumin, microscopy, culture and sensitivity of any wound or sinus discharge, and peripheral blood cultures.

Imaging

Imaging plays an essential role in the evaluation of patients with suspected arterial graft infection. In particular, it can potentially confirm the presence of infection or the development of local complications, e.g., false aneurysm formation, hydronephrosis. In addition, information can be obtained regarding proximal and distal vessels for planning reconstruction.

Ultrasound

Often useful in situations where a graft is placed superficially, ultrasound can quickly and easily detect the presence of perigraft collections and the presence or absence of false aneurysms. In the carotid territory, a distinct rippling of the surface of an infected patch has been reported as being visible on ultrasound. Ultrasound guided aspiration of a peri-graft collection may provide the opportunity for microbiological confirmation of infection. In the absence of overt clinical signs of local infection, one has to consider the possibility of introducing infection into an otherwise sterile field or precipitating other local complications and such aspiration should only take place under the guidance of a vascular surgeon.

Computed tomography (CT)

For intracavity grafts, CT remains the most useful method of imaging currently in use. The presence of a gas-filled fluid collection adjacent to the graft more than 3 months after implantation can be considered pathognomonic of infection. Such collections may be present in the first few weeks following implantation, and at these times interpretation needs to be carefully considered alongside the clinical features. In these circumstances and if time allows, serial scans may be helpful in distinguishing normal post-operative change, which should progressively resolve vs. progressive post-operative infection. Other features that may suggest infection include simple fluid collections, 'streaking' of surrounding fat planes or the presence of adjacent complications such as an anastomotic aneurysm.

In addition to confirming the diagnosis, CT angiography also offers the opportunity to outline the inflow and run-off vessels, thus avoiding the need for supplementary vascular imaging (Fig. 1).

Angiography

Digital subtraction angiography provides little information on the presence or extent of infection. It can be helpful in providing detailed images of the run-off vasculature and may show false aneurysms, but rarely adds significantly more than CT.

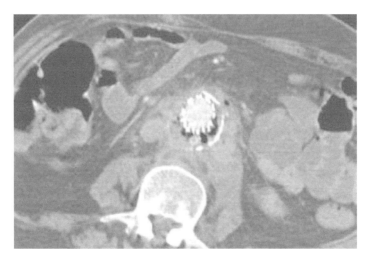

Figure 1.   CT showing an infected aortic stent graft 2 years after insertion. Note the presence of gas within the aortic sac.

Magnetic resonance (MR) scanning

Magnetic resonance offers many of the advantages seen with CT scanning, including the diagnosis of intracavity graft infection and imaging of adjacent vasculature. T2 weighted images may be more sensitive in identifying perigraft oedema prior to the development of a frank collection. There is, however, little firm data to support its use in place of CT, which is currently the more commonly utilised modality in UK practice.

FDG-PET and PET/CT scanning

FDG-PET imaging is based on the uptake of radiolabelled glucose in metabolically active cells, which includes inflammatory cells such as neutrophils and lymphocytes. To increase its sensitivity in diagnosing vascular graft infection, FDG-PET images can be fused with CT and MR images enabling the precise localisation of any abnormal FDG uptake. Focal or heterogeneous uptake with a projection over the graft on CT is highly suggestive of infection. Further work is required to define thresholds for positives, and clinical correlation should be applied when assessing uptake as diffuse uptake around a graft can be a normal finding.

Labelled white cell scans

Radionuclide-labelled white cell scintigraphy with technetium-99 and indium-111 have both been used in the diagnosis of vascular graft infection. They may be a useful adjunct to CT, particularly in confirming early graft infection although the results need to be interpreted with caution as although sensitive, the technique suffers from relatively low specificity.

Treatment strategies

In many instances, the ideal treatment strategy is excision of the infected prosthesis (if one is present), debridement of adjacent involved arterial wall and adjacent tissues and *in situ* reconstruction with autogenous vein. In the case of the infected lower limb prosthetic graft, the autologous LSV is the most obvious choice, although in many cases the reason for implanting a prosthetic graft in the first place has been the unsuitabil-ity of the saphenous vein. Consideration should be given to the contralat-eral LSV, if present, as well as short saphenous veins and upper limb veins.

In situ vein graft

Where the LSV is going to be of insufficient calibre, the superficial femo-ral veins (SFVs) can be successfully utilised. This is particularly so in replacing aortic grafts. The SFVs are frequently 10–12 mm in diameter, and there are now a number of series that have demonstrated success in replacing infected aortic prostheses. As well as aortic replacement, the SFV is also a useful conduit when replacing infected femoro-femoral crossover grafts. The SFVs can be harvested down to popliteal level and may even be harvested when the LSV has already gone. At the proximal end, particular care should be taken to ensure that the profunda vein remains intact. Some leg swelling may occur after harvest of the SFV, but this is rarely severe.

Excision and extra-anatomic bypass

In many instances, excision and extra-anatomic bypass would be consid-ered the conventional approach to managing prosthetic graft infection. It has the advantage of removing the infected prosthesis whilst providing revascularisation without placing the new graft in the infected bed. In most instances, it is necessary to use a second prosthesis for the extra-anatomic bypass, and there remains a relatively high rate of subsequent infection of the new prosthetic conduit.

Infected aortic grafts

Infection of a prosthetic aortic graft is invariably a catastrophic complica-tion following aortic aneurysm repair. Presentation often occurs rela-tively late after the original surgery and may represent haematogenous seeding of the prosthetic graft or low-grade contamination from the time of implantation. Presentation varies. In some cases, patients present with features of chronic sepsis, including general malaise, pyrexia of unknown origin and weight loss. Back pain and abdominal pain may be present, but are not invariable and the diagnosis is frequently delayed. More acutely, patients may present with signs of gastrointestinal (GI) bleeding either from an aorto-duodenal fistula (with or without false aneurysm formation) or more commonly an erosion of the duodenum by the body of the graft. In this instance, the arterial anastomosis is not involved, but bleeding is from the eroded edges of the duodenum. In all patients with upper GI bleeding and a history of previous aortic surgery, the diagnosis of aorto-duodenal fistula should be considered until proven otherwise.

In patients presenting less acutely, time should be spent not only in investigation, but also in attempting to optimise the patient's status for surgery. Any surgery for an infected aortic graft is going to be a major undertaking and any time spent improving the patient's general condition will ultimately pay dividends. Positive blood cultures may allow administration of appropriate antibiotics and attention should be given to the patient's nutritional status, which may well be depleted by the effects of chronic sepsis.

The surgical strategy will to a large extent be determined by the general condition of the patient and the urgency for operative intervention (principally the presence of life-threatening haemorrhage). The key elements of the surgical approach are the safe excision of the infected graft and the provision of distal revascularisation.

Any revisional aortic surgery is demanding, but particularly so in the presence of infection or when dealing with a proximal anastomotic false aneurysm. The ease by which proximal control can be established is largely determined by the length of aorta between the prosthetic graft and the origin of the renal arteries. In order to safely secure proximal control, some surgeons prefer to expose the aorta at the level of the diaphragm prior to dissecting out the infrarenal aorta. The lesser sac is entered by dividing the lesser omentum, and the left lobe of the liver is retracted upwards to expose the crus of the diaphragm. In the emergency situation this can be split bluntly with scissors, but in the elective setting can be progressively divided with diathermy. This exposes the most distal thoracic aorta above the coeliac axis, where a clamp can be placed without closing it. Attention can then be turned to the infrarenal aorta, safe in the knowledge that if major haemorrhage is encountered, proximal control can be easily achieved. An alternative means of securing rapid proximal control is to expose a more distal portion of the aortic graft and introduce an aortic occlusion balloon through a small arteriotomy in the graft.

Having achieved proximal control, distal control is generally more straightforward. If it is not possible to dissect out the iliac vessels, the graft can be divided and the iliac arteries controlled with Pruitt occlusion catheters or Fogarty type catheters fitted with 3-way taps.

Having excised the graft, the decision needs to be made about subsequent reconstruction. In the emergency setting, where the patient has been operated on for life-threatening haemorrhage, the decision will be dictated by the condition of the patient at this stage. If the patient is in extremis, the aortic stump should be over sewn and the patient returned to the intensive care unit in an attempt to stabilise them. If they recover sufficiently in the next few hours, they may be returned to the operating theatre for lower limb revascularisation although it has to be accepted that if they survive many will face bilateral lower limb amputation.

In dealing with the infrarenal aortic stump, sufficient tissue should be debrided to allow safe ligation of the aorta and minimise the risk of the aorta subsequently giving way and leading to stump blow-out. The aortic stump is most securely closed in two layers with a non-absorbable monofilament — a layer of interrupted mattress sutures and a second layer of continuous suture. If there has been a fistula to the duodenum the duodenum, will need to be repaired or controlled with an external drain. Failure to adequately control the duodenum, allowing a localised leak and collection to develop, is probably one of the factors which can lead to subsequent aortic stump blow-out — a condition that is usually fatal.

Where revascularisation is deemed appropriate, two options are available — extra- anatomic bypass or *in situ* replacement. The conventional approach is extra-anatomic bypass. Controversy exists as to whether this is by axillo-bifemoral or bi-axillo-femoral bypass. Furthermore, some authors advocate performance of the extra-anatomic bypass prior to graft excision to avoid the otherwise potentially prolonged period of lower limb ischaemia that occurs and the subsequent reperfusion effects. Others argue that pre-emptive insertion of the extra-anatomic grafts risks bacteraemia seeding at the time of excision of the infected aortic grafts and contributes to the 25% infection rate amongst extra-anatomic grafts inserted in the treatment of aortic graft infection. The other major concern with this approach is the risk of aortic stump blow-out. Historic series have reported blow rates of up to 40% although more recent practice would indicate a rate closer to 10%.

In situ graft replacement avoids the issue of an aortic stump and is thus particularly applicable when there is only a short infrarenal aortic segment although it does necessitate placing a graft in an infected bed. A number of series have reported good outcomes utilising prosthetic grafts treated to resist infection. The commonest way of doing this is to soak a polyester graft for 20 min in a rifampicin solution (60 mg mL^{-1}). The relative rarity of aortic graft infection means that most evidence comes from single-centre retrospective case series. One of the largest series of *in situ* prosthetic replacement reported on 52 patients with *in situ* prosthetic replacements although this included a mix of rifampicin-bonded grafts and other means of providing autogenous cover, e.g., omental patches [3]. Peri-operative mortality was 9% with 11% of patients developing recurrent infection of the aortic graft.

More recently, attention has turned to using autologous material for *in situ* replacement. Obviously, the LSV is of too narrow a calibre to be practicable, but a number of series have now reported good outcomes using SFV [4]. The vein can readily be harvested from the subsartorial canal. Proximally, it is divided immediately distal to its confluence with the profunda vein where the common femoral vein is formed. Distally, it is easiest to divide it just above the adductor hiatus — below this level there is an increasing number of geniculate branches to deal with, although if it is essential to obtain the maximum length then it is quite safe to harvest the entire above-knee popliteal vein in continuity. Post-operative leg swelling is reported to be minimal, even in cases where the LSV has been previously removed. In an adult, the femoral vein is generally 10–12 mm in diameter and can readily be fashioned to allow anastomosis with the aorta. If necessary, both femoral veins can be harvested to allow construction of a Y-graft and it can also prove useful in the replacement of an infected femorofemoral crossover graft (Fig. 2).

Another alternative to the autologous vein is fresh cryopreserved human tissue. This is available from a number of sites around the UK

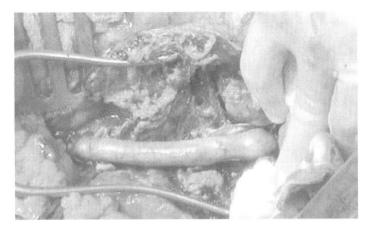

Figure 2.   *In situ* reconstruction of a mycotic aortic aneurysm with SFV.

including Oxford, Liverpool and Birmingham. The largest experience is with ascending aorta and aortic arch, which has been extensively used in paediatric cardiac surgery, but material is now available from more distal aorta and superficial femoral artery. There is, as yet, little experience in the UK of using such grafts for the replacement of infected peripheral vascular grafts, but reports from elsewhere suggest results comparable with autologous material [5].

Infected aortic endovascular grafts

Aortic stent grafts are not immune to infective complications [6]. A number of series have reported incidences of around 1%, similar to that seen following open aortic surgery. The mechanisms of presentation are also similar to those seen in infected open aortic grafts and include aortoenteric fistula. Furthermore, the same principles of treatment apply — removal of the infected prosthesis, debridement of infected tissue and, where possible, distal revascularisation. In most cases, removal of the infected stent graft is relatively straightforward as they do not become incorporated in the same manner as an open graft. Care must be exercised however when removing grafts with suprarenal fixation. It is easy to damage the suprarenal aorta whilst attempting to remove these devices and in some cases it is more judicious to detach and leave *in situ* the uncovered bare metal portion of the graft, which extends above the renal arteries.

Infected carotid patches

As with peripheral infection, infection related to a prosthetic carotid patch is generally a straightforward diagnosis. Presentation may be in the form of clear signs of acute infection with pain, swelling and erythema overlying the patch. In some cases, the presentation is less acute and manifests as a discharging sinus or the presence of a false aneurysm. Rupture of a prosthetic patch is fortunately rare, as are recurrent neuro-logical symptoms.

In most cases, first-line imaging is with Duplex scanning, to look for local features of infection and to confirm whether the internal carotid artery (ICA) remains patent — an occluded internal carotid is obviously considerably easier to manage. Magnetic resonance (MR) or computed tomography angiography (MRA/CTA) will give details about the distal carotid circulation. It can be very helpful to have an indication of the likely consequences of occlusion of the ICA as this is a very real risk fol-lowing revisional surgery for infection. Information gathered at the time of the original operation can be helpful, e.g., if performed under local anaesthetic, did the patient tolerate the procedure without the need for a shunt? If this information is not available, then angiog-raphy with a trial balloon occlusion of the ICA can provide useful information.

As with infection of an arterial prosthesis elsewhere, the treatment strategy has to be considered in light of the patient's status, but success-ful eradication of infection generally requires removal of the infected patch. The operation should only be undertaken by surgeons with consid-erable experience of carotid surgery. The patient should be warned of the relatively high risk of cranial nerve injury. The most difficult part of the procedure is usually obtaining adequate distal exposure to safely allow reconstruction. In patients with a low bifurcation and a short patch this is not too difficult, but if difficulty is anticipated, nasotracheal intubation allows the mandible to fully close and provides more room to manoeuvre than conventional intubation. When further access is required, some surgeons advocate approaching the distal internal carotid via an infratemporal fossa approach, usually in conjunction with an ear, nose and throat (ENT) surgeon.

Having established control proximally and distally, and following heparinisation of the patient, the patch can be opened and a suitable shunt inserted. In most cases, we plan to attempt reconstruction with autologous vein and this can be reversed and 'pre-loaded' onto the distal limb of the shunt prior to insertion. In some circumstances and even with good distal exposure, the accessible part of the ICA proves too friable to safely reconstruct. It is then necessary to ligate the artery and it is when faced with this situation that knowledge of the patients' likely tolerance of internal carotid ligation can aid the decision-making process as up to 50% of patients will suffer a stroke following acute ligation of the ICA.

In those patients where reconstruction is feasible, the choice between utilising the vein as a patch or interposition graft is largely determined by the amount of ICA wall left following adequate debridement of the edges of the original anastomosis. In a large proportion of cases, a patch is feasible and this is the simpler option. The vein that was loaded onto the shunt can be opened longitudinally and following excision of any valve leaflets can be used as a patch in the conventional manner.

If only a thin strip of back wall of the ICA remains, it is better to use the vein as an interposition graft. The distal ICA is transacted and the distal anastomosis fashioned first. Following completion of this anastomosis, the distal limb of the shunt is withdrawn into the vein graft and the anastomosis tested for adequate haemostasis. It is important to ensure this is satisfactory prior to undertaking the proximal anastomosis, as access to the deep aspect of the graft is subsequently very difficult. The proximal anastomosis can then be completed, ideally incorporating the origin of the external carotid artery, although this is not always practicable, in which case the orifice of the external carotid can be oversewn.

Infected Peripheral Grafts

The diagnosis of peripheral graft infection is generally more straightforward than is the case with intracavity grafts. Patients generally have signs of localised sepsis including pain, swelling and erythema over the graft/anastomosis. There may be a purulent discharge from a wound sinus, and any blood staining of the sinus should alert the surgeon to the possibility of incipient major haemorrhage. Anastomotic false aneurysm development is not always related to infection, but even in the absence of other signs of sepsis, the possibility should always be borne in mind.

In most cases of peripheral graft infection, the underlying graft is prosthetic and successful treatment ultimately requires removal of the infected prosthesis. The anastomosis may be quite friable or there may have been false aneurysm development. It is therefore generally wise to ensure adequate proximal control prior to exposure of the anastomosis. With infrainguinal grafts in the groin, it is often possible to expose the inguinal ligament, the lower margin of which can then be carefully dissected upwards to provide exposure of the distal external iliac artery. If there is any doubt about the ability to safely gain control by this route (e.g., with extensive scarring, in very obese patients or with haemorrhage requiring rapid control), then an extraperitoneal approach to the external iliac artery should be followed.

Having achieved proximal and distal control, the graft can then usually be detached from its anastomoses and removed. In some cases, the graft infection has resulted in the graft failing to become incorporated and removal from its track is relatively straightforward. It is often the case, however, that the graft has remained incorporated along a large proportion of its length. One useful technique is to utilise a Codman-style varicose vein stripper to remove the graft, however, one has to weigh up the risk of ongoing infection in a graft remnant against that of damaging adjacent structures, e.g., the femoral vein, in attempting to remove a well incorporated graft.

Revascularisation

In any case of arterial graft infection, amongst the most feared complications is that of recurrent infection with the possibility of life-threatening haemorrhage. Careful consideration therefore needs to be given as to whether the risks inherent in further attempts at arterial reconstruction are justified. In a proportion of cases, the limb in question will survive without further revascularisation. Experience of patients with infected false femoral aneurysms as a complication of drug misuse has shown that limb salvage can be maintained even following acute ligation of the common femoral artery. Factors that may indicate the possibility of achieving limb salvage without distal grafting include an already occluded graft, patients whose grafts were originally inserted for claudication and the ability to preserve flow down the profunda artery. Having taken down an infected common femoral anastomosis, it is necessary to excise a reasonable portion of the adjacent arterial wall. The atherosclerotic artery can harbour organisms, and failure to adequately debride the artery wall can result in late haemorrhage, even when closed primarily. If necessary, the artery can be closed with a patch although this should ideally be autologous material. In many cases, it is possible to find a short segment of vein to do this or alternatively, if the superficial femoral artery is occluded (which frequently it is) a segment can be excised, opened longitudinally and fashioned into a patch by removal of the occluded intima. Failing this, bovine pericardium may be used if no autologous material is available. Repair with further prosthetic material is a very high risk strategy (even if soaked in antibiotics or silver nitrate) and should be avoided.

It can be difficult to achieve sound wound closure of the groin, particularly when there has been extensive scarring. Detachment of sartorius from the anterior superior iliac spine and mobilisation of its lateral border (to avoid devascularising it) allows the muscle to be 'rolled over' and tacked down to cover the common femoral artery.

Should distal revascularisation be deemed necessary, then a number of options are available. Our own practice has changed over the years such that in nearly all cases prosthetic grafts are only utilised where no autologous material is available. There are however still some patients with an infected prosthetic infrainguinal graft in whom the LSV is still present and suitable to use as a conduit. This includes a number of patients in whom the original operation record makes note of an 'unsuitable' vein! It is always worth re-examining the vein with duplex to assess its suitability. Obviously, the search for a suitable vein should not stop at the ipsilateral long saphenous. The contralateral leg, short saphenous and upper limb veins should all be considered if necessary.

Interventional radiology techniques have advanced considerably over the years. Subintimal angioplasty, atherectomy catheters and remote endarterectomy have all increased the scope of disease that can be treated, but by whole or partial endovascular means, and these can all be considered in cases where re-do bypass grafting with autologous vein is not feasible.

In cases where sepsis is confined to the groin and with no other options available, consideration may be given to extra-anatomic bypass. Iliopopliteal bypass via the obturator canal and axillopopliteal bypass have both been utilised in these circumstances and it is worth remembering that both the above- and below-knee popliteal arteries can be approached from the lateral aspect of the limb.

Many of the same principles apply to other peripheral grafts as apply to infrainguinal grafts. Extra-anatomic grafts in particular have a relatively high incidence of graft infection. Although it is generally considered most appropriate to remove an infected graft, there have been some reports of successfully managing grafts *in situ*. This should ideally only be entertained when the infecting organism is of low virulence and the infection is confined to the mid portion of the graft, not involving the anastomoses. Surgical management includes adequate debridement of infected tissues, local application of antibacterial agents and adequate coverage of the graft, which may necessitate a vascularised myocutaneous flap.

Infected femoral pseudoaneurysms

Infected primary false aneurysms of the common femoral artery are perhaps worth a special mention. Invariably, a consequence of intravenous drug abuse, they typically present as an apparent acute abscess in the groin. This can be a real trap for the unwary and in all such cases an underlying false aneurysm should be positively excluded prior to incision and drainage. There is often a mixed growth of organisms although staphylococci and Gram negative species are most common.

Direct exposure of the artery is potentially hazardous and made all the more difficult by the indurated and thickened tissues. The judicious approach is to establish proximal control via an extraperitoneal approach to the external iliac artery. On exposure, there is often found to be a large defect in the anterior wall of the common femoral artery, which precludes primary repair. The very real risk of ongoing sepsis and recurrent haemorrhage means that in most cases the only prudent course of action is to ligate the common femoral artery without reconstruction. Contrary to expectations, the majority of patients will tolerate this with the affected limb surviving on a collateral circulation. In the unusual event of limb-threatening critical ischaemia developing, consideration may be given to an extra-anatomic ilio-popliteal bypass via the obturator canal although the safe option is a primary amputation.

Mycotic aneurysms

The term mycotic aneurysm is generally applied to any aneurysm with an infective aetiology. Historically, the commonest cause was septic embolisation in patients with infective endocarditis. Now a relatively rare cause, other aetiological mechanisms have come to the fore. There are a number of pathogenetic mechanisms including septic embolisation (into a small branch vessel or into the large vasa vasorum in the aorta), seeding of an established atherosclerotic plaque, secondary infection in an established aneurysm and rarely contiguous spread from local septic focus. Ultimately, the infective process results in progressive destruction of the arterial wall with eventual aneurysm formation. Once established, the natural history of mycotic aneurysms is to progressively enlarge and eventually rupture.

As with graft infection, an appropriate index of suspicion is essential in making the diagnosis. In many patients, the 'vascular' presentation may occur some time after the initial septic episode, or indeed a particular septic episode may not be apparent. In these cases the clue to the diagnosis often lies in the morphology of the aneurysm, which is frequently (but not invariably) saccular rather than fusiform (Fig. 3).

The commonest causative organism seen in modern vascular practice is salmonella species although staphylococci, streptococci, haemophilus

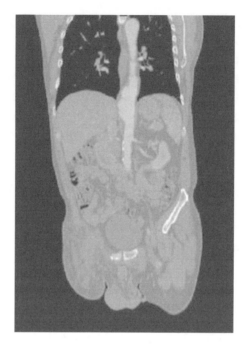

Figure 3.   CT showing a saccular aneurysm of the distal thoracic aorta, strongly suggestive of a mycotic aetiology. The aneurysm was excised and repaired with an *in situ* cryopreserved aortic arch homograft.

and pseudomonas are not infrequently cultured. Management is along similar lines to those for an infected prosthetic graft in the same anatomical location. One possible exception is the use of endovascular stents to treat mycotic aneurysms. This is a potentially attractive option in what is often a debilitated patient; published results demonstrate acceptable early outcome results [7]. There is, however, obvious concern about the development of late graft infection and as yet there is little long-term follow-up data.

References

1. Health Protection Agency. Surveillance of Surgical Site Infection in England: October 1997–September 2005. London: Health Protection Agency, 2006.
2. Szilagyi DE, Smith RF, Elliot JP *et al*. Infection in arterial reconstruction with synthetic grafts. *Ann Surg* 1972;176:321–332.

3. Oderich GS, Bower TC, Cherry KJ *et al*. Evolution from axillofemoral to in situ prosthetic reconstruction for the treatment of aortic graft infections at a single center. *J Vasc Surg* 2006;43:1166–1174.

4. Gibbons CP, Ferguson CJ, Figelstone LJ *et al*. Experience with femoro-popliteal vein as a conduit for vascular reconstruction in infected fields. *Eur J Vasc Endovasc Surg* 2003;25:424–431.

5. Brown KE, Heyer K, Rodriguez H *et al*. Arterial reconstruction with cryopreserved human allografts in the setting of infection: A single-center experience with midterm follow-up. *J Vasc Surg* 2009;49:660–666.

6. Sharif MA, Lee B, Lau LL *et al*. Prosthetic stent graft infection after endovascular abdominal aortic aneurysm repair. *J Vasc Surg* 2007;46:442–448.

7. Clough RE, Black SA, Lyons OT *et al*. Is endovascular repair of mycotic aortic aneurysms a durable treatment option? *Eur J Vasc Endovasc Surg* 2009; 37:407–412.

8. Teebken OE *et al*. Recommendations for reporting treatment of aortic graft infections. *Eur J Vasc Endovasc Surg* 2012;43:174–181.

Chapter 24

Management of Patients with Bleeding Diathesis

Saroj Das and Katherine Gardner

Key Points

- Assessment of haemorrhage should include classification of haemorrhage severity and checking blood parameters including full blood count (FBC), coagulation parameters, fibrinogen level, renal function and liver function tests.
- Peri-operative management of haemorrhage includes activation of the major haemorrhage protocol, administration of oxygen and IV fluids and early surgical or endovascular intervention to stop the bleeding.
- Acidosis and hypothermia are confounding factors which can exacerbate bleeding and should be addressed.
- Targeted procoagulation interventions should be considered, which include administration of fibrinogen, cryoprecipitate, FFP and platelets.
- Antifibrinolytic agents and recombinant factor VIIa can have a role.
- Antidotes are now available for most of the antithrombotic drugs including the new oral anticoagulants (NOACs).
- Post-operatively, antithrombotic therapy or venous thromboembolism (VTE) prophylaxis should be recommenced once haemostasis has been achieved.

Introduction

Management of patients who are bleeding is a routine part of the procedure for most surgeons, cardiologists and radiologists, however, when bleeding is out of proportion to what is expected, particular management is required. The majority of cases of haemorrhage and its complications occur in trauma, and it is the staff working in the Accident and Emergency Department who frequently manage such patients initially [1]. Traumatic injury is the commonest cause of death worldwide in persons between 1 and 44 years of age [1].

Haemorrhagic shock is the cause of up to 50% of deaths in the first 24 h after traumatic injury and 80% of deaths in the operating theatre [1], therefore it carries a significant mortality. The mechanism by which haemorrhage can lead to death is via a loss of intravascular volume, which can subsequently lead to hemodynamic instability, decreased tissue perfusion, cellular hypoxia, organ damage, and subsequently death [1].

The American College of Surgeons Advanced Trauma Life Support have developed a classification of haemorrhage severity to help guide clinicians towards the best management of patients with haemorrhage complications. There are four different groups: from class 1 (where there is no evidence of shock, such as which occurs when donating a unit of blood) to class 4 (a life-threatening event requiring immediate treatment) [2] (Table 1).

Table 1. American College of Surgeons advanced trauma life support classification of haemorrhage severity [2].

	Class of haemorrhage shock			
	I	II	III	IV
Blood loss (mL)	Up to 750	750–1500	1500–2000	>2000
Blood loss (% blood volume)	Up to 15	15–30	30–40	>40
Pulse rate (per min)	<100	100–120	120–140	>140
Blood pressure	Normal	Normal	Decreased	Decreased
Pulse pressure (mmHg)	Normal or increased	Decreased	Decreased	Decreased
Respiratory rate (per min)	14–20	20–30	30–40	>35
Urine output (mL/h)	>30	20–30	5–15	Negligible
Central nervous system/ mental status	Slightly anxious	Mildly anxious	Anxious, confused	Confused, lethargic

In this chapter, evidence-based recommendations are made, which address all aspects of bleeding in the acute situation, including in the pre-operative, peri-operative and post-operative contexts.

Pre-operative Preventative Measures

Identification of anaemia

Pre-operative identification of anaemia is important prior to surgery [3]. In major surgery, peri-operative blood loss and reduced post-operative erythropoiesis may lead to acute anaemia, particularly in patients presenting with pre-operative anaemia [3]. Preexisting anaemia can be identified via history, examination and laboratory FBC measurement, followed by implementation of strategies to correct it [3].

Guidelines regarding antithrombotic therapy

The management of antithrombotic therapy peri-operatively is a frequent challenge. Haemorrhagic risk with continued treatment must be balanced against thrombotic risk when antithrombotics are discontinued for surgery [4].

Following are the guidelines regarding vitamin K antagonist (e.g., warfarin) therapy management pre-operatively:

- In low-risk patients, e.g., patients with atrial fibrillation, warfarin can be safely stopped 3 days before surgery [4].
- In intermediate risk patients, e.g., patients with a history of venous thromboembolism (VTE), either:
  (1) give unfractionated heparin 5,000 units tds until 2 h post-operatively [4], or
  (2) give LMWH at a prophylactic dose until 12 h pre-operatively [4].

- In high-risk patients, e.g., patients with mechanical heart valves, infusion of unfractionated heparin should be started when INR is <2.5 at a dose depending on APTT to achieve an APTT ratio of 2.5–3.5 [4].

Several new oral anticoagulants (NOACs), namely apixaban, rivaroxaban, and dabigatran etexilate are currently licensed in UK and

Europe for various thromboembolic indications and provide some advantages over existing agents [5–10]. The following are the recommendations regarding NOAC therapy management pre-operatively:

- NOACs can be stopped ~24 h (2–3 half-lives) before a procedure that has a low bleeding risk, but 5 days before procedures with a medium or high bleeding risk, depending on which NOAC is used and on the patient's renal function [11,12].
- Other expert consensus documents recommend 24- to 48-h discontinuation windows [13]. Additional studies remain ongoing [13].

Guidelines Regarding antiplatelet drugs

- Aspirin can be continued for most surgical procedures [14]. The bleeding risk for patients prescribed dual antiplatelet treatment is increased, and it is prudent to defer elective surgery until monotherapy can be prescribed [15,16]. Platelet transfusion is an option for bleeding secondary to antiplatelet drugs [17]. Regarding Clopidogrel, Prasugrel and Ticagrelor, discontinuation is advised 5–7 days before the procedure in patients who are undergoing high-bleeding-risk surgery [18].

Peri-operative Measures

General rules of management (Table 2)

- Hospitals must have a major haemorrhage protocol in place, which is to be mobilised immediately when a massive haemorrhage situation is declared (the definitions of 'massive haemorrhage' do vary however and are felt to be of little value) [1]. The major haemorrhage protocol includes clinical, laboratory and logistic responses from a multidisciplinary team [1].
- High flow oxygen should be applied to maintain adequate oxygenation [1].
- Large bore IV access should be obtained and central access considered [1].
- Baseline bloods should be obtained for full blood count (FBC), prothrombin time (PT), activated partial thromboplastin time (APTT), urea and electrolytes and for cross-match [1].

Table 2.   General rule of management.

- Initial fluid replacement
- Resuscitation and prevention of further bleeding
- Transfusion triggers
- Oxygen fraction
- Monitoring tissue perfusion (lactate, base excess)
- Transfusion of labile blood products
- Cell salvage
- Avoidance of hypothermia
- Multidisciplinary approach (involve haematologist)

- Fluid replacement/resuscitation is required — a target systolic Bp of 80–100 mmHg should be utilised until major bleeding has been stopped [19].
- Transfusion triggers: Red blood cell transfusion should be given to achieve a target Hb of 7–9 g/dL [19]. Blood group O negative is the quickest blood to obtain (2 units' maximum can be transfused [4]), followed by group specific, then cross-matched blood [1]. Transfusion of Labile Blood Products is preferable.
- The haematologist on call should be consulted regarding emergency management of haemorrhage [1].
- Early surgical or endovascular intervention as appropriate should be considered [19].
- The theatre team should be advised about the need for cell salvage autotransfusion — this is encouraged in all cases of massive haemorrhage [1].
- Patients presenting with haemorrhagic shock and an unidentified source of bleeding should undergo immediate further investigation [19]. This may be via focused assessment with sonography for trauma scanning and/or early whole body CT if the patient is sufficiently stable [1].
- Acidosis can be a confounding factor. Serum lactate and base excess measurements should be taken (via blood gases) to estimate and monitor the extent of bleeding and shock [19]. Treatment of acidosis is mainly achieved via restoration of the patient's circulating volume to maintain tissue perfusion [20]. Recombinant Activated

Coagulation factor (rFVIIa) can be considered but only alongside pH correction [21].

- Hypothermia can also be a confounding factor. Actively warm the patient as well as all transfused fluids [1]. rFVIIa may be used in the treatment of patients with hypothermic coagulopathy [21].

Surgical management

- In the pre-hospital setting, control of obvious bleeding points can be attempted via pressure or a tourniquet [1].
- 'Patients presenting with haemorrhagic shock and an identified source of bleeding should undergo immediate bleeding control procedure unless initial resuscitation measures are successful' [19]. However, surgery may have to be interrupted and limited to essential 'damage control' initially in the severely injured patient [1].
- 'Patients with pelvic ring disruption in haemorrhagic shock should undergo immediate pelvic ring closure and stabilisation' [19].
- 'Patients with ongoing haemodynamic instability despite adequate pelvic ring stabilisation should undergo early pre-peritoneal packing, angiographic embolisation and/or surgical bleeding control' including packing [19].
- In abdominal bleeding, early control should be achieved using packing, direct surgical bleeding control and local haemostatic procedures. In the exsanguinating patient, aortic cross-clamping may be employed [19]. Endovascular approach using intra-aortic balloon occlusion technique (REBOA) has replaced aortic cross-clamping by open surgery (Fig. 1). Embolisation of target vessels has replaced open surgery in the control of bleeding in most situations.

Principles of Coagulation Management — Targeted Procoagulant Interventions

- Recent guidelines in 2013 recommend supplementation of fibrinogen if significant bleeding is accompanied by a plasma fibrinogen level of <1.5–2.0 g L [19,22]. Fibrinogen concentrate or cryoprecipitate are the recommended options for fibrinogen supplementation [19,22].

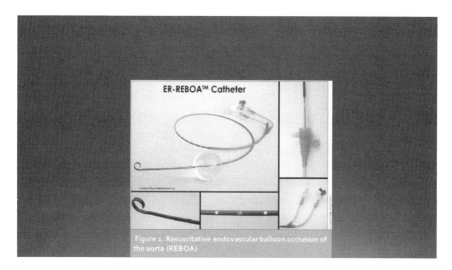

Figure 1.   Resuscitative endovascular balloon occlusion of the aorta (REBOA).

An initial Fibrinogen concentrate dose of 3–4 g or 50 mg/kg of Cryoprecipitate is recommended, which is approximately equivalent to 15–20 single donor units in an adult weighing 75 kg [19]. Repeat doses may be given depending on the laboratory assessment of fibrinogen levels and viscoelastic monitoring [19].

- Thawed FFP can also be used as a source of fibrinogen and clotting factors [19]. If bleeding continues after large volumes of IV fluids, red blood cells and platelets have been transfused, FFP and cryoprecipitate may be given so that the PT and APTT ratios are <1.5 [23].
- Platelet count should not be less than $50 \times 10^9/L$ in the acutely bleeding patient [23]. A dose of four to eight units of platelets can usually provide haemostasis in a thrombocytopenic, bleeding patient and typically increases the platelet count by $30–50 \times 10^9/L$ [25].

Antifibrinolytic agents

- Tranexamic acid is recommended for the trauma patient who is bleeding or at risk of significant hemorrhage, at a loading dose of 1 g infused over 10 min, followed by an intravenous infusion of 1 g over 8 h [19].

- E-aminocaproic acid is a potential alternative if tranexamic acid is not available, however its potency is 10 times weaker than that of Tranexamic Acid [19]. It is administered at a loading dose of 150 mg/kg followed by a continuous infusion of 15 mg/kg/h [19].
- The use of aprotinin is now contraindicated in bleeding trauma patients, since tranexamic acid has been shown to be efficacious and safe in trauma, and there have been concerns about the safety of aprotinin in other settings [26].

Recombinant factor VIIa replacement

Recombinant factor VIIa is not a first-line treatment for bleeding, however, once major bleeding from damaged vessels has been stopped, rFVIIa may be helpful to induce coagulation in areas of diffuse small vessel coagulopathic bleeding [19]. Recombinant factor VIIa should be considered only if first-line treatment with a combination of surgical and medical approaches fails to control bleeding [19].

Specific management of patients on anticoagulation (Table 3)

- Stop warfarin if not done so already [27].
- To reverse warfarin, give 25–50 IU/kg of four factor prothrombin complex concentrate (PCC) and 5 mg intravenous vitamin K [27] (which will switch on hepatic synthesis within a few hours) [28].
- Fresh frozen plasma produces suboptimal anticoagulation reversal and should only be used if PCC is not available [27].

Table 3.   Antidotes for anticoagulants.

- Oral anticoagulants (warfarin) — Vitamin K, PCC
- Unfractionated heparin — Protamine
- LMWH — Protamine, repeated dose
- Fondaparinux — Factor VIIa
- NOACs
   - Dabigatran — Idarucizumab (praxbind)
   - Rivaroxaban, apixaban, edoxaban — Andexanet alfa

- Unfractionated heparin can be reversed by protamine (1 mg protamine reverses 100 units of heparin) [1].
- LMWH can be partially reversed with protamine [1].
- Idarucizumab (praxbind) a specific antidote for direct thrombin inhibitor (dabigatran) is now available and has been approved by NICE. The recommended dose of idarucizumab is 5 g given intravenously as two consecutive infusions of 2.5 g/50 mL over 5–10 min each or as two consecutive 2.5 g bolus injections. Administration of a second 5-g dose of idarucizumab may be considered in any of the following clinical situations:
  - recurrence of clinically relevant bleeding together with prolonged clotting times,
  - if potential rebleeding would be life-threatening and prolonged clotting times are observed,
  - patients require a second emergency surgery or urgent procedure and have prolonged clotting times.

  Andexanet, a recombinant, modified factor Xa molecule developed as a direct reversal agent for patients receiving a Factor-Xa inhibitor with a major bleeding episode or requiring emergency surgery. The compound is under development and is an antidote for Apixaban, Edoxaban and rivaroxaban.
- Factor VIIa may be used for fondaparinux.
- For life-threatening bleeding, the off-label therapeutic use of PCC may be considered to attempt to overcome the anti-FXa or anti-FIIa activities of NOACs by increasing the plasma concentration of these clotting factors, although clinical evidence is lacking [29].
- Specific antidotes for NOACs are in development currently, namely, a specific reversal agent for factor Xa inhibitors (andexanet alfa) [30], and a potent monoclonal antibody directed against dabigatran, called idarucizumab [31].

Specific conditions and their management

- Patients with inherited coagulation disorders such as haemophilia require concentrated factor infusion to cover the peri-operative period under guidance from a haematologist [4].

- Management of traumatic bleeding may require management different from that of peri-operative bleeding through a different surgical cause.
- Management of haemorrhage in different surgeries, and for elective vs. emergency surgeries, follows different principles.

Post-Operative Management

Following treatment for massive haemorrhage, the patient must be admitted to a critical care area for monitoring and observation [1].

Reintroduction of anticoagulants post haemorrhage

- If warfarin is to be reintroduced, unfractionated heparin 5000 units tds should be administered after surgery until warfarin has been recommenced and the INR has been established at 2.5 for 2 days [4].
- Where the patient is prescribed LMWH, this should be continued post-operatively with warfarin until the INR is satisfactory [4].
- If the patient's risk of thrombosis is high and anticoagulation after peri-procedural cessation is required, NOAC administration can be resumed 12–24 h after procedures associated with rapid and complete restoration of hemostasis [32]. In general, evidence suggests that NOACs may be resumed within 24 h for a procedure with a low risk of bleeding, and within 48–72 h for a procedure with a high risk of bleeding [13].
- Standard venous thromboprophylaxis should be commenced as soon as possible after haemostasis has been achieved, as patients develop a prothrombotic state following massive haemorrhage [1].

References

1. Thomas D, Wee M, Clyburn P, Walker I, Brohi K, Collins P, Doughty H, Isaac J, Mahoney PF, Shewry L. Blood transfusion and the anaesthetist: Management of massive haemorrhage. *Anaesthesia.* 2010;65(11):1153–1161.
2. Committee on Trauma. *Advanced Trauma Life Support Manual.* Chicago: American College of Surgeons; 1997. pp. 103–112.

3. Muñoz M, Gómez-Ramírez S, Campos A, Ruiz J, Liumbruno GM. Pre-operative anaemia: Prevalence, consequences and approaches to management. *Blood Transfus* 2015;13(3):370–379.
4. *Blood Transfusion and the Anaesthetist — Blood Component Therapy*. AAGBI: http://www.aagbi.org/publications/guidelines/docs/bloodtransfusion06.pdf.
5. APIXIBAN — Bristol-Myers Squibb, Pfizer EEIG. Eliquis (apixaban) Summary of Product Characteristics. 2014. Available at: http://www.ema.europa.eu/docs/en_GB/document_library/EPAR_-Product_Information/human/002148/WC500107728.pdf.
6. APIXIBAN Bristol-Myers Squibb Company, Pfizer Inc. Eliquis (apixaban) Prescribing Information. 2014. Available at: http://packageinserts.bms.com/pi/pi_eliquis.pdf.
7. RIVAROXIBAN Bayer Pharma AG. Xarelto (rivaroxaban) Summary of Product Characteristics. 2014. Available at: http://www.ema.europa.eu/docs/en_GB/document_library/EPAR_-Product_Information/human/000944/WC500057108.pdf.
8. RIVAROXIBAN Janssen Pharmaceuticals Inc. Xarelto (rivaroxaban) Prescribing Information. 2014. Available at: http://www.xareltohcp.com/sites/default/files/pdf/xarelto_0.pdf.
9. DABIGATRAN Boehringer Ingelheim International GmbH. Pradaxa (dabigatran etexilate) Summary of Product Characteristics. 2014. Available at: http://www.ema.europa.eu/docs/en_GB/document_library/EPAR_-_Product_Information/human/000829/WC500041059.pdf.
10. DABIGATRAN Boehringer Ingelheim Pharmaceuticals Inc. Pradaxa (dabigatran etexilate) Prescribing Information. 2014. Available at: http://bidocs.boehringer-ingelheim.com/BIWebAccess/ViewServlet.ser?docBase=renetnt&folderPath=/Prescribing Information/PIs/Pradaxa/Pradaxa.pdf.
11. Gogarten W, Vandermeulen E, Van Aken H, Kozek S, Llau JV, Samama CM. Regional anaesthesia and antithrombotic agents: Recommendations of the European Society of Anaesthesiology. *Eur J Anaesthesiol* 2010;27:999–1015.
12. Sié P, Samama CM, Godier A *et al*. Surgery and invasive procedures in patients on long-term treatment with direct oral anticoagulants: Thrombin or factor-Xa inhibitors. Recommendations of the working group on perioperative Hemostasis and the French study group on thrombosis and haemostasis. *Arch Cardiovasc Dis* 2011;104:669–676.
13. Spyropoulos AC, Douketis JD. How I treat anticoagulated patients undergoing an elective procedure or surgery. *Blood* 2012;120:2954–2962.

14. van Veen JJ, Makris M. Management of peri-operative anti-thrombotic therapy. *Anaesthesia* 2015;70:58–e23.
15. Sørensen R, Hansen ML, Abildstrom SZ *et al*. Risk of bleeding in patients with acute myocardial infarction treated with different combinations of aspirin, clopidogrel, and vitamin K antagonists in Denmark: A retrospective analysis of nationwide registry data. *Lancet* 2009;374:1967–1974.
16. Ernst A, Eberhardt R, Wahidi M, Becker HD, Herth FJF. Effect of routine clopidogrel use on bleeding complications after transbronchial biopsy in humans. *Chest* 2006;129:734–737.
17. Scharbert G, Wetzel[1] L, Schrottmaier WC, Kral JB, Weber T, Assinger A. Comparison of patient intake of ticagrelor, prasugrel, or clopidogrel on restoring platelet function by donor platelets. *Transfusion* 2015;6:1320–1326.
18. Rahman A, Latona J. New oral anticoagulants and perioperative management of anticoagulant/antiplatelet agents. *Aust Fam Physician* 2014; 43(12):861–866.
19. Spahn DR, Bouillon B, Cerny V *et al*. Management of bleeding and coagulopathy following major trauma: An updated European guideline. *Crit Care* 2013;17:R76.
20. Mohamed El Sayad, Hussein N. Recent advances of hemorrhage management in severe trauma. *Emergency Med Int*, 2014; 2014. DOI:10.1155/2014/638956.
21. Sibylle A. Kozek-Langenecker, Management of severe perioperative bleeding. Guidelines from the European Society of Anaesthesiology. *Eur J Anaesthesiol* 2013;30:270–382.
22. Rossaint R, Bouillon B, Cerny V *et al*. Management of bleeding following major trauma: An updated European guideline. *Crit Care* 2010;14:R52.
23. O'Shaughnessy DF1, Atterbury C, Bolton Maggs P, Murphy M, Thomas D, Yates S, Williamson LM. British Committee for Standards in Haematology, Blood Transfusion Task Force. Guidelines for the use of fresh-frozen plasma, cryoprecipitate and cryosupernatant. *Br J Haematol* 2004;126:11–28.
24. British Committee for Standards in Haematology, Blood Transfusion Task Force. Guidelines for the use of platelet transfusions. *Br J Haematol* 2003; 17:10–23.
25. Kashuk JL, Moore EE, Sawyer M, Le T, Johnson J, Biffl WL, Cothren CC, Barnett C, Stahel P, Sillman CC, Sauaia A, Banerjee A. Post injury coagulopathy management: Goal directed resuscitation via POC thrombelastography. *Ann Surg* 2010;17:604–614.

26. Fergusson DA, Hébert PC, Mazer CD, Fremes S, MacAdams C, Murkin JM, Teoh K, Duke PC, Arellano R, Blajchman MA, Bussières JS, Côté D, Karski J, Martineau R, Robblee JA, Rodger M, Wells G, Clinch J, Pretorius R. BART Investigators. A comparison of aprotinin and lysine analogues in high-risk cardiac surgery. *N Engl J Med* 2008;17:2319–2331. DOI:10.1056/NEJMoa0802395.

27. Joint United Kingdom (UK) Blood Transfusion and Tissue Transplantation Services Professional Advisory Committee http://www.transfusionguidelines.org.uk/transfusion-handbook/7-effective-transfusion-in-surgery-and-critical-care/7-1-transfusion-in-surgery.

28. Hanley JP. Warfarin reversal. *J Clin Pathol* 2004;57(11):1132–1139.

29. Greinacher A, Thiele T, Selleng K. Reversal of anticoagulants: An overview of current developments. *Thromb Haemost* 2015;113(5):931–942.

30. Lu G, DeGuzman FR, Hollenbach SJ *et al.* A specific antidote for reversal of anticoagulation by direct and indirect inhibitors of coagulation factor Xa. *Nat Med* 2013; 19:446–451.

31. Schiele F, van Ryn J, Canada K *et al.* A specific antidote for dabigatran: Functional and structural characterization. *Blood* 2013;121:3554–3562.

32. Direct Oral Anticoagulants Jerrold H. Levy MD, Alex C. Spyropoulos MD, Charles M. Samama MD, PhD and James Douketis MD. *JACC: Cardiovasc Interven* 2014;7(12):1333–1351.

Chapter 25

Vascular Malformations

George Hamilton and Jocelyn Brookes

Key Points

- In the neonate, differentiate between haemangioma and vascular malformation.
- Clinical assessment is of prime importance.
  - Is intervention or simple reassurance required?
  - Realistically manage patient and parent expectations.
- Investigate by ultrasound, Duplex and magnetic resonance imaging (STIR, T1 and T2 with selective use of magnetic resonance angiography and magnetic resonance venography).
- Invasive angiography rarely indicated except for complex arteriovenous (AV) malformations and planned embolisation; identify the nidus.
- Classify the malformation — extra-truncular or truncular, high or low flow, ISSVA Classification?
- The majority of congenital vascular malformations (CVMs) are venous
  - Investigate for coagulopathy (DIC) in diffuse extensive capillary/venous malformations in the young child and adult.
- Malignant vascular malformations are rare.
- Tailor treatment to the severity of the lesion
  - Cosmesis, pain, function, asymmetry, tissue damage, etc.

- Foam sclerotherapy will be suitable and repeatable for the majority of venous malformations.
- Klippel–Trénaunay and Parkes-Weber syndromes and high flow malformations will need multidisciplinary input
  — Vascular and endovascular, orthopaedic, plastic surgeons, paediatrician and dermatologist.
- Look for and ablate ectatic and aneurysmal lateral marginal and deep veins because of risk of thromboembolic disease and death.
- Ethanol sclerotherapy and surgery for the minority, usually high flow AV malformations.
- The best care for patients of all age groups with CVMs is provided by multidisciplinary groups (including plastic surgery) with a special interest.

Introduction

Vascular malformations, currently most commonly termed congenital vascular malformations (CVMs), have a wide spectrum of clinical presentation and behaviour, ranging from simple birthmarks to massive disfiguring lesions, which in a minority of patients can be life-threatening. Understanding the pathophysiology and anatomy of CVMs has been poor, resulting in clinical confusion with regard to treatment strategies and resulting poor out comes. Since the 1990s, there has been a significant advancement in the understanding of the variety of CVMs by the introduction of clinically relevant and useful classification systems leading to significant improvement in their management.

Definition/Classification of Congenital Vascular Malformations

Neonatal/infantile haemangioma

Infantile and neonatal haemangioma usually appears after birth and rather than being a malformation is a vascular tumour arising from endothelial cells. Infantile haemangioma is characterised by early proliferation, and growth can be rapidly followed by spontaneous involution between 3 and 10 years. Haemangioma is relatively common with an incidence of 2–3% in newborn infants. The incidence of CVM is lower, about 1%; because of its presentation also during the neonatal period, it is important to distinguish clinically between CVM and haemangioma. CVM is characterised by malformed blood vessels while haemangioma is a localised vascular tumour behaving as described above.

Congenital vascular malformations

CVMs can be classified according to their make up, as either arterial, venous, arteriovenous, lymphatic, capillary, and often combined or mixed vascular malformation. Venous malformations are the most common form of CVM, with 15–20% being mixed lesions, constituted of the Klippel–Trénaunay syndrome and Parkes-Weber syndrome [1].

Eponymous syndromes

Early in the last century, before angiography was available, several clinical syndromes were described and named according to the clinician. Two eponymous syndromes, namely Klippel–Trénaunay and Parkes-Weber, continue to be identified in modern times. This is largely because the syndromes describe the primary vascular malformation together with the secondary non-vascular pathologies.

Klippel–Trénaunay syndrome has venous, lymphatic and capillary components associated with overgrowth — soft tissue swelling, long bone growth, leg discrepancy and gigantism [2]. Parkes-Weber syndrome has clinically similar capillary, venous and lymphatic malformation with overgrowth, but is also characterised by extensive, mostly microscopic, arteriovenous shunting throughout the affected limb (Table 1) [3].

The development of imaging modalities has led to a better understanding and classification of CVMs.

Hamburg classification

This classification was based on a consensus established at the International Workshop in Hamburg in 1998 with subsequent regular

Table 1.   Eponymous malformations.

Klippel–Trénaunay syndrome

- Predominantly haemolymphatic (HLM)
- Venous, lymphatic and capillary malformation
- Vascular bone syndrome

Parkes-Weber syndrome

- Capillary, venous and lymphatic
- Multiple arteriovenous shunting malformation (AVM)

---

modifications. The classification system is based on insights achieved in understanding the underlying pathophysiology, anatomical distribution, both macroscopic and microscopic, the resulting underlying haemodynamic effects and further differentiation relating to their time of development in the embryo. The classification is summarised in Table 2 with the first component (A) being classification into one of five types based on the vascular pathophysiology, namely arterial, venous, lymphatic, arteriovenous and combined vascular malformations.

The second very important component of the classification (B) is based on the embryological stage at which the malformation develops, dividing malformations into either extra-truncular or truncular.

This part of the classification is particularly important in terms of management and prognosis in that the clinical behaviour of the two forms is predicated at the embryological stage at which the malformation develops and at which development arrest occurs.

Extra-truncular congenital vascular malformations

Extra-truncular cardiovascular malformations arise during the earlier phase of embryological development. At this stage, vascular cells are primarily angioblasts derived from mesenchymal cells. These are similar to stem cells, which at any stage of life can be stimulated to proliferate. These stimuli can be hormonal, such as menarche, adolescence and pregnancy, or as a response to trauma or surgical intervention.

Table 2.   The Hamburg classification of CVMs.

A: Anatomical types

- Predominantly arterial defects
- Predominantly venous defects
- Predominantly arteriovenous (AV) shunting defects
- Predominantly lymphatic defects
- Combined vascular defects (Klippel–Trénaunay and Parkes-Weber syndromes)

B: Embryological types

- *Extra-truncular forms* — Infiltrating, diffuse limited, localised
- *Truncular forms* — Aplasia, hypoplasia, hyperplasia, stenosis, membrane, congenital spur
- *Dilation* — Localised (aneurysm), diffuse (ectasia)

Extra-truncular malformations most commonly are diffuse and infiltrating in nature, less commonly more localised, but typically having compressive effects on adjacent tissues and organs. A further clinically important feature is their high propensity for recurrence if treatment is suboptimal. In general, extra-truncular malformations are high flow, have greater morbidity, worse prognosis and present a greater therapeutic challenge.

Truncular congenital vascular malformations

These malformations develop later in embryological vascular development. They are therefore constituted of cells that have lost their pluripotential stem cell-like properties, in particular the potential to proliferate. These malformations may present as persistent foetal remnants, such as the sciatic vein, or a defectively developed structure, often occlusive, with a combination of stenotic, aneurysmal or web-like vessel disease. The classification therefore further subdivides truncular lesions into obstructive or dilated. Truncular lesions are much less likely to recur when treated.

Mulliken classification of cardiovascular malformations

This is a different system that characterised malformations as either slow flow or fast flow. This further haemodynamic classification is clinically useful particularly to the vascular specialist, but the Hamburg classification remains predominant, particularly with its ability to predict the clinical outcome for treatment according to the malformation being either extra-truncular or truncular.

International Society for the Study of Vascular Anomalies (ISSVA) Modified Classification

The ISSVA introduced in 2014 a modification of its previous classification with the purpose of improved application to clinical reporting and guidelines. This further classification is increasingly used [4] (Table 3).

Differential diagnosis

Most commonly, presentation takes place in the perinatal period. A CVM having developed in the later stages of foetal development presents as an abnormal vascular lesion at birth. A haemangioma is most commonly

Table 3.   2014 ISSVA classification of vascular anomalies.

Simple	Combined	Of major named vessels	Associated with other anomalies
CM	CM + VM	Artery, vein lymphatic	Klippel–Trénaunay Syndrome
LM	CM + LM	Large calibre	Parkes-Weber Syndrome
VM	CM + AVM	Axial/conducting	Sturge–Weber Syndrome
AVM	LM + VM	Aplasia, hypoplasia	Servelle-Martorell Syndrome
AV fistula	CM + LM + VM	Ectasias, aneurysm	Mafucci Syndrome
	CM+LM+AVM	Valvular dysfunction/ aplasia	CLOVES Syndrome
	CM+VM+AVM	Persistent embryonic vessels	Proteus Syndrome
	CM+LM+VM+AVM	(truncular)	

Note: M = malformation, C = capillary, L = lymphatic, AV = arteriovenous, V = venous.

Table 4.   Differential diagnosis.

- Haemangioma occurs in 2–3% of neonates, rising to 10% at the end of the first year
  - Vascular tumour
- CVM occurs in 1%
  - Congenital stable malformation that grows commensurately
- Venous malformations are the most common CVMs
  - 15–20% are mixed lesions (Klippel–Trénaunay and Parkes-Weber syndromes)

---

not present at birth, but develops suddenly within the first 4 weeks of the neonatal period with rapid early growth, stimulation and then regression between the ages of 3 and 10 years. The first step in the differential diagnosis is therefore to exclude the diagnosis of haemangioma (Table 4).

Classification of a CVM is the next step in the process of differential diagnosis and as described above is made by applying the Hamburg or more commonly the ISSVA classification. The presence of an arteriovenous component predicts a more virulent and unpredictable clinical course with higher morbidity. It is therefore also extremely important to investigate every vascular malformation for the possibility of an arteriovenous component. Initially this may not be clinically obvious, but declares itself during follow up.

Diagnosis

After the initial steps of clinical assessment by history taking and examination, the first step in the diagnostic process is by non-invasive assessment, primarily in the vascular laboratory. Duplex ultrasonography based on colour Doppler imaging and spectral waveform analysis primarily provides anatomical and haemodynamic information. This methodology can reliably demonstrate arterial and venous components, and define the anatomy and extent of the lesion, in particular the presence of feeding arteries and draining veins. When there is deeper involvement of anatomical structures, such as in the chest, abdomen or pelvis, or involvement of long bones, duplex sonography may be limited in its diagnostic potential (Table 5).

Table 5.   Investigation.

• *Ultrasound/duplex*
— Excellent screening tool, central to correct diagnosis
• Flow characteristics of the lesion can be defined
• Arterial, venous or combined
— High flow or low flow
— Confirms complications, such as thrombosis, phleboliths, etc.
• *Computed tomography (CT)*
• Excellent anatomical detail with contrast for arteriovenous (AV) malformations
• *Magnetic resonance imaging (MRI)*
— Excellent anatomical detail of surrounding tissues
— Confirms venous and/or arterial nature of the lesion
— Excellent for picking up complications or occult features

Magnetic resonance imaging is the second component of the initial diagnostic process for all malformations. STIR, T1 and T2 weighted studies will provide excellent anatomical detail of the extent of the cardiovascular malformation, differentiate between high and low flow lesions and is particularly valuable in the diagnosis of venous malformations. In addition, MR angiography and venography can be added to the above MRI investigation for further anatomical detail. Computed tomography contrast scans are also valuable for assessment, in particular of malformations involving bone, the thorax, abdomen and pelvis. Three-dimensional reconstruction of CT angiograms is particularly useful in the diagnosis treatment planning of arteriovenous malformations (Fig. 1).

Lympho-scintigraphy is the investigation of choice for assessment of lymphatic or haemo-lymphatic malformations and MR lymph-angiography may also be used to provide further anatomical detail of the extent of the lymphatic malformation.

Simple bone X-ray is indicated where there is limb asymmetry in the presence of vascular-bone syndrome, and MRI can confirm the presence of bony or articular involvement.

In cases of deep seated haemangioma or CVMs, MR and CT imaging are important. This will be needed to differentiate between various

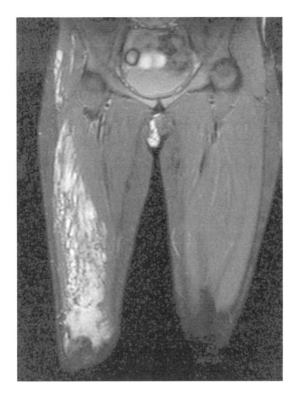

Figure 1. MRI revealing the extent of a venous malformation with diffuse involvement of the thigh muscles and the right labium majorum.

hamartomatous pathologies and most importantly to exclude the possibility of sarcoma. Where there is still doubt, CT-guided needle biopsy is of value in these cases.

Angiography and venography are important, more invasive investigations currently used in planning interventional or surgical treatment of symptomatic vascular malformations such as complex AVM and venous aneurysm or stenosis.

Basic haematological investigations are of course important, but should include coagulation studies, initially D-dimer and fibrinogen, to detect the possible presence of a consumptive coagulopathy, in extensive lesions. Large marginal veins and venous aneurysms have a high risk of venous thrombosis. Coagulopathy is found in children with extensive haemangiomas and malformations, and in these children, anticoagulation might be required.

Diagnosis summary

Diagnosis in the vast majority of malformations is based on careful clinical assessment and examination, Duplex sonography with STIR, T1 and T2 weighted MRI. In very young children, more complex investigations, which require sedation or general anaesthesia, can be delayed where the malformation is clinically assessed as unlikely to be aggressive [5]. Earlier management principles focused on aggressive surgical excision of these lesions. The poor outcomes in the absence of the clinical insight given by the classifications resulted in a move to more conservative treatment. Currently, treatment outcomes are much improved and are focused on a multidisciplinary approach. This will involve disciplines such as paediatric dermatology, vascular and endovascular surgery, plastic and reconstructive surgery, orthopaedic surgery, head and neck surgery, and ENT surgery. The outcome of multidisciplinary assessment will focus primarily on dealing with the malformation and subsequently on dealing with the secondary components, particularly on the musculoskeletal system and cosmesis.

Indications for Treatment

Many malformations presenting in children will not need initial treatment, but rather careful monitoring of their development and or regression. This will require careful documentation of clinical history, photographic and non-invasive assessment.

Absolute indications for intervention are in most cases clear and include bleeding from arteriovenous or venous malformations, progression of high output heart failure in arteriovenous malformations, persistent lymphatic leakage with infection or sepsis from lymphatic or haemo-lymphatic malformations, and chronic venous insufficiency secondary to venous or haemo-lymphatic malformations. Vascular malformations situated in potentially life-threatening regions such as next to the airway or significantly compromising limbs, or vital functions such as seeing, hearing, eating, are also indications for intervention. Relative indications for treatment include severe unremitting pain, non-healing ulceration, lesions causing deep vein thrombosis, such as in the marginal vein with its associated risk of thromboembolic disease, haemarthrosis where the lesions involve joints in particular the knee, and cosmetically unacceptable lesions.

In venous malformations (the most common presentation), early aggressive treatment is only indicated in situations as highlighted above, particularly for pain but also where the vascular bone syndrome results in limb gigantism. The treatment plan for diffuse extra-truncular lesions has to be very carefully formulated because of its progressive nature and high potential for recurrence (Table 6).

In treatment of all malformations, the management of expectations of the patient and parents is key. It must be made clear that multiple interventions may be required to control and deal with the effects of the malformation, and it is also important to stress that control rather than cure is the likeliest outcome in the majority of patients [6].

Table 6.   Indications for intervention.

Prevention of harm
— Heart failure
— Consumptive coagulopathy
— Ischaemia of limb, skin, etc.
— Compression of airway, etc.
— Bleeding

Treatment of symptoms
— Pain
— Unpleasant pulsation— tinnitus or bruit

Treatment of signs
— Unsightly vessels or swelling
— Limb or facial asymmetry
— Cosmesis

Surgical treatment

The old principle of surgical ligation of a feeding or draining vessel very rarely applies and indeed ligation of a feeding artery is absolutely contraindicated since this will deny the possibility of endovascular treatment to future interventions or recurrences. Surgical treatment may be combined with embolisation in extensive arteriovenous malformations, or may be required after sclerotherapy in predominately venous malformations. The advent of successful embolo-sclerotherapy allows treatment of complex and infiltrating CVMs that previously were beyond surgical therapy (Fig. 2).

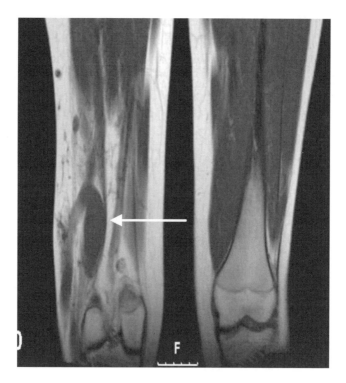

Figure 2.   The aneurysmal marginal vein in the lateral aspect of the right leg of this young woman was removed with preoperative marking and intraoperative duplex localisation of the deep draining veins for ligation. These venous ectasias have significant potential for thromboembolic complications [7].

In general, the low flow truncular forms are primarily treated by scle-rotherapy, but surgery remains important, particularly in venous malfor-mations such as the lateral marginal vein in the Klippel–Trénaunay syndrome and in venous aneurysms [7]. Surgery to vascular malforma-tions can be either haemodynamic or ablative. Haemodynamic surgery is designed as the first step in dealing with the vascular malformation where restoration of arterial blood flow around an infiltrating lesion, e.g., a femoropopliteal bypass graft, or a venous bypass to restore venous drainage, is required. After haemodynamic surgery has been successfully achieved excisional or ablative surgery can be performed. Complete abla-tive resection of CVMs has greater success when the malformation is superficial to the deep fascia and not invading into major muscles, bone or into the thorax, abdomen or pelvis [8]. Secondary surgery to correct limb length discrepancy (epiphysiodesis) can then take place, usually between the ages of 3–7 years, by the orthopaedic service.

The more extensive excisional surgery will in many cases involve the reconstructive plastic surgeons. Where there is gross deformity and marked compromise of function in a limb, then primary amputation may be the best option, resulting in early optimisation of function (Fig. 3).

Endovascular therapy

Embolisation using coils or liquid embolic agents such as glues and Onyx™ is useful in dealing with the arterial component of arteriovenous malformations. In extensive venous malformations, coils and glues are relatively contraindicated because of the diffuse nature of the lesion. The high propensity for these structures to be flushed out of the malforma-tion. Although glue and Onyx can be effective, a hard cast within the obliterated malformation may be uncomfortable or unsightly. Coil and glue embolisation will rarely be effective in the more diffuse extra-truncular lesions. Sclerotherapy by injection of various agents is of value in many malformations, arteriovenous, venous, truncular and extra-truncular. These sclerosants act by their toxic effects, resulting in endothelial destruction, thrombosis and fibrosis. The important factors to be considered are the strength of the sclerosant, the length of time

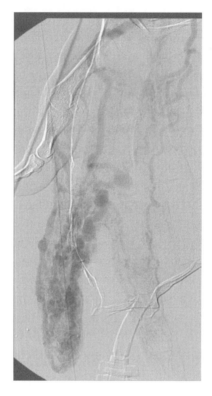

Figure 3.   This extensive and progressive extra-truncular malformation flared up after trauma; primary amputation of the index finger resulted in an excellent symptomatic and functional outcome.

that the sclerosant is in contact with the vein wall and the area of contact between sclerosant and endothelium. A mainstay of treatment with sclerosants is post-injection compression. There are several sclerosants in use [9].

Ethanol

Absolute ethanol has been used for many decades. It is a very potent sclerosant, so much so that it can cause vessel necrosis and have local toxic effects. These include severe pain, swelling with compartment syndrome, damage to surrounding structures, in particular nerves and in more superficial lesions, overlying skin necrosis. In addition, ethanol has potent systemic side effects including cardiac arrhythmias and pulmonary hypertension secondary to pulmonary vasospasm. The reported incidence of complications including cardiovascular collapse and death has been reported to be as high as 28%, but in experienced centres is very low.

Ethanol is therefore a very powerful sclerosant but with potentially devastating side effects and should only be used in more aggressive generally extra-truncular malformations and after experienced multidisciplinary assessment of the therapeutic options. Ethanol injection is particularly useful in dealing with diffuse extra-truncular lesions causing significant complications. The core or nidus of the lesion must be identified and targeted with the ethanol injection to achieve a good result.

The ethanol is injected either directly under careful fluoroscopic control or by a catheter. General anaesthesia is required and careful attention to postoperative monitoring and analgesia is essential. The maximum dose of ethanol should not exceed 1 mL kg^{-1} of body weight, but can be repeated after 10 min.

Other sclerosing agents

Polidocanol, tetradecyl sulphate, sodium morrhuate and ethanolamine have been used in the treatment of cardiovascular malformations. They are particularly valuable in dealing with venous malformations, and treatments can be repeated many times, in many cases without general anaesthesia.

Technique

In arteriovenous malformations catheter delivery is most commonly used. In venous malformations direct-injection sclerotherapy is used. Duplex ultrasonography is very useful in imaging the malformation and very frequently multiple needles are used. Under fluoroscopy, contrast is injected to define the extent of the malformation and also to assess its volume. The volume identified of sclerosant is injected — it is important to be able to monitor the spread of the sclerosant, into the malformation.

This is not a problem with the foam sclerosant, but when a neat sclerosant solution is being used, this should be mixed with contrast. The aim is to compress the draining vein and then to inject additional sclerosant to fill as much of the malformation as possible. With the use of multiple needles injections continue until the sclerosant begins to drain from the other needles (Fig. 4). Compression is then applied. Using foam, intravenous sedation and pain relief may be all that is required. With the injection of neat sclerosants and certainly ethanol, general anaesthesia will be required. More recently, with major venous malformations, a transvenous placement of an occlusion balloon catheter into a large draining vein has been used. Alternatively, in more superficial lesions tourniquets are useful for occluding draining veins. These manoeuvres aid in maximal filling of the malformation with the sclerosant.

The results of injection sclerotherapy have been good with the modern focus being on the use of foam sclerosant (this is prepared by mixing neat sclerosant with either air or carbon dioxide at a ratio of 1:10). There are several outcome reports with success, particularly in reduction of the pain associated with venous malformations. The complication rate is low, mainly with transient skin pigmentation and a very low incidence of skin necrosis. Multiple episodes of injection sclerotherapy are required in the majority of patients with venous malformations [10].

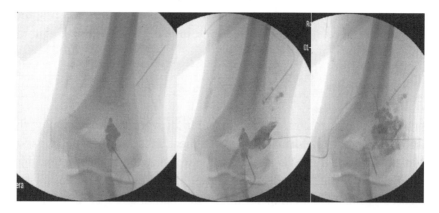

Figure 4.   Using three separate needles the components of this venous malformation of the elbow were sequentially filled with foam sclerosant to treat the entire malformation; immediate compression was applied.

The 'Nidus' concept in ablation of high flow malformations

The nidus is the junction between high flow arteriolar and venular components of arteriovenous malformations, constituted of minute primitive dysfunctional vascular cells. The connection can be single as in an arteriovenous fistula, or multiple as in a diffuse extra-truncular AVM (Fig. 5). Radiological identification of the nidus, single or multiple, is key to successful management of high flow lesions (ref). Occlusion of the nidus once identified can be achieved by direct injection of ethanol or in

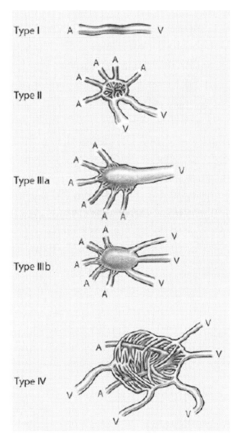

Figure 5.   Yakes classification of arteriovenous malformations (extra-truncular); multiple nidus morphology in all except type I, with type IV having diffuse dysmorphic pattern and most difficult to control.

simpler AVMs of sclerosant foam. Slowing of flow by a combination of pre-nidus arterial balloon occlusion and tourniquet or finger pressure post-nidus venous occlusion will optimise the sclerosant effect. In addition, directed stick puncture to the venous side of the identified nidus facilitates successful closure [11].

Summary

Over the last decade, there have been significant advances and improvements in the management of the difficult condition of CVMs. Central to this success is the clinical classification of these disorders, in particular into truncular and extra-truncular, and high or low flow lesions. The multidisciplinary approach is of absolute importance with the vascular/endovascular surgeon and interventional radiologist central to the team. Embolosclerotherapy has proved to be a major advance in the management of these conditions, particularly venous malformations. It has also revolutionised the approach to high flow and extensive malformations, facilitating surgical excision in around 15% of patients of life-threatening lesions or those associated with severe complications. Advances in devices and agents such as coils, glues and sclerosant foam have also reduced the morbidity of treatment and widened the indications. Ethanol remains the most effective sclerosant but is toxic and has significant side effects, in inexperienced hands. The current drive is towards finding alternatives to ethanol, but remains important in treating complex high flow malformations.

Most patients referred to a multidiscipline unit will not require treatment, but benefit from the reassurance that their disease is unlikely to progress, that it is not a tumour and that if symptoms do develop they have established contact with a unit that is able to deliver all aspects of the care that they may need.

References

1. Lee BB, Laredo J, Lee TS, Huh S, Neville R. Terminology and classification of congenital vascular malformations. *Phlebology* 2007;22:249–252.
2. Gloviczki P, Driscoll DJ. Klippel–Trénaunay syndrome: Current management. *Phlebology* 2007;22:291–298.

3. Comi AM. Update on Sturge–Weber syndrome: Diagnosis, treatment, quantitative measures, and controversies. *Lymphat Res Biol* 2007;5:257–264.

4. Wassef M, Blei F, Adams D, Alomari A, Baselga E, Berenstein A, Burrows P, Frieden IJ, Garzon MC, Lopez-Gutierrez JC, Lord DJ, Mitchel S, Powell J, Prendiville J, Vikkula M; ISSVA Board and Scientific Committee. Vascular Anomalies Classification: Recommendations From the International Society for the Study of Vascular Anomalies. *Pediatrics* 2015;136(1):e203–214.

5. Lee BB, Laredo J, Lee SJ, Huh SH, Joe JH, Neville R. Congenital vascular malformations: General diagnostic principles. *Phlebology* 2007;22:253–257.

6. Lee BB, Laredo J, Kim YW, Neville R. Congenital vascular malformations: General treatment principles. *Phlebology* 2007;22:258–263.

7. Mattassi R, Vaghi M. Management of the marginal vein: Current issues. *Phlebology* 2007;22:283–286.

8. Maftei N, Howard A, Brown LC, Gunning MP, Standfield NJ. The surgical management of 73 vascular malformations and preoperative predictive factors of major haemorrhage — a single centre experience. *Eur J Vasc Endovasc Surg* 2009;38:488–497.

9. Lee BB, Baumgartner I, Berlien P, Bianchini G, Burrows P, Gloviczki P, Huang Y, Laredo J, Loose DA, Markovic J, Mattassi R, Parsi K, Rabe E, Rosenblatt M, Shortell C, Stillo F, Vaghi M, Villavicencio L, Zamboni P. International Union of Phlebology. Diagnosis and Treatment of Venous Malformations. Consensus Document of the International Union of Phlebology (IUP): Updated 2013. *Int Angiol* 2015;34(2):97–149.

10. Bergan J, Cheng V. Foam sclerotherapy of venous malformations. *Phlebology* 2007;22:299–302.

11. Lee BB, Baumgartner I, Berlien HP, Bianchini G, Burrows P, Do YS, Ivancev K, Kool LS, Laredo J, Loose DA, Lopez-Gutierrez JC, Mattassi R, Parsi K, Rimon U, Rosenblatt M, Shortell C, Simkin R, Stillo F, Villavicencio L, Yakes W; International Union of Angiology. Consensus Document of the International Union of Angiology (IUA)-2013. Current concept on the management of arterio-venous management. *Int Angiol* 2013;32(1):9–36.

Chapter 26

Vasospastic Disorders and Vasculitis

Muhammed Anees Sharif, Bridget Griffiths and
Gerard Stansby

Key Points

- Understanding of the nomenclature used for the classification of vasospastic disorders into primary and secondary Raynaud's phenomena (RP) is essential.
- The management of these disorders requires a multidisciplinary team approach involving physicians, rheumatologists and vascular specialists.
- Treatment of Raynaud's includes general supportive measures, pharmacotherapy and correction of underlying disorders.
- Vasculitis is associated with a range of medical conditions and can present as digital ischaemia.
- A diagnosis of vasculitis is suggested by constitutional symptoms and confirmed by raised inflammatory markers, the presence of autoantibodies, targeted radiological imaging and biopsy of skin lesions or other involved organs.
- Immunosuppressive therapy is the mainstay of treatment in vasculitic disorders.

Introduction

Raynaud's phenomenon (RP) refers to a clinical state characterised by episodic vasospasm, usually involving the distal small arteries of the upper limbs although sometimes toes and feet are also affected. In addition, there are other vascular disorders characterised by inflammatory changes in the arterial wall, known as the 'vasculitides', which can present with digital ischaemia.

Vasospasm (Raynaud's Phenomenon)

Maurice Raynaud first described this clinical picture in 1862 [1]. The classical presentation of RP is characterised by a sequence of colour changes in the following order:

- pallor, reflecting initial vasospasm,
- cyanosis as a result of deoxygenation of stagnant blood during maximum vasospasm,
- rubor, representing inflow of oxygenated blood and reactive hyperaemia as the vasospasm subsides.

Episodes usually last for 30–60 min. However, some patients present with only cold hands and do not exhibit the classical triphasic/triple colour response (white, blue and then red) although they demonstrate a similar blood flow pattern to classical vasospasm. The factors triggering these changes and the parts of the body affected are listed in Table 1.

Epidemiology

The overall incidence of RP is 11.8% with women affected 9 times more often than men. In certain geographical areas that are prone to a cold and damp climate, 20–30% of the population is affected. A familial predisposition has also been reported, which is more likely if the age at onset is less than 30 years.

RP has particularly been described as a complication of occupations involving vibrating tools such as pneumatic drills and vibrating saw

Table 1.   Triggering factors and the parts of the body affected by RP.

Factors provoking a vasospastic episode

- Cold exposure
- Emotional stress
- Vibration — hand arm vibration syndrome (HAVS)
- Industrial chemicals
- Tobacco smoke
- Trauma
- Drugs, e.g., β-blockers

Parts of the body affected by vasospasm

- Fingers (commonest)
- Toes
- Nose
- Ear lobes
- Tongue
- Nipples

chains, in which context it is also referred to as 'vibration white finger'. Over 50% of people using these tools may ultimately show symptoms of the disease. The underlying mechanism appears to be a high-frequency vibration, which exposes the small digital arteries in the fingers to severe stress. This leads to inflammatory changes and fibrosis in the arterial wall. Since 1985, HAVS has been listed as an industrial disease in the UK, and these patients might be eligible for compensation provided they fulfil disease specific criteria.

Chronic exposure to cold temperature at the industrial level has also been associated with vasospastic disorder, and up to 50% of workers dealing with alternate cold and hot water manifest some symptoms of vasospasm.

Nomenclature Used in Vasospastic Disorders

- RP — A blanket term used to describe all vasospastic disorders.

- Primary Raynaud's phenomenon (PRP) — Vasospastic symptoms manifested on their own without any underlying systemic disease process.
- Secondary Raynaud's phenomenon (SRP) — Vasospasm associated with another known disease entity, e.g., rheumatoid arthritis, systemic sclerosis.

Most people with mild symptoms would usually present to their general practitioner and usually have PRP. Those with more severe forms are more likely to have SRP. It should be noted that sometimes the symptoms of vasospasm are present for many years in advance of diagnosis of the associated SRP cause. The differentiation between PRP and SRP is helpful in planning the initial treatment, but is sometimes difficult, requiring a sound clinical knowledge of the diseases associated with SRP as listed in Table 2.

Table 2.   Disorders associated with SRP.

Autoimmune connective tissue diseases (CTDs)

- Systemic sclerosis (SSc or scleroderma) — both limited and diffuse cutaneous subtypes (limited cutaneous SSc formerly known as CREST)
- Polymyositis and dermatomyositis
- Mixed CTD
- Systemic lupus erythematosus
- Rheumatoid arthritis
- Primary Sjögren's syndrome
- IgA nephropathy (formerly known as Henoch–Schönlein purpura)

Vasculitides

- Large vessel vasculitis, e.g., Takayasu arteritis
- Medium vessel vasculitis, e.g., polyarteritis nodosa
- Small vessel vasculitis, e.g., granulomatosis with polyangiitis

Obstructive

- Atherosclerosis
- Buerger's disease (thromboangitis obliterans)

(Continued)

Table 2.   (*Continued*)

- Microemboli
- Thoracic outlet syndrome (cervical rib/band)

Myeloproliferative disorders

- Leukaemia
- Myeloid metaplasia
- Polycythaemia rubra vera

Drugs

- β-blockers
- Cytotoxic drugs
- Antimigraine drugs including ergotamine

Industrial

- HAVS
- Vinyl chloride
- Frozen food workers

Circulating globulins

- Malignancy
- Multiple myeloma
- Cryoglobulinaemia

Miscellaneous

- Chronic renal failure
- Reflex sympathetic dystrophy
- Hypothyroidism

Note: CREST = calcinosis cutis, Raynaud's phenomenon, oesophageal dysfunction, sclerodactyly, telangiectasia.

Pathophysiology

Although the exact mechanism of RP is not completely understood, a number of key factors are implicated in its aetiology and pathogenesis. These include the following:

(i) neurogenic alterations,
(ii) haemodynamic changes,

(iii) inflammatory and immune dysregulation,
(iv) mechanical,
 (v) genetic predisposition.

For simplicity, we have described these different mechanisms separately. However, in actual practice, there is likely to be a complex interaction between them.

Neurogenic alterations

Patients with RP have an increased sensitivity to cold and show increased vasospastic tone in response to cold exposure and other triggering factors. This vascular neurogenic response can occur in the absence of an obstructive arterial lesion. The vasospastic response is explained on the basis of enhanced sensitivity of both alpha and beta adrenergic receptors in the peripheral sympathetic nervous system controlling the arterial tone.

Haemodynamic changes

Normal vascular tone depends on interactions between the flowing stream of blood (cellular and plasma components) and the endothelial lining of the vessel wall. Patients with RP show changes in these microvascular components, which trigger an obstructive and vasospastic response. These include the following:

- Changes in blood and blood components:
  - Platelet activation and aggregation leads to formation of platelet plugs, causing obstruction to the blood flow and release of thromboxane A2 resulting in vasospasm.
  - Activated leukocytes release free radicals causing further vasoconstriction.
  - Red cells become stiff and obstruct the vessel lumen resulting in further obstruction to microcirculation.
  - Plasma viscosity is increased as a result of an increase in plasma proteins.

- Changes in endothelial function:
  - Patients with RP show signs of endothelial dysfunction, such as activation of von Willebrand factor (VWF), which promotes clotting and activates platelets.
  - Tissue plasminogen activator (tPA) activity is reduced, resulting in less effective fibrinolysis and a prothrombotic state in patients with RP.

Inflammatory and immune dysregulation

Patients with an underlying autoimmune connective tissue disorder or vasculitis manifest the most severe symptoms of RP. It is a reflection of an intense systemic inflammatory and immune response involving the connective tissues in general including the connective tissue in the arterial wall. The vessel wall in these cases shows a mixture of inflammatory cells including neutrophils, lymphocytes and plasma cells.

Mechanical

Vibration white finger disease seen in patients exposed to high-frequency vibration tools is associated with mechanical damage to vessel wall and secondary inflammatory changes.

Genetic predisposition

RP is reported in patients with scleroderma and shows a familial association with the MHC class II antigens. In addition, primary RP has been seen in monozygotic twins.

Clinical Presentation

Key points in the clinical assessment and diagnosis are as follows:

- The clinical picture is episodic with each episode lasting from a few minutes to an hour.
- RP is usually triggered by exposure to cold or emotional upset.

- Usually fingers and sometimes toes are affected. The distribution of involved digits could be asymmetrical with one or more digits affected at one time, although all digits can be affected in one particular patient.
- Involvement of one limb only suggests a possible local cause such as a cervical rib.
- Patients either show a biphasic or triphasic response of colour changes.
- The first phase is observed after initial exposure to the triggering factor and is associated with vasospasm characterised by clinical feature of pallor. Some patients would experience cold hands and numbness at this stage as a result of reduced blood flow to the digital arteries.
- The initial phase is followed by cyanosis and/or rubor because of reperfusion and is sometimes associated with pain and paraesthesia.
- Other parts of the body can be affected as described earlier, including ear lobes, nose and nipples.
- A cyanotic episode without preceding pallor is not usually because of RP.

Laboratory Investigations

A number of laboratory tests including blood flow measurement, blood tests and radiological investigations can be helpful during investigation of patients with RP (Table 3).

- The diagnosis of RP is mainly clinical, based on a history of biphasic/triphasic colour changes in response to cold exposure or emotional upset, along with physical examination if the presentation is during an acute episode.
- Laboratory investigations are mainly aimed at differentiating PRP from SRP by identifying any underlying systemic disease.
- Nail-fold capillaroscopy has been established as a corner stone in the diagnosis of autoimmune CTD, particularly scleroderma, in patients with RP.

Table 3.   Investigative techniques used for the assessment of blood flow in patients with RP.

Investigation	Technique	Interpretation
Nail-fold capillaroscopy	Microscopic examination of the nail bed for abnormal blood vessels.	Abnormally enlarged, dilated and tortuous blood vessels indicate possibility of CTD, particularly scleroderma.
		Beware that similar changes can occur in diabetes mellitus and nail-fold trauma.
Computerised thermography	Skin temperature is assessed as a marker of blood flow during different phases of RP.	Caution is required in interpreting the results as both the arterial as well as venous flow can affect the skin temperature.
Mild cold challenge	Hands are immersed in cool water at a regulated temperature for a defined period and then rate of rewarming is assessed over next 10 min.	Slow rewarming may be consistent with RP.

- The relevant blood tests include the following:
  o Full blood count, urea and electrolytes, creatinine, C-reactive protein (CRP), erythrocyte sedimentation rate (ESR) and urinalysis to detect renal dysfunction.
  o An autoantibody screen, which should include rheumatoid factor/ anti-CCP, antinuclear antibodies (ENA antibodies and anti-dsDNA antibodies) and ANCA.
  o Cryoglobulins and cold agglutinins are required only if there is a clinical suspicion of a prothrombotic state.
  o Thyroid function test, if suspecting hypothyroidism as an underlying cause of RP.
- Abnormal nail-fold capillaroscopy combined with an abnormal autoantibody test predicts an underlying CTD in 90% patients with RP.
- A baseline upper extremity arterial Duplex scan should be carried out to exclude an underlying occlusive arterial disease.
- A plain chest radiograph can demonstrate a cervical rib if present and sometimes can demonstrate basal pulmonary fibrosis, which is sometimes seen in a CTD.

Management

Patients with primary RP usually have mild or moderate symptoms and do not require specific drug treatment. However, they should be given general advice such as keep warm, wear multiple layers and stop smoking, reassurance and written information such as that provided by the charity and patient support group Scleroderma and Raynaud's UK. Any causative drug, such as β-blockers, should be replaced with alternatives and any underlying disease such as hypothyroidism should be treated. Good symptomatic control is possible with these measures, despite the non-availability of a definite cure. Figure 1 outlines the management algorithm in patients with RP.

General supportive measures

These are suitable for patients with RP showing mild to moderate symptoms without an underlying disease process. The key points are as follows:

- reassurance, explanation and information leaflets,
- stop smoking,
- wear multiple layers, use hand warmers, electric gloves and socks,
- special shoes with broad and padded fitting (Abel shoes) — these are available from the hospital appliance departments,
- meticulous attention to areas of skin breakdown, ulcers and infection.

Pharmacological therapy

This should be reserved for more severe symptoms, which affect quality of life or work, as outlined in Fig. 1. The commonly used drugs are listed in Table 4.

Calcium channel blockers

Nifedipine and amlodipine are the most effective and commonly used vasodilators. Other drugs include diltiazem, but they may be less effective.

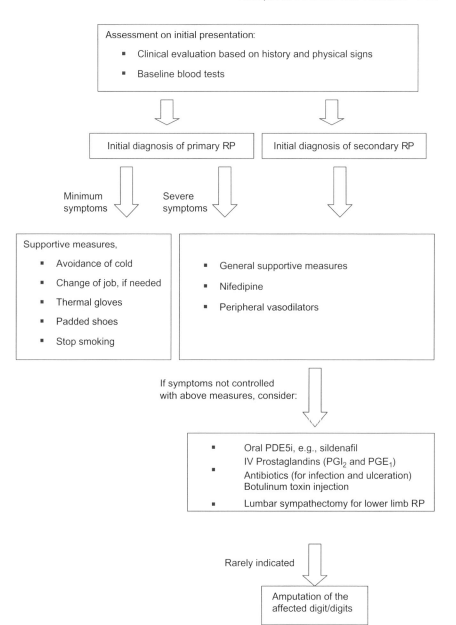

Figure 1.   Algorithm for the management of RP. PDE5i (phosphodiesterase inhibitor).

Table 4. Modified Ishikawa classification for the diagnosis of Takayasu arteritis (TAK) [6].

Three major criteria

1. Left mid-subclavian artery lesion

2. Right mid-subclavian artery lesion

3. Characteristic symptoms and signs of at least 1 month duration

Ten minor criteria

1. High ESR (>20 mm h^{-1})

2. Carotid artery tenderness

3. Hypertension

4. Aortic regurgitation or annuloaortic ectasia

5. Pulmonary artery lesion

6. Left mid common carotid lesion

7. Distal brachiocephalic trunk lesion

8. Descending thoracic aorta lesion

9. Abdominal aorta lesion

10. Coronary artery lesion

ESR, erythrocyte sedimentation rate

Note: The presence of two major or one major and two to four minor criteria suggests a high probability of TAK.

Peripheral vasodilators

These include pentoxifylline, naftidrofuryl inositol nicotinate, moxisylyte and botulinum toxin injections. Patients with PRP benefit more from these agents than those with SRP. A combination of low dose nifedipine and one of the peripheral vasodilators may avoid the adverse effects of both, while achieving maximum symptomatic relief.

Phosphodiesterase-type 5 inhibitors (PDE5 inhibitors)

If a patient has persistent moderate to severe symptoms despite employing the above supportive and therapeutic measures, then it may be appropriate to try one of the oral PDE5 inhibitors, e.g., sildenafil. The dose is typically 25 mg 3 times per day. However, the patient may not be able to tolerate this dose so a lower dose should be used, or their disease may not be adequately treated and so they will require a higher dose. Some medications such as nitrates should not be coprescribed with sildenafil due to a significant risk of profound hypotension and a rare risk of blindness.

Prostaglandins (PGI2 and PGE1)

These are powerful vasodilatory agents with additional antiplatelet activity and cytoprotec-tive effects. Iloprost and epoprostenol are synthetic analogues with a longer half-life and are commonly used as intravenous infusion over a period of 6 h for 3–5 days during the course of one treatment. The dose is titrated against the individual response and the maximum dose is adjusted at a rate lower than the dose causing headache, hypotension and flushing (maximum permissible daily dose is 2 ng kg^{-1} min^{-1}). A single course of treatment may provide relief for several months.

Endothelin Receptor Antagonists (ERAs)

This class of drug causes vasodilatation and is licensed for use in pulmonary arterial hypertension. Bosentan, an oral endothelin antagonist, is also licensed for use in patients with systemic sclerosis and severe digital ulcers. In England, its use is permitted in patients who have failed treatment with a combination of sildenafil and IV prostaglandins [2].

Sympathectomy

Cervical and lumbar sympathectomy using phenol injection can sometimes relieve symptoms of upper and lower extremity RP, respectively. However, it should be reserved only as a last option for those with severe symptoms who do not respond to other methods of treatment. The results of sympathectomy are not always predictable. Thoracoscopic cervical sympathectomy, in particular, is less effective and is associated with a higher rate of relapsing symptoms with only one-third achieving a long-term benefit [3]. In addition, there are frequent side effects and for this reason it is not recommended as routine. Digital sympathectomy can be helpful in alleviating the symptoms associated with chronic digital ischaemia in patients with severe RP [4].

Vasculitides

Vasculitis is characterised by inflammatory changes in the vessel wall, which can affect either the arteries or veins and results in destruction of the normal architecture of the vessel wall. The three commonest vasculitic disorders that vascular surgeons may be involved with are Takayasu arteritis, Giant cell arteritis and Buerger's disease. In this section, we will consider these vasculitides.

Takayasu arteritis

Takayasu arteritis (TAK) produces segmental and patchy granulomatous inflammation of the arterial wall. The condition was first described by Mikito Takayasu in 1908, and is of unknown aetiology. The inflammatory process produces medial thickening and intimal kinking. These changes result in stenoses, occlusion and aneurysmal dilatation. Takayasu arteritis predominantly affects the aorta and its major branches and is therefore categorised as a large vessel vasculitis [5].

Clinical presentation

Takyasu arteritis classically affects young females (90% females, and most are aged between 15 and 30 years at onset). The condition usually presents with systemic symptoms and loss of normal supra-aortic pulses — hence the term 'pulseless disease'. In simple terms, the condition evolves from an acute pre-pulseless phase to a chronic pulseless phase, although not all patients progress on to the chronic phase. The prepulseless phase can be divided into the early prodrome followed by the occlusive phase. The subclavian vessels are most commonly affected followed by the aorta and carotid vessels. RP is commonly associated with TAK.

Diagnostic and classification criteria

Various diagnostic and classification criteria have been designed to aid the early diagnosis of TAK. These include the 1990 American College of Rheumatology (ACR) criteria, the 1988 Ishikawa classification and the 1995 modification of the Ishikawa classification (Table 4). The modified classification had a sensitivity of 92.5% with a specificity of 95% for the diagnosis of TAK in 106 patients who had TAK, as shown on angiograms, compared to 20 control subjects [6].

Investigations

Clinical diagnosis of TAK can pose diagnostic difficulty in view of its varied presentation. Various non-invasive imaging studies can help not only in making an early diagnosis, but are also helpful in monitoring the progress of the disease and response to treatment. Conventional angiography, on the other hand, can only provide luminal details. Ultrasound can identify the early morphological changes in the vessel wall characterised by cir-cumferential thickening. Oedema or enhancement of the vessel wall on computed tomography (CT), magnetic resonance imaging (MRI) or [18]Fluorodeoxyglucose positron emission tomography scan ([18]FDG PET CT scan) is considered a sign of active inflammation. However, this may not lead to the characteristic morphological changes of TAK and, on the other hand, vessels showing no inflammatory changes can later develop TAK.

Treatment

Takayasu arteritis is initially managed with highdose corticosteroids, with or without immune modifying drugs such as intravenous cyclophospha-mide, azathioprine or methotrexate. A quarter of the patients do not enter into remission. Where surgical intervention is being contemplated, the patient should ideally be in remission, although if this cannot be achieved surgery may be necessary to prevent end-organ damage. Bypass surgery should be performed to and from disease free areas of the artery, with biopsies taken from anastomotic sites. Aneurysm forma-tion tends to occur at a later stage, and the indications for intervention will depend on conventional factors such as aneurysm size, rate of growth and the presence of distal embolisation.

Restenosis after intervention has been observed in up to one third of the patients with TAK. This can be minimised by delaying the intervention until the patient is in remission and starting immunosuppressive treatment after the intervention [7].

Giant cell arteritis (temporal arteritis)

A surgeon's most frequent encounter with giant cell arteritis (GCA) is during the request for temporal artery biopsy. GCA is a systemic inflammatory vasculitis predominantly affecting extra-cranial medium- and large-sized arteries. The inflammatory infiltrate consists predominantly of mononuclear cells with giant cell formation. Although a variety of causative factors have been implicated (genetic, immune, infective), the exact aetiology for GCA remains unknown. The inflammation can be segmental in distribution, and for this reason the biopsy should be at least 1 cm in length and the results should be interpreted with caution. The vertebral, superficial temporal and ophthalmic arteries are the vessels most commonly, involved. Less commonly, the disease affects larger vessels such as the aorta, subclavian arteries and branches of the abdominal aorta [8].

Clinical presentation

The condition rarely presents before the sixth decade and affects females twice as often as males. Involvement of the ophthalmic artery can result in ischaemic optic neuropathy, which can result in sudden blindness and hence the condition is treated as a medical emergency. Presenting symptoms often include the following:

- fever,
- new onset headache often seen as the hallmark symptom (usually temporal or occipital in location),
- scalp tenderness,
- jaw or tongue claudication,

- visual disturbances,
- tinnitus
  - polymyalgia,
- peripheral neuropathy,
- aneurysm formation, if a large vessel is affected.

Investigations

The majority of patients with GCA have an elevated ESR and CRP (C-reactive protein). Traditionally, temporal artery biopsy has been performed to confirm the diagnosis, although a negative biopsy does not exclude the disease. Ultrasound imaging of the temporal arteries is becoming more widely available as a diagnostic tool as a possible alternative to biopsy. It shows a dark halo (oedema) surrounding the diseased vessel — 'halo sign'. Although still not universally accepted, the combination of ultrasound evidence of inflammatory process plus a good clinical history is taken by some clinicians to be diagnostic.

Management

GCA is managed with highdose corticosteroid therapy to induce remission and to reduce the inflammatory changes in the vessel wall. The presence of visual symptoms warrants immediate treatment with corticosteroids, as prompt treatment reduces the risk of permanent visual impairment. Constitutional symptoms, vascular symptoms, and inflammatory markers (ESR, CRP) can guide immunosuppressant therapy. Therapeutic surgical intervention is confined to managing consequences of the disease, such as aneurysm formation.

Buerger's disease

Buerger's disease (thromboangiitis obliterans) is an inflammatory disease that predomi- nantly affects medium- and small-sized arteries. Leo Buerger first described the condition in 11 amputated limbs of patients of Jewish descent in 1908, and he termed the disease thromboangiitis obliterans. The special features of the disease [9] include the following:

- The pathological changes are distinct from atherosclerosis with minimal atheroma formation and more cellular infiltrate along with a striking perivascular inflammatory reaction resulting in occlusion of the vessel lumen.
- These inflammatory changes can be observed in both the arterial as well as the venous system.
- Both the upper and lower extremities can be affected, although lower limb disease occurs more frequently.
- Tobacco exposure is strongly associated with the initiation and progression of Buerger's disease, although the exact pathological mechanism is not known.
- Smoking cessation is the only way to stop the disease progression and nearly half of those who continue to smoke end up with a major amputation.

Clinical presentation

The disease usually affects men at the age of <45 years. Unlike patients with atherosclerotic disease, patients with Buerger's usually present with rest pain and tissue loss, rather than claudication. This reflects the involvement of more distal vessels. The prevalence of Buerger's disease is higher in patients of Middle or Far Eastern descent. The disease is historically rare in women, although this pattern is changing as is reflected by the increasing proportion of female smokers.

The tissue loss typically involves painful ulceration or necrosis of the digits of the hands and feet. As the disease progresses it may involve more proximal vessels, although it would be very unusual to lose proximal pulses from Buerger's disease alone. Involvement of the small vessels results in vasospastic symptoms. Patients may also present with sepsis or extensive foot infections where local infections of necrotic tissue are neglected. The venous inflammatory changes can cause a superficial thrombophlebitis.

Several diagnostic criteria have been suggested to aid correct diagnosis. These include the following:

- exclusion of other causes of limb ischaemia (hypercoagulability, emboli, diabetes etc.),

- tobacco use (previous or current),
- the presence of distal extremity arterial disease,
- young age of onset (<45).

The presence of additional features such as upper limb disease, phlebitis migrans, RP, and radiological signs strengthen the diagnosis.

Investigations

The radiological appearance of Buerger's disease comprises of relatively normal arteries to the knee level, abrupt occlusions of the tibial vessels and 'corkscrew' collateral feeding the distal vessels at the ankle. It is often helpful to look at the images of the unaffected limb, as these hallmark radiological features may already be present in the asymptomatic limb. It should be remembered that the similar angiographic features could also be seen in diabetes and other CTDs.

There are no specific laboratory tests for Buerger's disease. The primary role of laboratory tests is to exclude other causes of occlusive arterial disease. Likewise, echocardiography is useful to exclude a proximal embolic source.

Management

Medical

The absolute goal in managing Buerger's disease is to stop smoking completely and permanently. Aspirin should be prescribed for its antiplatelet effects, and analgesics for pain control. Prostaglandin infusions (e.g., iloprost) may help to control the symptoms. However, it is uncertain if it could alter the progression of tissue loss. Patients should be educated about foot care, prevention of injury and avoidance of cold exposure.

Surgical

Given the pattern of small- and medium-vessel occlusive disease, the options for surgical revascularisation in Buerger's are extremely limited. Any significant co-existing proximal atherosclerotic arterial disease should be treated to improve the inflow. Attempting to intervene with revascularisation is probably futile whilst the patient continues to smoke. Local amputation is often required to treat necrosis, non-healing ulcers or intractable pain. Distal ischaemic lesions will often auto-amputate, and it is usually helpful to await demarcation even if surgery is planned. Antibiotics may be needed intermittently for any infective episodes.

Behçet's Disease

Behçet's disease (BD) is a multisystem inflammatory condition that can affect both arteries and veins [5]. The disorder was first publicised by the Turkish dermatologist Hulusi Behçet in 1937, who described a syndrome of aphthous ulceration, genital ulceration and uveitis. Behçet's disease has historically been noted to occur more frequently along the old silk trading routes of the Middle East and in Central Asia, hence the name 'Silk Road' disease. No specific causative factor has been noted, although it is seen more commonly in individuals with the HLA-B51 gene.

Veins are affected more often than arteries. When large arteries are involved, inflammatory changes affect the vasa vasorum, resulting in medial destruction and fibrosis. Subsequent damage to the arterial wall can lead to aneurysm formation.

Clinical presentation

Behçet's disease is a chronic inflammatory condition characterised by episodes of recurrence and remission. International diagnostic guidelines emphasise the importance of the following features for the diagnosis:

- oral (aphthous) ulcers,
- genital ulcers,
- skin lesions,
- uveitis.

Venous involvement is manifested by thrombophlebitis of the superficial and deep veins. These changes are not wholly confined to the peripheral vasculature and can also involve the visceral and central veins. Arterial involvement may be manifested by aneurysmal disease, which necessi-tates intervention due to the risk of rupture. Occlusive disease can occur in BD and tends to affect medium- and small-sized arteries.

Investigations

There is no specific diagnostic test for BD. The disease occurs more com-monly in HLA-B51 individuals, and this gene is more prevalent in the Middle East. The 'pathergy' test can be helpful in the diagnosis of BD, but is not 100% specific. The test involves a needle prick to the forearm. The presence of a papule (measuring >2 mm in diameter) 1 to 2 days after the test constitutes a positive result. Investigation for aneurysmal or venous disease would follow standard investigative pathways.

Management

Steroid therapy is utilised to ease the symptoms and reduce the inflam-matory changes of the disease. Immunosuppressive drugs, including antitumour necrosis factor alpha (anti-TNFα) therapy, is beneficial in the management of uveitis, skin and mucosal symptoms. Aneurysm forma-tion in BD necessitates surgical intervention due to the risk of rupture. False aneurysms at the anastomotic sites are more common in BD as compared to atherosclerotic disease. Similarly, inflammatory changes can occur at the site of previous arterial surgery.

Inherited Connective Tissue Disorders

In this section, we will discuss some common inherited connective tissue disorders affecting the vascular system, including Marfan's syndrome and Ehlers–Danlos syndrome.

Marfan's syndrome

Marfan's syndrome is an autosomal dominant connective tissue disorder. One quarter of the affected population has a new genetic mutation. The underlying genetic defect arises from mutations of the fibrillin-1 (FBN1) gene based on chromosome 15. Fibrillin is a complex structural protein that serves as substrates for elastin in the aorta and other connective tissues. Abnormalities of these microfibrils results in weakening of the aortic wall and cardiac valves. In addition, the normal fibrillin-1 protein has a role in vascular smooth muscle development by binding to trans-forming growth factor beta (TGF-β). The role of angiotensin II receptor blockers has been investigated in modifying the vascular changes induced by TGF-β.

Clinical presentation

The major manifestations of Marfan's syndrome include the following:

- mitral valve prolapse,
- aortic root dilatation,
- aortic aneurysm formation,
- aortic dissection,
- dural abnormalities,
- lens dislocation (ectopia lentis).

External features include tall stature, arachnodactyly, dolichosteno-melia (limbs disproportionately long compared with trunk), joint hyper-mobility, scoliosis, pectus excavatum, high arched palate and dental crowding.

Investigations

Genetic investigations have a limited role in the diagnosis of Marfan's syndrome as not all FBN1 mutations are associated with Marfan's syn-drome. In addition, genetic testing is not available in all centres. The diagnosis is currently made on the basis of family history and clinical features, with or without molecular testing if available. The 'Ghent' diag-nostic criteria consist of major and minor features based on the systems involved. To be diagnosed with Marfan's syndrome using the Ghent crite-ria requires two major criteria and one minor criterion affecting different systems or, if there is a family history, one major criterion and one minor criterion.

Major criteria include the following:

- aneurysmal aorta,
- dissection of aorta,
- dislocation of the lens,
- family history of the syndrome,
- at least four skeletal problems, such as:
  - pectus carinatum or pectus excavatum,
  - arm span greater than height,
  - reduced upper to lower segment ratio. This is when the length of the torso (from shoulders to legs) is shorter than the length of the legs,
  - positive wrist sign. This is when the thumb and little finger overlap when you grasp the other wrist,
  - positive thumb sign. This is when you put your thumb on your hand and it extends beyond the palm,
  - curvature of the spine (scoliosis) with a curve greater than 20°,
  - spondylolisthesis,
  - flat feet (pes planus),
  - protrusio acetabuli on hip X-ray,
- dural ectasia of spinal cord — shown on CT or MRI, minor criteria include the following:
  - myopia,
  - unexplained stretch marks,
  - loose joints,
  - long, thin face,
  - high, arched palate.

Patients with Marfan's syndrome should be regularly screened for cardiac complications and aortic dilatation to allow prophylactic intervention against potentially fatal complications.

Management

Open surgical repair of descending thoracic and abdominal aortic dilatation is considered a reliable treatment option in patients with Marfan's syndrome and has resulted in improved survival based on studies carried out over the last decade. It still remains the first choice of treatment. Thoracic endovascular stenting for aneurysmal disease and dissection in patients with Marfan's syndrome has been increasingly used in recent years, but the published studies in this area are limited to small numbers. Further, larger studies are required with long-term follow up to show a conclusive benefit of thoracic endovascular stenting in Marfan's syndrome [10]. In particular, there is a worry about the durability of endografting since the majority of these patients are young. It is also essential that the follow up in these patients should include monitoring for new aneurysmal disease or anastomotic aneurysms.

Loeys–Dietz syndrome

Loeys–Dietz (LD) syndrome is a recently discovered autosomal dominant disorder with many of the clinical features of Marfan's syndrome. The disorder originates from a defect in the gene responsible for coding the transformation of growth factor β-receptors (TGF-β 1 or 2). The two genetic defects result in a similar syndrome and the condition was previously considered to be a subtype of Marfan's syndrome.

Clinical presentation

The main clinical features of LD syndrome include the following:

- arterial aneurysms,
- arterial tortuosity (often in the carotid vessels),
- hypertelorism (widely-spaced eyes),
- bifid or broad uvula.

This combination of major features is usually seen together in other inherited connective tissue disorders. As with Marfan's syndrome, aneurysms occur at a young age and frequently involve the aortic root. LD syndrome has been classified into two subtypes, depending on the craniofacial involvement. Many of the other features seen in LD are also seen in Marfan's syndrome, as previously described.

Ehlers–Danlos syndromes

Ehlers–Danlos syndromes (EDSs) are a heterogeneous group of inherited connective tissue disorders that result in impaired strength, elasticity and healing of the tissues. The condition is thought to have an incidence of 1:10,000, and is usually inherited as an autosomal dominant disease. EDS is caused by abnormalities of collagen synthesis. The clinical picture depends on the type of collagen defect and the distribution of that type of collagen in the individual tissues. There are at least thirteen phenotypes with considerable overlap between them [11]. This often makes the exact categorisation difficult in up to half of the patients. Vascular EDS (vEDS, formerly known as type IV EDS) is of most relevance to the vascular surgeon and it usually involves an abnormality of type III collagen (e.g., variant in one allele of COL3A1) and sometimes type I collagen, e.g., COL1A1.

Clinical presentation

vEDS often presents with arterial rupture at a young age or visceral rupture, e.g., spontaneous sigmoid colon perforation in the absence of known diverticular disease or other bowel pathology, uterine rupture during the third trimester in the absence of previous C-section. Sometimes the diagnosis is only made during post mortem. An arterial rupture is either spontaneous or follows minor trauma, with or without the presence of an underlying aneurysm. Aneurysms often involve multiple sites and arterial dissection is common. There is a high risk of bleeding complications and aneurysm formation following surgical intervention in these patients, in view of the tissue friability.

Clinical findings include the following:

- arterial rupture at a young age,
- spontaneous sigmoid colon perforation in absence of known bowel pathology,
- uterine rupture during third trimester in absence of previous C-section,
- carotid-cavernous sinus fistula in the absence of trauma,

516 *Postgraduate Vascular Surgery (Second Edition)*

- thin translucent skin with increased venous visibility,
- easy bruising with no identified trauma and/or in unusual sites, e.g., cheeks,
- hyperextensible skin:
  - spontaneous pneumothorax,
- hypermobile joints:
  - talipes equinovarus,
  - congenital hip dislocation,
- high and narrow palate,
- dental crowding,
- abnormal wound healing and scars ('tissue paper scars'),
- aneurysm formation,
- early onset varicose veins (<30 years and nulliparous if female),
- arteriovenous fistulae.

Investigations

The combination of the clinical features listed above, particularly arterial rupture or dissection in individuals less than 40 years of age, unexplained sigmoid colon rupture or spontaneous pneumothorax, in addition to a family history of the disease or history of a family member unexpectedly dying at a young age should alert the clinician to the possibility of EDS. To confirm the diagnosis, collagen typing can be performed on cultured skin fibroblasts to look for mutations in COL3A1 and COL1A1. Investigations for vascular involvement should be non-invasive, as conventional diag-nostic angiography carries an unacceptably high risk of haemorrhagic complications.

Management

Treatment for EDS is currently confined to the identification and treat-ment of complications. Patients should also receive lifestyle advice to avoid trauma. As previously noted, surgical or endovascular intervention should be avoided unless absolutely necessary due to the friability of the tissues and bleeding complications.

Investigations for inherited CTDs

The characteristic facial features and clinical findings will usually suggest the diagnosis. Genetic tests provide more definitive confirmation of the disease. Patients with LD syndrome should be placed under long-term CT or MR follow up to detect aneurysm formation at an early stage.

Management

Murine laboratory research has suggested that angiotensin II receptor blockade can reduce the formation of aortic aneurysms in Marfan's syndrome. This observation is particularly relevant in LD, where the abnormality in TGF-β activity is the fundamental defect. Therapy with angiotensin II receptor blockers such as losartan reduces the potential complications caused by increased TGF-β.

Pseudoxanthoma elasticum

Pseudoxanthoma elasticum (PXE) is a rare genetic condition with an incidence of 1:50,000. The condition involves progressive calcification and fragmentation of elastic fibres contained within the dermis of the skin, retina and cardiovascular system. More recent studies have suggested that this may be a systemic metabolic condition. The cardiovascular and gastrointestinal complications are the major causes of morbidity and mortality. Vascular calcification involves the intimal and medial layers of the vessel wall containing the elastic fibres. The cardiovascular complications of PXE often occur later than the cutaneous and haemorrhagic complications. The gastrointestinal bleeding complications result from the fragility of the calcified submucosal vessels.

Clinical presentation

The condition is usually first manifested with cutaneous lesions on the lateral part of the neck (often symmetrical). These lesions have the appearance of small yellow papules and occur in a linear or reticular pattern. The lesions can coalesce and form plaques and take on the appearance of 'plucked chicken' skin. The skin lesions also commonly occur in the folds of major joints such as the axillae. As the skin disease progresses, it often becomes lax, wrin- kled and hangs in the form of thick folds. Other clinical features of PXE include the following:

- gastrointestinal haemorrhage,
- intermittent claudication,
- ischaemic heart disease,
- retinal haemorrhages,
- haematuria.

Investigations

Blood tests are carried out for anaemia, renal impairment and baseline lipid levels. Urine should be tested for haematuria. Whenever possible, vascular imaging should follow a non-invasive course because of the risk of haemorrhagic complications after conventional angiography. The cardiac function should be assessed before vascular intervention in view of the high risk of cardiac complications.

Management

Patients should be counselled regarding changes in lifestyle to reduce the risk of complications. There is no specific treatment at present to halt or reverse the disease progression. Best medical therapy should be instituted to reduce the cardiovascular risk, although caution should be exercised with antiplatelet therapy due to the haemorrhagic risk.

References

1. Wigley FM, Flavahan NA. Raynaud's Phenomenon. *N Engl J Med* 2016;375: 556–565.
2. Hughes M, Ong V, Anderson M *et al.* Consensus best practice pathway of the UK Scleroderma Study Group: Digital vasculopathy in systemic sclerosis. *Rheumatology* 2015;54:2015–2024.
3. Thune TH, Ladegaard L, Licht PB. Thoracoscopic sympathectomy for Raynaud's phenomenon — A long term follow-up study. *Eur J Vasc Endovasc Surg* 2006;32:198–202.

4. Kotsis SV, Chung KC. A systemic review of the outcomes of digital sympa-thectomy for treatment of chronic digital ischaemia. *J Rheumatol* 2003;30: 1788–1792.

5. Jennette JC, Falk RJ, Bacon PA *et al.* 2012 revised international chapel hill consensus conference nomenclature of vasculitites. *Arthritis and Rheumatism* 2013;65:1–11.

6. Sharma BK, Jain S, Suri S, Numano F. Diagnostic criteria for Takayasu's arte-ritis. *Int J Cardiol* 1996;4:S141–S147.

7. Park MC, Lee SW, Park YB, Lee SK, Choi D, Shim WH. Post-interventional immunosuppressive treatment and vascular restenosis in Takayasu's arteri-tis. *Rheumatolgy* 2006;45:600–605.

8. Weyand CM, Goronzy JJ. Giant-cell arteritis and polymyalgia rheumatica. *N Eng J Med* 2014;371:50–57.

9. Małecki R, Zdrojowy K, Adamiec R. Thromboangiitis obliterans in the 21st century — A new face of disease. *Atherosclerosis* 2009;206:328–234.

10. Cooper DG, Walsh SR, Sadat U, Hayes PD, Boyle JR. Treating the thoracic aorta in Marfan syndrome: Surgery or TEVAR? *J Endovasc Ther* 2009;16:60–70.

11. Malfait F, Francomano C, Byers P, *et al*. The 2017 international classification of the Ehlers–Danlos syndromes. *Am J Med Genet Part C Semin Med Genet* 2017;175C:8–26.

Chapter 27

Access Surgery

Monica Hansrani

Key Points

- The population requiring dialysis is increasing by 5–6% worldwide and costs the NHS more than £1 billion per year.
- Therapy includes transplantation, peritoneal and haemodialysis (HD).
- Adequate HD requires relatively painless, durable, problem free access.
- This chapter aims to give a framework for assessment, planning best access and dealing with complications.

Introduction

Management of patients with chronic kidney disease costs the NHS in excess of £1.45 billion per year, which is 1.3% of the annual NHS expenditure. More than half of this is spent on renal replacement therapy, which is provided for 2% of the CKD population. Renal replacement is provided by kidney transplant, haemodialysis (HD)/haemofiltration or peritoneal dialysis (PD). The population requiring dialysis is increasing worldwide by 5–6% per annum and has a bleak 50% 5-year survival.

Peritoneal Dialysis

PD was first described in 1959. In 1968, Henry Tenckhoff developed the concept of the intraperitoneal indwelling catheter. PD has several advantages over HD including the fact that it is cheaper, simple to use, leads to improved quality of life due to increased independence and mobility as well as maintaining residual renal function and lower mortality. Evidence would suggest this physiological effect may only be advantageous for 12 months of use. Unlike the HD, PD delivers steady-state treatment avoiding wide fluctuations of plasma volume and solutes. The disadvantage of PD is poor blood pressure control due to fluid overload, and peritonitis (see Table 1).

The process of PD is most commonly performed by continuous ambulatory peritoneal dialysis (CAPD) in which dialysate is placed in the abdomen (fill), remaining there for 4–6 h (dwell) before being removed (drain) and replaced with fresh solution. In continuous cycling peritoneal dialysis (CCPD), a machine automatically fills and drains the dialysate over 10–12 h and is usually performed at night.

The peritoneal catheter is composed of a flexible silicone tube with an open-end port and multiple side holes distally. They come in various lengths and configurations (straight, swan-neck or pigtail) with varying

Table 1.   Indications for PD.

Strong indication for PD	PD preferred
Vascular access not possible or failed	Bleeding diathesis
Intolerance to HD	Multiple myeloma
Congestive cardiac failure	Labile diabetes mellitus
Prosthetic valvular disease	Chronic infections
Patient preference	Temporising therapy whilst awaiting transplantation
Poor cardiac function	Needle phobia
Children 0–5 years	Active lifestyle
	Children aged between 6 and 16 years

numbers of dacron cuffs. Though originally described by Tenckhoff using an open technique, the catheter can be placed laparoscopically or percutaneously under local anaesthetic using a Seldinger technique, allowing placement by interventional nephrologists. The catheter is placed obliquely through the abdominal wall with a proximal subcutaneous cuff holding the catheter in place whilst the distal cuff (if present) lies in the pre-peritoneal space acting as a barrier to infection. The distal hole laden tip is placed in the pouch of Douglas. It is recommended that the wound heals for a minimum of 2 weeks prior to use.

Potential complications include bleeding, bowel perforation, catheter occlusion due to thrombus, fibrin, omental wrapping or kinking, leakage of dialysate, hydrothorax (1.6–10%), hernia formation, wound infection and peritonitis. A late complication is the development of peritoneal sclerosis with an estimated incidence of 1.5–4.6 cases per 1,000 patient years and in its most severe form, called encapsulated peritoneal sclerosis, has a 50% mortality at 12 months. The mean time to developing a hernia is 1 year after initiation of PD with the risk increasing 20% per annum for patients on CAPD. Peritonitis occurs approximately once per patient year. Mortality for patients with peritonitis is 4% (see Table 2).

Table 2. Contraindications to PD.

Contraindications	Relative contraindications	Not ideal, but possible
Ultrafiltration failure	Multiple adhesions	Obesity
Severe inflammatory bowel disease	Presence of a stoma	Multiple herniae
	Severe malnutrition	Severe backache
Active acute diverticulitis or intraabdominal sepsis	Proteinuria >10 g/day	Battlefield abdomen
Active ischaemic bowel	Poor personal hygiene	Impaired manual dexterity
Severe active psychotic disorder	Dementia	Blindness
Significant intellectual disability	Physical disability such that patient unable to perform exchanges	Poor home situation
Pregnancy	Homelessness	Depression

Haemodialysis

The first human HD was performed in Germany in 1924. Technical and anticoagulation problems limited the treatment and the patients died after temporary improvement in their uraemia. The first patient saved by HD was a woman in the Netherlands in 1943, who presented with acute renal failure. However, there were still problems with vascular access which meant that patients could only use HD for a very limited time. In 1960, the arteriovenous cannula system, an extra corporeal system, was introduced by Scribner. Brescia and his team published his research on the surgically created arteriovenous fistula (AVF) in 1966, which finally allowed for permanent access and the ability for patients with chronic renal failure to remain on long-term HD (Fig. 1).

AVF is the recommended access due to its association with low mortality and morbidity and cost compared to other access types, however, following creation, 20–60% are unsuitable for HD and an AVF will require on average 1.5–3.3 interventions to facilitate usability for HD. Central

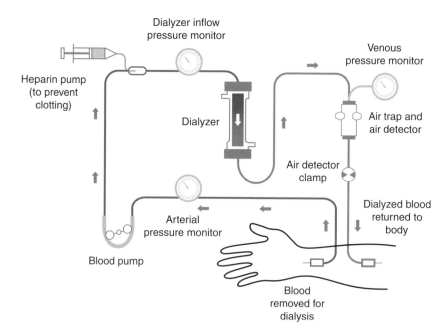

Figure 1.   Diagram of a HD circuit.

venous catheters (CVCs) should only be used when the options for an AVF or arteriovenous graft (AVG) have been exhausted or when HD is only required for a short-term. The UK Renal Association also recommends that 60% of patients approaching HD should start their treatment using an AVF or AVG, and that 80% of patients established on HD should already be using an AVF or AVG. A systematic review of 67 studies (62 cohort studies) found patients dialysing through a central venous catheter had a higher risk of all-cause mortality, fatal infection and cardiovascular events when compared to the use of an AVF and when compared to the use of a prosthetic graft. Prosthetic grafts were associated with higher all-cause mortality and fatal infections when compared to autologous fistulas. The increased relative risk is in the order of 1.5–2.3 (although some studies suggest that it may be as high as RR 7.6) for catheters vs. 1.2 for AVG when compared to those dialysing via AVF. This is supported by the UK Department of Health, who attach a decreased tariff for HD via a central catheter compared to an AVF or AVG to encourage their use.

Initial Patient Assessment

Early referral of a patient with CKD to a nephrologist is needed to facilitate CKD therapy with medications and diets that preserve kidney function.

Table 3 shows the Kidney Disease Outcome Quality Initiative (KDOQI) recommended guidelines for assessment of patients. The Kidney Foundation recommends pre-operative ultrasound assessment and vein mapping as using an artery with a diameter >2 mm and a vein with a diameter >2.5 mm significantly improves success rates. It is recommended that all patients with a history of central venous catheters or pacemakers should have their central veins assessed either indirectly by ultrasound, or directly by MRA, CT or invasive venography.

Education of patients regarding fistulae, protection of vessels, vessel mapping, and sufficient lead-time for fistula maturation has significantly improved the rate of fistula placement. Native fistulae should be created 6 months before need, to allow for maturation and revision if necessary, and grafts 6–8 weeks prior to need.

Table 3. NKF KDOQI Guidelines (2006) for patient assessment for HD access. Patient evaluation prior to access placement.

Consideration	Relevance
Patient history	
History of previous CVC	Previous placement of a CVC is associated with central venous stenosis.
Dominant arm	To minimise negative impact on quality of life, use of the non-dominant arm is preferred.
History of pacemaker use	There is a correlation between pacemaker use and central venous stenosis.
History of severe CHF	Accesses may alter hemodynamics and cardiac output.
History of arterial or venous peripheral catheter	Previous placement of an arterial or venous peripheral catheter may have damaged target vasculature.
History of diabetes mellitus	Diabetes mellitus is associated with damage to vasculature necessary for internal accesses.
History of anticoagulant therapy or any coagulation disorder	Abnormal coagulation may cause clotting or problems with hemostasis of accesses.
Presence of comorbid conditions, such as malignancy or coronary artery disease, that limit patient's life expectancy	Morbidity associated with placement and maintenance of certain accesses may not justify their use in some patients.
History of vascular access	Previously failed vascular accesses will limit available sites for accesses, the cause of a previous failure may influence planned access if the cause is still present.
History of heart valve disease or prosthesis	Rate of infection associated with specific access types should be considered.
History of previous arm, neck, or chest surgery/ trauma	Vascular damage associated with previous surgery or trauma may limit viable access sites.
Anticipated kidney transplant from living donor	Catheter access may be sufficient.

Physical examination

Physical Examination of Arterial System

Character of peripheral pulses, supplemented by hand-held	An adequate arterial system is needed for access; the quality of the arterial system will influence the choice of access site.
Doppler evaluation when indicated	Abnormal arterial flow pattern to the hand may contraindicate the creation of a radial-cephalic fistula.
Results of Allen test	Pressures determine suitability of arterial access in upper extremities.
Bilateral upper extremity blood pressures	Pressures determine suitability of arterial access in upper extremities.

Physical Examination of Venous System

Evaluation for edema	Edema indicates venous outflow problems that may limit usefulness of the associated potential access site or extremity for access placement.
Assessment of arm size comparability	Differential arm size may indicate inadequate veins or venous obstruction which should influence choice of access site.
Examination for collateral veins	Collateral veins are indicative of venous obstruction.
Tourniquet venous palpation with vein mapping	Palpation and mapping allow selection of ideal veins for access.
Examination for evidence of previous central or peripheral venous catheterisation	Use of CVCs is associated with central venous stenosis, previous placement of venous catheters may have damaged target vasculature necessary for access.
Examination for evidence of arm, chest, or neck surgery trauma	Vascular damage associated with previous surgery or trauma may limit access sites.

Cardiovascular Evaluation

Examination for evidence of heart failure	Accesses may alter cardiac output.

Post-operative Assessment of the Patient

Clinical assessment of a patient post the creation of a fistula should include the following:

- history to elicit possible ischaemic complications, neurological change, functional change or pain in the limb, breathlessness/symptoms of heart failure, episodes of infection/bleeding, needling history of the fistula,
- haemodynamic status of the patient — do they maintain an adequate blood pressure to maintain adequate flow to the limb and fistula, evidence of heart failure, are they adequately hydrated?
- palpation of the fistula vein along its length to assess volume filling and the presence, change or absence of thrill which may indicate good flow, a significant tributary that is diverting flow and diluting the volume, or occlusion of the fistula,
- palpation of the fistula to assess for heat to suggest infection or phlebitis,
- palpation of the fistula to feel for thickening to suggest fibrosis/stenosis or abnormal dilatation, haematomas or (pseudo)aneurysms and general size to assess development,
- assessment of pulses in the limb and neurological status,
- assessment for signs of central vein stenosis with limb swelling and dilated collateral veins,
- assessment of the wound if needed.

Indications for ultrasound assessment include the following:

- poorly filling fistula suggesting poor arterial inflow,
- poorly matured fistula,
- loss of thrill,
- distal limb ischaemia or neurological symptoms,
- clinical signs of infection,
- peri-fistula/graft mass, (pseudo)aneurysm, thickening,
- increased bleeding time/high pressure in fistula to suggest distal stenosis,
- difficult cannulation,

- thrombus aspiration,
- increased recirculation time of 15% or greater,
- reduced clearance rate of <60%.

The role of surveillance of fistula is currently unclear. Although recommended by the Kidney Foundation, there is currently no agreed standardised time interval for duplex surveillance. Evidence has shown that surveillance leads to early intervention and increased secondary patency particularly in grafts, however, as yet there is no evidence to suggest that this translates into increased use of the fistulae for dialysis. There is, however, strong evidence of the effectiveness of clinical examination in finding >80% of problems. This highlights the importance of well-trained dialysis staff in the maintenance of patency both from good needling techniques and regular assessment and escalation of concerns.

Central Venous Catheters

Central venous catheters (CVCs) for HD may be non-tunnelled — designed for acute episodes and temporary duration, ideally less than 3 weeks — or tunnelled, used for longer duration, and sometimes for years. Acute catheters are designed to be placed with a minimum amount of effort. They generally have double lumens, no subcutaneous cuff or locking device and have a short linear tunnel (see Table 4).

Tunnelled catheters (TNLs) are most commonly dual lumen, may be composed of silicone, polyurethane, polyethylene or polytetrafluroethylene (PTFE) and contain a subcutaneous Dacron cuff, or a plastic 'grommet' to immobilise the catheter below the skin surface. The red port identifies the 'arterial' lumen that draws blood from the body (proximal/ side opening) and the blue port identifies the 'venous' lumen for return of blood from the dialysis machine to the patient (the distal opening). Some have end-holes only and some have end- and side-holes. Side-holes can be in linear or in spiral array. Arterial inlet and venous outlet holes in different double-lumen catheters have different distances between them. These variables in design have never been investigated systematically to assess their influence on catheter function, recirculation, and occlusion rates. Double-lumen TNLs, are felt to reduce recirculation

Table 4. Complications of inserting catheters for vascular access.

Acute	Long-term
• Pneumothorax	
• Vascular damage (e.g., perforation, dissection)	• Infection and sepsis
• Air embolism	• Thrombotic complications (e.g., DVT, pulmonary embolus)
• Aberrant catheter placement	• Phlebitis of the cannulated vessel
• Damage to the thoracic duct	• Superior vena cava syndrome
• Cardiac complications (e.g., cardiac irritation, cardiac perforation)	• Catheter dislodgement and migration
• Local tissue trauma or damage (e.g., bleeding into surrounding tissues, nerve injury)	

rates compared to single-lumen, however, there is no evidence to support this. The balance for such hypothetical benefit is greater acute trauma during implantation and greater chronic trauma due to enhanced catheter stiffness. Simultaneous implantation of two ('twin') catheters does not reduce surgical trauma and complication rates.

TNLs are typically placed percutaneously into a large central vein (internal jugular, subclavian vein or femoral) through the vena cava with the goal of placing the tips of the catheter at the junction of the SVC and the right atrium. Placement of femoral catheters has the distinct drawback of restricting the mobility of the patient during walking and exercise. The IJVs are superficial and have the largest radii of the neck veins, making them the easiest veins to access technically and have the lowest thrombosis rate. Some of the major reasons for catheter malfunction are fibrin sheath formation, catheter kinking or malposition, and thrombosis, both acute and chronic. Central vein stenosis due to endothelial injury, associated with the placement of central venous catheters, can endanger AVFs or AVGs in either extremity. Usually asymptomatic, these manifest clinically when challenged by increased flow, commonly from AVFs or AVGs. The risk factors include multiple catheters, longer duration, subclavian venous location, and placement on the left-hand side of neck. Thrombosis in the internal jugular veins is often not clinically apparent as the thrombus is isolated from the high outflow drainage of the arms, and there is prompt development of collaterals. However, access through the internal jugular veins is associated with central venous stenosis. The right IJV is preferred as it provides a short direst route the right atrium. The use of ultrasound guidance has reduced the risk of inadvertent carotid artery puncture from 7–10% to virtually 0%.

The KDOQI recommends avoiding the subclavian vein when upper limb options remain for arteriovenous access as occlusion/stenosis occurs commonly (in 40–50% of patients after 2–3 weeks of insertion) and results in clinically symptomatic venous outflow obstruction in the arm and loss of future access options. Another major complication is pneumothorax (0.1–15%). Alternative sites of access include external jugular vein, saphenous vein, translumbar IVC, hepatic veins and catheterisation of small supradiaphragmatic chest collaterals in the event of central vein stenosis (see Table 5).

Catheters allow immediate access for HD, however, in addition to the risk of central vein stenosis and thrombosis, there is often inadequate blood flow and an increased mortality risk, usually sepsis-related. TNL-related bacteraemia averages between 3.4 and 5.5 incidences per 1000 catheter days. Catheters are also associated with increased hospitalisation rates due to sepsis, and intervention rates making them overall costlier.

Fully subcutaneous catheters have been developed with a fully subcutaneous port accessing the catheter including the Hemasite, Bentley DiaTAP button, Lifesite and Dialock systems. Initial studies would suggest that they do have high-flow rates and low complication rates in comparison to TNL, but do not yet match AVF or AVG outcomes.

Arteriovenous fistula and grafts

The ideal access for HD allows easy, repeated cannulation, is comfortable for the patient, provides adequate flow rates that allow rapid clearance and has long-term patency without the need for further interventions. The 'Rule of 6's' describes the ideal AVF conduit — it should provide a flow rate of at least 600 mL/min, should lie less than 6 mm below the surface of the skin and have a minimum diameter of 6 mm. It should also have adequate straight and accessible length (ideally 10–5 cm) to allow the placement of two dialysis needles.

Table 5.   Pros and cons of sites of insertion of central venous catheters.

Venous access	Advantages	Disadvantages	Comments
Internal jugular veins	• Superficial end Easily accessible: US guided access ideal. • Largest redii–low risk of stenosis.	• Central vein stenoses–can jeopardize functioning AVG/AVF. • IJV thrombosis. Usually asymptomatic.	'Preferred' site of vascular access RIJV preferred over IJV specially in left AVF/AVG.
External jugular vein	• Superficial location. • Straight path to RA. • Empties into the SCV. not get affected in IJV thrombosis.	• Small radii– challenging access in inexperienced hands. • Thrombosis.	REJV especially useful in occluded RIJV and left AVF/AVG.
Femoral vein	• Superficial and Easily accessible.	• Prone to infection: addressed by a lateral tunnel. • Prone to occlusion: Addressed by placement of tip beyond confluence of CIV. • Restricted mobility.	'Operators choice' in many after occlusion of IJV's.
Subclavian vein	• Large radius.	• Pneumothorax. • Subclavian vein thrombosis and stenosis excludes use of arm veins for AVF/AVG.	Infrequently used — not recommended by DOQI guidelines specially when AVF/AVG In arm is planned.
Collateral veins	• Direct path to RA. • Catheter care easy. • Patient comfort.	• Technical difficulties including accessibility. • Complications like hemorrhage.	Most compelling reason for use is preservation of other access sites for future use.
Translumbar inferior vena cava	• Large radius. • Thrombosis rare. • Anatomic position reliable. • Safe procedure.	• Technically challenging and time consuming. • Frequent exchanges due to poor blood flow and catheter-related infection. • Catheter dislodgement- due to adipose tissue along tract.	Safe, alternate access for short-term bridge to dialysis.
Hepatic vein	• Useful last resort option in IVC occlusions.	• Technically challenging and time consuming. • Frequent exchanges due to poor blood flow and catheter-related infection. • Catheter dislodgement- due to respiratory excursions of liver. • Hemorrhage during access.	Safe, alternate access for short-term bridge to dialysis in case of complete IVC obstruction.

The KDOQI suggested order of placement for arteriovenous access is upper limb AVF before upper limb AVG before lower limb AVF and AVG. For the upper limb, the non-dominant limb is preferred and access initially created as distally as possible to preserve future options for access as well as reducing the risk of steal. In the upper limb, the most distal fistula being the 'snuff box' fistula is formed using the thenar branch of the radial artery and the most distal cephalic vein. Early thrombosis, high rate of failure to mature and difficulty in accessing for rescue endovascular therapy, as well as the rarity of adequately sized vessels means that this fistula is not common. Common sites include the wrist radio-cephalic (Brescia-Cimino fistula), wrist ulnar basilica, transposition of the basilic vein across the forearm to form a radio-basilic wrist fistula, forearm radiocephalic and ulnar basilic, brachiocephalic, brachio-median cubital vein (Gracz fistula) and brachiobasilic (see Fig. 2). Current KDOQI guidelines suggest that when an upper limb AVG is required, the configuration of choice should be a forearm loop first, followed by an upper arm graft (either straight or curved), then an upper arm loop configuration. A comparison between

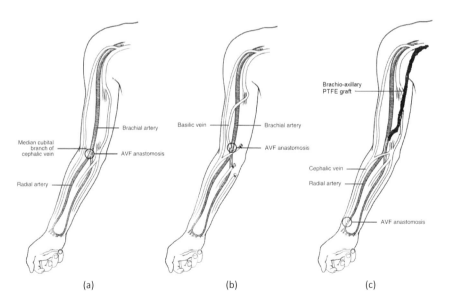

(a)   (b)   (c)

Figure 2. Diagrams demonstrating the anatomy of common upper limb fistulae (a) brachio-median cubital vein (Gracz) fistula, (b) brachio-basilic vein with vein transposed anterolaterally, (c) radiocephalic fistula and brachio-axillary graft.

Table 6.   Literature reported patency for fistulae of various sites.

Fistula site	Primary patency at 12 months (%)	Secondary patency at 12 months (%)
Snuff box	72–78	65–93
Radiocephalic	33–54	52–74
Ulnarbasilic	43–71	54–85
Radiobasilic	50	—
Brachiocephalic	46–68	74–84
Brachiobasilic	40–68	70–84
SFV translocation brachio-axillary	79–83	93–100
Forearm loop graft	43–44	67–79
Upper arm graft	48–70	69–87
Femorofemoral loop	38–54	80
Femoral vein transposition	73–83	86–93
Femorosaphenous (loop + straight)	70	80
Upper thigh graft	48	62–69
Mid-thigh graft	43–83	62–97

forearm and upper arm graft, however, has shown no difference in primary unassisted patency or cumulative primary graft failure rates, based on either the graft location or its configuration (see Table 6).

Surgical considerations

When forming a radio-cephalic fistula, an end-to-end or end-to-side anastomosis is used, with the literature reporting success in both techniques. The end-to-side approach has been reported to give a higher primary and secondary patency rate and a lower rate of thrombotic complications. The anastomosis should be 12 mm in small distal vessels, but no more than 6 mm in the brachial artery/femoral to avoid the risk of steal. Anastomoses made with an acute angle appear to elicit less neointimal hyperplasia and is the only technical aspect that statistically improves patency. Grade of the surgeon performing the procedure had no impact.

The anastomosis is performed using a non-dissolvable synthetic suture material. Suture-less techniques utilising micro-clips which are applied to the everted vessel edges with a special clip applicator have been studied, and show comparable primary patency rates with a shorter operating time when compared to a sutured anastomosis in both AVF and AVG.

Other novel surgical techniques in AVF formation include the use of a 'piggy-back' anastomotic technique, where the vein is divided and the cut end over-sewn (see Fig. 3). The vessels are then laid beside each other and the anastomosis is formed between a posterior incision on the vein and an anterior incision made on the artery. In the formation of the radio-cephalic AVF, this technique has been shown to significantly reduce the rate of juxta-anastomotic stenosis and to decrease fistula failure rates.

The possibility of creating an AVF entirely percutaneously is also under evaluation, in theory reducing vascular trauma, improving patency and improving patient compliance. The EverlinQ endoAVF system consists of 2 6F catheters that contain a magnetic end. One catheter is placed in the artery, and the other in the neighbouring vein. The magnets when aligned, attract each other and juxtapose the vessels, aligning a radiofrequency electrode in the venous catheter to a ceramic backstop in the arterial catheter. The electrode is then fired for 2 s, creating an approximately 5 mm × 1 mm anastomosis. Studies have demonstrated its efficacy, with 96% able to dialyse within 1 month of creation. The Ellipsys

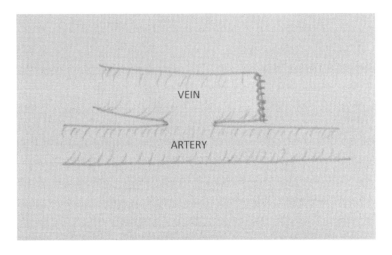

Figure 3.   Diagrammatic representation of a piggy-back anastomosis.

system utilises ultrasound to guide passage of a catheter into the vein which then exits the vein and enters a neighbouring artery with a single system. The system then aligns the vessels and a DC current creates thermal energy that then creates a hole and fuses the vessels together. Large-scale studies are awaited.

Average patency for a distal AVF is estimated at 7 years whilst for an AVG it is 2 years.

Access Conduit

Another avenue in the pursuit of improvements to vascular access is the use of biological grafts. These include the use of cryopreserved femoral vein allografts, and the use of xenografts such as bovine carotid artery, bovine mesenteric vein and bovine ureteric grafts. The use of bovine carotid artery grafts has been associated with a high complication rate, particularly that of pseudo-aneurysm formation, late infection, haematoma formation and significant oedema. Like bovine carotid artery, bovine ureter has been associated with significant aneurysm formation. Complications such as dilation, seroma formation, infection and thrombosis were all reduced with the use of bovine mesenteric vein when compared to AVG.

In hopes of providing a biologically equivalent conduit to native vein, attention has more recently turned to the use of grafts from bioengineered blood vessels. Veins can be constructed from cultivated donated human cells seeded onto a tubular bioresorbable 'scaffold'. The tissue has a decellularised collagen structure which does not trigger an immune response. These are currently being evaluated in studies in the USA. Investigation is currently underway of the use of entirely biological grafts, where the scaffold of the graft itself is formed from autologous cells. Further research is also ongoing into the *in vitro* creation of tissue-engineered blood vessels, including a promising early study of their use in human subjects which showed a primary patency rate of 60% at six months. A comparison of primary and secondary patency rates biological grafts can be found in Table 1.

Prosthetic AVG are typically created using a polytetrafluoroethylene (PTFE) conduit anastomosed directly between the artery and vein. These grafts can be especially thinned, ring reinforced or tapered.

In the elective setting, an AVF can take approximately 6 weeks to mature, and most synthetic AVG's are left for approximately 2 weeks before first cannulation to allow formation of a fibrous sheath to enhance sealing after needle puncture. In the emergency setting, these delays prohibit their use, and until recently, a central venous catheter would be necessary to initiate emergency dialysis. Recent advances in graft technology now allow immediate (within hours) graft cannulation after the formation of an AVG. These grafts have a multilaminated structure, often with a silicon self-sealing middle layer, and include the Acuseal, Flixene, Avflo and Rapidax grafts. Primary and secondary patency rates with these grafts are summarised in Table 7.

Table 7.   Reported primary and secondary patency of novel fistulae.

Novel AVF/AVG type	Primary patency at 12 months (%)	Secondary patency at 12 months (%)
AVF	60	71
Endoscopic basilic vein transposition	58	96
Brachial vein	40–100	92
PTFE graft	45	65
Immediate cannulation grafts		
Acuseal graft	33–68	40–93
Flixene and Rapidax grafts	30–66	63–83
Avflo graft	75	81
Biological grafts		
Cryopreserved femoral vein	42–49	68
Bovine carotid artery	75	—
Bovine mesenteric vein	36	60
Bovine ureter	14	75
Autologous bioresorbable scaffold	70 (6 months)	—
Tissue engineered blood vessels	78 (1 month)	—
Hybrid grafts		
HeRO graft	22	60

New Approaches

The Optiflow device is a prosthetic implant composed of non-thrombogenic siliconised polyurethane that forms an anastomotic conduit from the artery to the vein. It requires full surgical exposure of the vessels, and effectively replaces the anastomosis with the device allowing for a standardised anastomosis and flow characteristics, potentially improving outcomes. A large-scale study is currently underway in USA to assess the clinical efficacy of the device.

Access Complications

Stenosis/Thrombosis

The formation of stenosis is initiated by endothelial cell injury which then leads to smooth muscle cell proliferation and neointimal hyperplasia, finally causing access thrombosis. Endothelial injury can occur due to shear stress from turbulent blood flow, mechanical trauma from venesection and angioplasties. In AVF, 80–85% of stenosis occur in the juxta-anastomotic site or outflow vein, and 15–20% in the arterial inflow, whilst in AVG, 80–85% occur at the graft-vein anastomosis, 2–5% at the graft-artery anastomosis and 11–15% intragraft.

The patient may present with failure to mature, decreased access flow on duplex, difficulty in needling, prolonged bleeding times or elevated venous or arterial pressures.

Percutaneous angioplasty has an initial 90% technical success rate with 1 year secondary patency rates of 82% in both AVF and AVG. Pre-emptive angioplasty of stenotic lesions does not appear to improve graft survival. The use of stents in peripheral veins and grafts does not appear to improve patency rates although they may have a role in treating central stenosis. Stents are also not licensed for use in areas of potential needling in fistulae.

Surgical revision with options including patch angioplasty, resection and re-anastomosis or interposition grafting, provides results that are comparable or better than angioplasty, but may not be readily available. It is more often used in recurrent stenosis or when angioplasty has failed (Table 8).

Table 8.   Incidence of common access complications.

Complication	Incidence (%)	Clinical features
Failure to mature	23–37	Fistula diameter and thickness remain inadequate for dialysis after 8–12 weeks, more common in elderly, female diabetics and distal fistulae
Thrombosis	17–25	Loss of thrill, palp thrombus, pain at site of thrombus
Stenosis	14–42	Difficulty needling, increased recirculation, decreased clearance, loss of thrill, prolonged bleeding time
Congestive cardiac failure	12–17	Dyspnoea, orthopnoea, oedema
Steal	2–8	Pale/blue cold distal extremity, ischaemic pain at rest, ulceration, gangrene, reversal of arterial flow
Ischaemic monomelic neuropathy	1–10	Severe pain distal to fistula immediately, sensory and/or functional loss, eventual paralysis, normal vascular examination
Aneurysm/ pseudoaneurysm	2–8	Diffuse progressive dilatation, palp thickening beyond suggesting stenosis, prolonged bleeding, overlying skin degeneration
Infection	2–3	Hot, red and painful, with or without systemic signs, 7–10× more common in AVG vs. AVF

Although the KDOQI guidelines suggest monthly surveillance and treatment of haemodynamically significant stenosis, growing evidence would suggest that this may not improve access survival, is costly and may even be harmful.

When an access thromboses, the outcomes are not as good. Ideally, intervention should occur within 48 h of occlusion for veins and 7 days for grafts. Success from surgical thrombectomy may be as high as 94% with 12-month patency of 68–88% for both AVF and AVG. Endovascular techniques include catheter-directed 'pulse spray' thrombolysis (thrombolytic agent is injected in a pulsed manner under high pressure directly into the thrombus) or the use of crossed catheters to thrombolyse from the centre outwards. Catheter-directed thrombolysis demonstrates success rates of between 73% and 95%. Mechanical intra-vascular devices include the Arrow-Trerotola that contacts the vessel wall and strips the thrombus directly from it; the Angiojet system, Hydrolyser catheter or Oasis catheter that uses hydrodynamics to create negative pressure suction that removes the thrombus without the device directly contacting the intima of the vessel (reported technical success of 82–89%) and the Amplatz device which uses a sharp, rotating blade that acts to break up the thrombus and disperse it into the circulation in microscopic particles (technical success rate of 83%). More recent developments in mechanical thrombectomy include the use of ultra-sound accelerated thrombolysis, where both local thrombolysis and high frequency ultrasound are delivered into the thrombus simultane-ously. Complications of mechanical thrombectomy include embolisation (which can occur to either the arterial circulation or to the venous circu-lation as a pulmonary embolism, and can also occur following pharma-cological thrombolysis), vessel injury (including dissection and rupture) and haemolysis.

The data on pharmacological agents that improve patency are con-tradictory and often confusing, however, as a brief summary: aspirin has been shown to significantly improve AVF patency and clopidogrel AVG patency, however, this has not translated into a statistically significant increase in the use of the access for HD overall or has not been reported as an outcome, and is still debated. The combination of aspirin and clopidogrel did not significantly improve patency beyond each agent alone and showed significantly increased bleeding complications. Dipyridamole also shows evidence of decreased thrombosis rate in AVG in a single study. Warfarin has not shown any promise and is associated with significant bleeding problems.

Statins and ACE inhibitor do not improve patency, although retro-spective studies have shown a higher intervention-free access survival rate in AVG patients in those on an ACE inhibitor. Despite fewer episodes of graft thrombosis in patients taking daily fish oil supplements, there was no overall difference in the proportion of grafts that lost patency within the first 12 months.

Central venous stenosis is managed with percutaneous angioplasty +/− stenting. However, a new device called the HeRO graft (Haemodialysis

Reliable Outflow device) combines a PTFE graft with a titanium connector to a 5 mm nitinol stent that can be placed over the wire through a central vein stenosis or occlusion so that the tip is placed at the right atrium. Initial patency has been encouraging with significantly better flows than a TNL. A new titanium connector that allows connection to any graft or vein is currently awaiting approval for use in the UK.

Infection

Infection in AVF is uncommon (2–3%), but may be 10 times more common in grafts, and can often lead to thrombosis of the access. Most graft infections occur within the first month after placement. Risk factors include poor patient hygiene, diabetes, older age, femoral access and previous bacteraemia. It is essential that patients and staff are educated in good aseptic technique to prevent infection. The most common organisms are *S. aureus*, *S. epidermidis*, *S. viridans* and *Pseudomonas aeruginosa*. Infection of a graft will require a protracted course of antibiotics and potentially surgical removal of the AVG.

Failure to mature

Most fistulae will develop increasing in diameter and wall thickness due to shear stress and hoop stress changes when they are initially fashioned. The length of time this can take is often related to initial vessel diameters, arterial and venous flow dynamics and venous outflow resistance, but is expected to take 4–8 weeks. Fistulae that show inadequate signs of development 'fail to mature'.

Arterial inflow is dependent upon an adequate systemic blood pressure and hydration. In >10% of patients, inadequate arterial inflow is due to a proximal arterial stenosis. Juxta-anastomotic stenoses (50%) and large or multiple accessory veins that 'syphon' off blood decreasing intravenous pressure are the most common causes and distal venous stenosis should also be sorted. Aggressive treatment of stenosis with endovascular angioplasty or surgical revision is associated with >95% initial success and 90% 1 year secondary patency in some studies. Venous mapping and ligation (or endovascular occlusion) of accessory veins also significantly improve patency. Management of persistent hypotension is often difficult.

Exercise and infrared therapy are being evaluated and may also improve fistula maturation.

Steal

Steal is defined as inadequate (hypo) perfusion of the distal limb in the presence of an arteriovenous fistula. It occurs when there is inadequate adaptation to compensate for the enhanced systolic AV flow and the diastolic retrograde flow. This may be due to inadequate inflow perfusion (arterial stenosis), inadequate collateralisation, increased systemic resistance in the limb distal to the fistula (peripheral vascular disease) or exceptionally high flow through the fistula especially during dialysis. It is often divided into four stages (Table 9). Differential diagnosis includes temporary nerve compression secondary to tissue swelling or haematoma (this usually resolves within 4 weeks), carpal tunnel syndrome, Sudeck's dystrophy, calciphylaxis or ischaemic monomelic neuropathy (see below).

Patients present with pain, duskiness of digits/distal limb, coolness, paraesthesia and paralysis which may worsen during dialysis.

The prevalence ranges from 0.25% to 20% depending upon the location of the anastomosis and the stage. Steal syndrome requiring

Table 9.   Grading of AV access steal.

Grading of AV access steal (Tordoir)	Findings on investigation
Stage 1: Pale/blue and/or cold hand without pain	Retrograde diastolic flow without complaints; steal phenomenon on duplex.
Stage 2: Pain during exercise and/ or HD	
Stage 3: Rest pain Stage 4: Ulcers/necrosis/gangrene	Transcutaneous oxygen partial pressure (tcpO2) is <30 mmHg, wrist or digital arterial pressures are below 50 mmHg and the digital (wrist)/brachial pressure index is below 0.6. With access compression, the respective values rise significantly, sometimes even to normal.

intervention (stage III or IV) varies between 1% and 2% in distal radio-cephalic AV fistulae, 5% and 15% in brachiocephalic/basilic fistulae and upper limb grafts and between 16% and 36% following the creation of a femoral (autogenous or allograft) access. Women, diabetics, smokers, elderly patients and patients with known coronary or peripheral arterial occlusive disease are at higher risk than the remaining HD population. Diabetics with Stage II steal should be regularly monitored for deterioration in their symptoms.

Proximal arterial stenosis has been demonstrated in 25–50% of patients with dialysis access-related ischaemia. Angioplasty +/− stenting of the lesion is associated with relief of symptoms in nearly all patients where it is the sole cause, however, in most patients it merely contributes.

Treatment for Grade III and IV steal is surgical, with treatment aimed at reducing the flow to the fistula and/or increasing flow preferentially to the limb. Steal can be divided into high flow where flow within the fistula >800 mL/min in AVF and >1200 mL/min in AVG, or low flow where the flow is <400 mL/min in AVF and <600 mL/min in AVG. Reducing flow to a fistula with low flow would lead to thrombosis, therefore the treatment needs to be tailored to the cause and all patients should undergo investigation to assess inflow arteries, distal arteries, fistula flow and limb veins by duplex, and MRA, CTA or intraarterial angiography.

Treatment options include the following:

Ligation — This leads to immediate relief of symptoms, but with loss of the access. It is the treatment of choice in suspected IMN, but must be balanced with the risk of steal developing when a new fistula is created.

Banding — This involves narrowing the proximal fistula close to or at the anastomosis by tying with non-absorbable suture, wrapping with dacron/PTFE cuff, or interposing a small calibre short segment graft with or without tapering. Initial studies showed poor durability, but were significantly improved with the use of intra-operative duplex or transcutaneous tissue oxygenation monitoring.

DRAL/DRIL (Distal radial artery ligation/distal revascularisation-interval ligation) —This involves ligation of the artery distal to the fistula to prevent retrograde flow. In wrist fistulae, due to collateral circulation, this is adequate, however, in more proximal fistulae an additional graft is taken from 8 to 10 cm proximal to the AV anastomosis to beyond the ligation.

PAVA/PAI (Proximal arteriovenous anastomosis/proximalisation of arterial inflow) — This involves ligating the anastomosis and placing a 4–5 mm interposition graft from the proximal artery (axillary/brachial) to the proximal fistula. This technique can be used to treat low flow steal (see Fig. 4).

RUDI (Revision using distal inflow) — This involves ligating the anastomosis and placing an interposition graft from a forearm artery, the flow has been shown to be reduced by 50%. It can be used as an alternate to

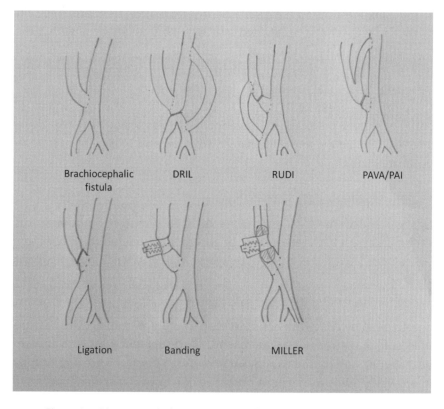

Figure 4.   Diagrammatical representation of surgical treatments for steal.

banding allowing an increased needling area, but requires good distal perfusion and is more invasive.

MILLER (Minimally invasive limited ligation endoluminal-assisted revision) — This involves endovascular placement of an inflated 4 or 5 mm balloon at the proximal fistula and tying a non-absorbable suture to gain a defined reduction in vessel diameter. It is a modified form of banding.

High-flow access and high-flow cardiac failure

High flow in an AV access is defined as >2 L/min and can lead to problems including post-dialysis bleeding, elevated venous pressures, pathologically accelerated access growth and cardiac overload. Cardiovascular disease (CVD) accounts for half of the deaths and one-third of hospitalisations of dialysis patients. High arteriovenous access flow is also often overlooked as a source of cardiac dysfunction. In bypassing the customary arteriole/capillary beds with a direct high-flow connection between the arterial and venous systems, an AVF can cause a precipitous drop in peripheral arterial resistance. The body compensates for this by increasing heart rate and stroke volume, which over time can lead to the development of congestive heart failure (CHF). Management of this follows the lines of management of steal, with an aim to increase resistance in the fistula and/or reduce flow. All of the above procedures used for management of steal have been used in the management of high-flow fistulae with excellent short-term symptomatic relief, and similar 1 year secondary patency (see Table 10).

Ischaemic monomelic ischaemia

First reported by Bolton *et al.* in 1979, IMN is a rare but serious complication of vascular access surgery and part of the spectrum of dialysis access-induced ischaemic syndromes (DAIIS). It is characterised by the *immediate* onset of severe neuropathic pain and neurological dysfunction in ipsilateral hand and forearm (or lower leg) affecting multiple nerves post the fistula creation. On examination, the limb is warm, well-perfused with pulses intact. They may have reduced sensation in fingers,

Table 10.   Outcome for procedures used to manage steal (and high-flow fistulae).

	Success rate (relief of symptoms) %	1 year patency %
Ligation	100	0
Banding	75–95	40–50
DRIL/DRAL	>90	85–100
PAVA/PAI	84	87
RUDI	80	74
MILLER	90	50–80

allodynia and hyperaesthesia, weakness of APB and intrinsic hand muscles. Wrist drop and claw hand can rapidly develop. Risk factors include female gender, diabetes, pre-existing neuropathy and peripheral vascular disease. It affects larger vessel fistulae and has not been reported in fistulae distal to the brachial artery. Initial investigations include duplex ultrasound and electrophysiology, but should not delay treatment. At present, there is evidence to suggest that ligation of the fistula (or DRIL with preservation of the fistula) if performed immediately — not more than 2 weeks post creation — can lead to significant symptomatic improvement, however, the evidence is weak. Prognosis for recovery depends on both severity of initial nerve injury and timing of any definitive intervention. Delay in diagnosis means patients are left with residual chronic symptoms such as sensorimotor deficits, contractures/'clawing' of hand or pain. Long-term supportive care for patients with IMN includes symptom control with analgesics including neuropathic adjuncts, physiotherapy, and psychological support. Both IMN and steal syndrome can have major medicolegal consequences (see Table 11).

Aneurysm/pseudoaneurysm formation

There is no true definition of a fistula aneurysm; and pseudoaneurysms are often reported together, making their true incidence difficult to judge. It may be anywhere from the reported 5–60%, though 2–8% is more likely. Repeated needling can lead to multiple small fibrous scars

Table 11. A comparison of steal syndrome and ischaemic monomelic neuropathy.

	IMN	Steal syndrome
Gender	Female	Male or female
Comorbidities	Diabetes (↑↑↑ risk) peripheral vascular disease pre-existing polyneuropathy	Diabetes (↑ risk) peripheral vascular disease smoking
Fistula site	Upper arm/forearm, never wrist (brachial artery)	Upper arm/forearm/wrist (any artery)
Onset of symptoms	Immediate	Progressive worse on dialysis
Tissues affected	Nerves	Skin, muscle and nerves
Ischaemia	Mild no tissue loss	Severe risk of ulceration/tissue loss
Neurological dysfunction	Severe	Variable
Pain	Severe out of proportion	Variable improved by occluding fistula flow
Examination findings	Warm hand normal capillary refill time good pulses digital pressures normal/slightly ↓	Cold hand prolonged capillary refill time diminished/absent pulses digital pressures ↓↓↓

which may expand with time resulting in localised aneurysmal dilatation. In areas where needling has not been performed, dilatation can occur due to high flow induced abnormal shear stress which promotes remodelling and gradual increased calibre of the vessel. In distal stenosis, the increased transmural pressure proximally can also result in remodelling of the vessel. These aneurysms and psuedoaneurysms (often secondary to repeated localised puncture in a prosthetic graft) have a low risk of rupture as they are thick walled. However, intervention with ligation, partial aneurysmectomy with reduction venoplasty, or graft interposition is indicated where there is rapid increase in size, pain, infection or obvious thinning or degeneration of overlying skin. Any causative stenosis must also be treated appropriately. Post-intervention patency at 12 months is reported as 57% overall, with AVF doing better than AVG, true better than pseudoaneurysms, better in patients with <3 previous aneurysms and in forearm than upper arm access.

Lower Limb Access

Currently, lower limb access is used for those patients unsuitable for upper limb arteriovenous access, often when all upper limb options have been exhausted or the patient has central vein stenosis. However, it can allow patients two-handed self-cannulation and often provides a better cosmetic appearance that can be easily hidden under clothes. The superficial femoral/popliteal vein (SFV/PV) can be transposed into a subcutaneous tunnel fashioned antero-laterally in the thigh and anastomosed to the superficial femoral artery (SFA) at the adductor hiatus, or looped to anastomose with the common femoral artery (CFA) at the groin to give a fistula with excellent patency rates, low rate of infection (1.6%), but has a significant risk of steal at 21%. The long saphenous vein (LSV) can also be mobilised, divided distally and either looped in the anterior thigh to anastomose with the CFA at the groin, or into a medial superficial tunnel to anastomose with the distal SFA or above knee popliteal arteries. Data are sparse, but these fistulae may have inferior patency with frequent early thrombosis and intimal hyperplasia due to the smaller diameter, but less risk of steal. Prosthetic grafts can be placed either in a subcutaneous anterior thigh loop between the common or superficial femoral artery (adductor loop graft) and the common femoral, proximal superficial femoral or long saphenous vein. Suprapubic CFA to contralateral femoral vein has also been described (bikini graft). Although prosthetic grafts have a low risk of steal at 7%, they have a significantly higher risk of infection (18%), a much higher secondary intervention rate and poorer patency — 68% secondary patency at 12 months.

Paediatric Patients

The preferred renal replacement for paediatric patients is transplant or PD. HD is seen as a bridge to transplant. The same considerations and assessments are required as for adults, however, there is a higher risk of non-maturation, which in smaller children can take 4–6 months. Using microsurgical techniques under tourniquet, 8-0 to 10-0 prolene and interrupted sutures may improve outcomes.

Further Reading

Dialysis Outcomes and Practice Patterns Study	www.dopps.org/
The National Kidney Foundation Kidney Disease Outcomes Quality Initiative	https://www.kidney.org/professionals/guidelines
KHA-CARI Guidelines Home Page	www.cari.org.au/
Current Guidelines — Renal Association	www.renal.org/guidelines/current-guidelines
Fistula First Breakthrough Initiative	www.fistulafirst.org

Chapter 28

Diagnosis and Management of Hyperhidrosis

Hassan Badri and Vish Bhattacharya

Key Points

- Postganglionic sympathetic C fibres supply control the sweat gland function.
- Primary hyperhidrosis can impair the social, professional, psychological and physical aspects of patients' lives.
- Local referral pathways and stepwise management protocols should be adopted by the multidisciplinary group.
- Conservative treatments such as topical treatment and iontophoresis should be tried first and patient compliance makes a difference.
- Botulin toxin injections are effective and well received by patients especially for the axillary and facial forms but repeated injections are required.
- Thoracoscopic sympathectomy of T2, T3 for palmar and T2, T3, T4 ganglia for axillary hyperhidrosis is effective and a lifelong solution.
- Extensive consultation should always take place and patients must be warned about complications especially compensatory sweating and the irreversibility of these procedures.
- Local surgical treatments such as elliptical excision, curettage and liposuction for axillary form are effective and less invasive.

Introduction

Sweating is a natural process and part of physiological responses of body thermoregulation but when the sweating is excessive and greater than what is needed for this physiological response, it is called hyperhidrosis. Hyperhidrosis may be primary or secondary.

It is caused by hyper-function of the exocrine sweat glands that are controlled by the sympathetic nervous system via postsynaptic cholinergic fibres. Secondary hyperhidrosis is related to other conditions such as hyperthyroidism, tuberculosis, lymphoma, or pheochromocytoma.

Primary hyperhidrosis affects around 2% of the general population. Patients are usually in their teenage years with a positive family history in up to 50% of cases. It is usually focal, bilateral, and symmetrical with the palms, soles, face, scalp, and axillae being the most commonly affected sites [1].

Symptoms

Patients suffer from excessive sweating in a localised area of their body, which often causes significant impairment in social, occupational, and emotional well-being restricting the patients' private and professional lives. Furthermore, the condition itself might cause bromhidrosis (unpleasant odour), dermal mycoses, and gram-negative infections of the feet or palmar and plantar warts [1].

Diagnosis

Diagnosis is usually clinical. The criteria for diagnosing hyperhidrosis include focal, visible, excessive sweating of at least 6 months' duration without apparent cause with at least two of the following characteristics:

- Bilateral and relatively symmetrical
- Impairment of daily activities
- At least one episode a week
- Age of onset less than 25 years

- Positive family history
- Cessation of focal sweating during sleep [2].

Minor *et al.* described a test in which 2% of iodine solution is applied to the affected area, allowed to dry and then sprinkled with starch powder. The hyperhidrotic skin then develops blue-black colouration as the sweat allows the iodine to mix with starch. Colorimetry is a similar procedure where the colour changes that occur on specially coated paper placed in contact with the sweat are analysed [1].

Management

Topical therapy

Aluminium chloride hexahydrate in absolute anhydrous ethyl alcohol is the most effective antiperspirant for treating hyperhidrosis. The product is applied on the affected areas every night until symptoms are controlled and then weekly or fortnightly to maintain control of sweating. However, it cannot be applied on irritated, broken or recently shaven skin [3]. It can also cause irritation, hypersensitivity, and staining of clothes. Boric acid, glutaraldehyde, formaldehyde, potassium permanganate and tannic acid have shown less satisfactory results.

Systemic therapy

Anticholinergic agents block sweat production at the level of the neuro-glandular junction by competing with acetylcholine. Glycopyrrolate therapy with a dose of 1–2 mg/day showed good results in around 75% of patients. Oxybutynin therapy improved symptoms in an average of 76% of patients and improved QOL in 76% of patients.

Methantheline bromide therapy was associated with a 41% reduction in axillary sweating, but only 16% reduction in palmar sweating.

However, systemic therapy is unpopular due to side effects such as dry mouth, blurred vision, mydriasis, urinary retention and constipation [4].

Iontophoresis

Iontophoresis treatment involves immersion of hands and feet in electrode — containing trays filled with tap water. A direct electrical current
of about 15 mA passes onto the skin for a period of 20–30 min. The
mechanism of action is poorly understood but thought to act by either
causing obstruction of sweat pores or impairment of the electrochemical
gradient of sweat secretion. It is effective for palmar and plantar hyperhidrosis and can be used in paediatric patients and is not associated with
rebound compensatory hyperhidrosis.

Repeated courses of treatment are usually required to prevent
relapse. Adverse effects include sensory disturbances, cracking and burns
of the treated skin [5]. It is impractical for treating the axillary area and is
contraindicated in patients with pacemakers and in pregnancy.

Botulinum toxin

Botulinum toxin A is a neurotoxin which acts at the acetylcholine pre-
synaptic nerve endings at the neuromuscular junctions of exocrine sweat
glands. Injections are placed intra-dermally and as the toxin works over an
area of approximately 1.2 cm diameter, the injections are spaced up to
2.5 cm apart. The duration of effect gradually wanes in 4–12 months and
repeated treatments are usually required. It is a very effective and acceptable modality for axillary disease, and can also be used in palmar, plantar
and facial forms with good results. However, injections at these sites are
more painful and local anaesthesia or nerve blocks may be needed [6].

Common side-effects include pain (usually transitory), intrinsic muscle wasting of the hand (with palmar treatment), haematoma and itching
and sweating. Recently, oral oxybutynin has shown promising results
with 63% and 50% of patients reporting excellent results [7].

Surgical treatment

Endoscopic sympathectomy

Sympathectomy is used to eliminate the sympathetic innervation of the
sweat glands and consequently reduce the amount of sweating.

Thoracoscopic sympathectomy has proved to be the most effective and durable treatment for patients suffering from severe hyperhidrosis. For palmar hyperhidrosis, it is recommended to restrict the sympathectomy to T2, T3 ganglia [8].

For axillary hyperhidrosis, the T2, T3 as well as the T4 ganglia are denervated. In the case of plantar hyperhidrosis, ablation of the lumbar ganglia L2, L3 and L4 is required.

Significant improvement is reported after surgery for the palmar hyperhidrosis with a satisfaction rate of 93% and improvement in quality of life of 100%. The axillary group showed slightly inferior results with figures of 67% and 83%, respectively. The satisfaction rate was lower (47%) after a mean follow-up of 12 years after surgery [8].

Another method of interrupting the sympathetic trunk is by applying clips. This method offers similar success rate and has an additional advantage that clips may be removed in patients who develop severe compensatory hyperhidrosis.

The commonest complication after sympathectomy is compensatory sweating which occurs in 33–87% of patients. Compensatory sweating affects previously unaffected areas such as trunk, chest, back, and lower limb and can be avoided by limiting the extent of sympathectomy.

Other surgical complications included pneumothorax (0.5%), segmental atelectasis (0.35%), haemothorax (0.1%), and mild wound infections (0.1%). Horner's syndrome is transitory in 0.8% and permanent in 0.1%.

The recurrence rates for palmar and axillary hyperhidrosis after surgery are 1.3% and 17% in the fifth year, respectively [1].

Percutaneous sympathectomy

Chemical sympathectomy under computed tomography (CT) guidance by injecting ethanol or phenol showed immediate success rate up to 96% and improvement in quality of life of 87% at 12 months [9]. Dorsal percutaneous stereotactic thermocoagulation sympathectomy is a newer alternative procedure. Retreatment is often required but final success rates of around 100% have been reported [10].

Local surgical procedures

Local surgical treatments have only been described for axillary region and include local excision of sweat glands, curettage and liposuction. They were found to be effective, less invasive and showed comparative outcomes to surgical sympathectomy. They are much less likely to cause compensatory sweating but are more associated with local skin or wound complications [11].

Future development

Microwave-based treatment and to a lesser extent lasers are new potential effective procedures for treating hyperhidrosis but evidence is still lacking in this area.

References

1. Togel B, Greve B, Raulin C. Current therapeutic strategies for hyperhidrosis: A review. *Eur J Dermatol* 2002;12(3):219–223.
2. Hornberger J, Grimes K, Neumann M, Glaser DA, Lowe NJ, Naver H *et al*. Recognition, diagnosis and treatment of primary focal hyperhidrosis. *J Am Acad Dermatol* 2004;51:274–286.
3. Stolman LP. Treatment of hyperhidrosis. *Dermatol Clin* 1998;16(4):863–869.
4. Cruddas L, Baker DM. Treatment of primary hyperhidrosis with oral anticholinergic medications: A systematic review. *J Eur Acad Dermatol Venereol* 2017;31(6):952–963.
5. Akins DL, Meisenheimer JL, Dobson RL. Efficacy of the drionic unit in the treatment of hyperhidrosis. *J Am Acad Dermatol* 1987;16:828–832.
6. Karamfilov T, Konrad H, Karte K *et al*. Lower relapse rate of botulinum toxin A therapy for axillary hyperhidrosis by dose increase. *Arch Dermatol* 2000; 136:487–490.
7. Millan-Cayetano JF, del Boz J, Rivas-Ruiz F, Blazquez-Sanchez N, Ibanez CH, de Troya-Martin M. Oral oxybutynin for the treatment of hyperhidrosis: Outcomes after one-year follow-up. *Austr J Dermatol* 2017;58(2):e31-e35.
8. Dumont P, Denoyer A, Robin P. Long-term results of thoracoscopic sympathectomy for hyperhidrosis. *Ann Thorac Surg* 2004;78(5):1801–1807.
9. Guo J, Yong Fei, Huang B, Yao M. CT-guided thoracic sympathetic blockade for palmar hyperhidrosis: Immediate results and postoperative quality of life. *J Clin Neurosci* 2016;34:89–93.

10. Chuang KS, Liu JC. Long-term assessment of percutaneous stereotactic thermocoagulation of upper thoracic ganglionectomy and sympathectomy for palmar and craniofacial hyperhidrosis in 1742 cases. *Neurosurgery* 2002; 51:963–970.

11. Heidemann E, Licht PB. Comparative study of thoracoscopic sympathectomy versus local surgical treatment for axillary hyperhidrosis. *Ann Thorac Surg* 2013;95(1):264–268.

Chapter 29

Critical Care Considerations and Pre-operative Assessment for General and Vascular Surgery

Ian D. Nesbitt and David M. Cressey

Key Points

- Peri-operative cardiac complications are the most serious risks to delineate and pre-emptively manage.
- Discussions between anaesthetists, surgeons and cardiologists are frequently required on a case-by-case basis.
- Critical care is an essential and rapidly developing support to many surgical procedures.

Introduction

'Good surgeons know how to operate, better surgeons know when to operate, and the best surgeons know when not to operate.' This aphorism reflects the intertwined nature of surgery, anaesthesia and critical care. Poor patient selection or preparation for a particular surgical procedure cannot be entirely compensated for by good anaesthesia or critical care. The purposes of pre-operative assessment include an identification and management of individual patient risks as well as appropriate resource allocation.

Sixty percent of patients undergoing major vascular surgery have significant coronary artery disease (CAD). Similarly, CAD is common amongst patients having non-vascular procedures, so an understanding of the important principles of investigation and management is important for all surgeons and anaesthetists. This section will therefore concentrate particularly on cardiovascular assessment, although other disease states are also considered.

Pre-operative Assessment

(1) General pre-operative assessment

When considering an individual patient, the degree of CAD is often difficult to adequately assess by history and examination alone (e.g., because of limitations in exercise capacity due to claudication, general fatigue or the time limited nature of an emergency presentation). However, a good history and examination can allow specific directed investigations to be carried out. Examples include: echocardiography for patients with suspected aortic stenosis and cardiopulmonary exercise testing for patients with poor functional reserve. Individual history taking can be combined with population based information such as the Heart Outcomes Prevention Evaluation (HOPE) study and Reduction of Atherothrombosis for Continued Health (REACH) registry, which show that a history of peripheral vascular disease strongly predicts adverse cardiovascular outcomes to help direct other investigations or management.

(2) Risk assessment and scoring systems for surgery

Aside from a general pre-operative assessment, more sophisticated investigations may have additional benefits. It is important to assess the risk of a particular procedure not only from a patient's viewpoint (adequate information is required for informed consent), but also from a medical and organisational perspective. This includes appropriate targeting of resource and therapy, e.g., pre-operative investigation and physiological optimisation; efficient use of critical care beds; consideration of conservative management rather than operative intervention and also comparisons of observed vs. expected outcomes, which may be used for wider comparative purposes (Table 1).

In all these scores, cardiac failure and recent myocardial infarction are the strongest indicators of post-operative cardiac complications. Aortic stenosis is a strong independent predictor of peri-operative complications — a gradient of 25–50 mmHg increases operative risk five-fold, and a gradient greater than 50 mmHg increases risk seven-fold.

The Revised Cardiac Risk Index (RCRI) performs best as a predictor of low risk in real life practice, and is detailed in Table 2. Higher risk patients usually require additional evaluation.

Table 1.   Some risk scoring systems.

Risk score	Comments
Association of anesthesiologists (ASA)	General scoring system with significant variation in scoring between different clinicians.
Goldman index	Developed >30 years ago: superseded by later systems.
Detsky score	Principally concerned with peri-operative cardiac event prediction.
Lee revised cardiac risk index	See Table 2 for additional details.
V-POSSUM	Specific vascular surgical score developed in UK.
Parsonnet score	Scoring system for cardiac surgery.

Table 2.   Revised cardiac risk index.

Revised cardiac risk index	Details
Ischaemic heart disease	Angina, myocardial infarction, previous PCI or CABG
Heart failure	History of or examination compatible with left ventricular failure. Paroxysmal nocturnal dyspnoea
Cerebrovascular disease	Previous TIA or CVA
Insulin dependant diabetes	—
Chronic renal impairment	Creatinine > 177 micromol/L (2 mg/dL)
High risk surgical case	Thoracic, abdominal or pelvic vascular operation

Notes: No RCRI criteria = Low risk (0.4–1% risk of cardiac complications), 1–2 RCRI criteria = intermediate risk (2–7% risk), 3 + RCRI criteria = high risk (>9% risk).

Ideally, a scoring system allows accurate and individualised prediction of the outcome from a particular operation for each patient, with low false positive and negative rates. No scoring system yet allows this. Some scoring systems (e.g., V-POSSUM) can be used to provide performance comparison between units, or within a unit over time, while others, (e.g., P-POSSUM) use population based historical outcomes to prospectively stratify patients. This can be useful to discuss general risks with patients, but are too imprecise to be used to attempt accurate individual prediction of specific outcomes.

Attempts to improve the prognostic ability of pre-operative investigations have yielded mixed results. It is increasingly recognised that static testing, such as resting echocardiography, may provide information on valvular anatomy or pulmonary artery pressures, but has little prognostic value in vascular surgery. Dynamic testing such as dobutamine stress echocardiography (DSE) adds value to pre-operative investigations, but even this has limited prognostic ability, and there is much current interest in cardiopulmonary exercise testing (CPX) [1].

CPX involves a combination of exercise ECG (usually on a bicycle) with concurrent measurement of exhaled CO_2 and oxygen consumption (Fig. 1). These allow calculations of anaerobic threshold (AT) and development of any myocardial ischaemia during exercise. An AT below 11 mL/min/kg is considered an indicator of high risk case, although more complex evaluations are increasingly being developed, based on nature of surgery, early vs. late ischaemic changes and absolute AT(1). It is likely that prognostic cut-off values will vary between population groups and surgical centres.

These investigations can be used to aid decision making regarding intra- and post-operative care. For example, a patient with a high AT having aortic reconstruction may be suitable for a level 2 (HDU type) bed post-operatively, while a patient with a poor AT having similar surgery may be much more likely to require a level 3 (ITU type) bed, with consequent implications for hospital resource management. In the UK, the National Emergency Laparotomy Audit uses pre-operative scoring with historical outcome data to aid contemporaneous decision making in this regard.

Pre-operative decision making requires more than simply assessing risk. If possible, the peri-operative risks should be reduced or eliminated.

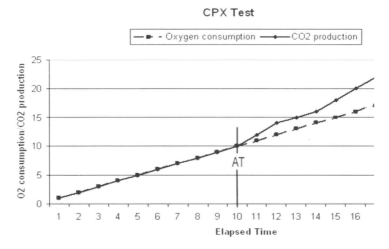

Figure 1.   CPX testing.

Notes: CPX testing: During gentle (aerobic) exercise, oxygen consumption and CO_2 production are similar, so the graphs have a similar slope.

During strenuous (anaerobic) exercise, CO_2 production is greater than O_2 consumption, so the CO_2 graph has a steeper slope.

The transition between aerobic and anaerobic metabolism is the anaerobic threshold (AT), and reflects the integrated ability of the cardio-respiratory and cellular mechanisms to manage an increased workload.

Aside from training and general conditioning, a variety of cardiac and respiratory disease states produce diagnostic patterns in CPX data.

This may involve optimising the patients' condition. Typically, this includes achieving control of comorbidities including blood pressure, diabetes, dyslipidaemia and consideration of β-blockade.

The actual investigative and management pathways will vary between institutions, but ultimately, success depends on good communications and relationships between radiology, anaesthesia, critical care and surgery. There is an increasing role for pre-assessment clinics (PAC) as a co-ordinator of investigations and optimisation, but to be successful, PAC requires a strong leadership and clear strategies. Agreed inter-departmental policies are an important part of this, e.g., anticoagulation, major bleeding, cross matching, etc., based partly on national recommendations such as National Institute for Health and Clinical Excellence (NICE) guidelines for pre-operative investigation.

Co-ordination of complex cases, e.g., decisions about staging of carotid and coronary surgery, proximal thoracoabdominal aortic aneurysms requiring partial or complete cardiopulmonary bypass, staged visceral revascularisation, etc., should be carried out in specialist centres with an adequate volume of work to achieve good results. Increasingly unfit patients are presenting for carotid, thoracic and abdominal endovascular procedures, and again require expert multidisciplinary team assessment if possible.

Specific Management of Other Comorbidities

(a) *Pulmonary disease*

Obstructive pulmonary diseases (asthma, emphysema and bronchitis) should have long-term drug therapy optimised. Typically, this is based on multimodal anti-inflammatory drugs and bronchodilators. Particular attention to pre-existing pulmonary disease is required if surgery involves deflating a lung for surgical access.

Restrictive lung disease may be intrinsic, e.g., fibrosis, or more commonly extrinsic, e.g., due to kyphosis or obesity. Treatment options for the specific restrictive lung disease may be limited, but may influence the choice of regional vs. local or general anaesthesia for a particular surgical procedure.

As with cardiovascular diseases, close liaison with the anaesthetist and intensive care team is required to optimally manage patients with significant lung disease. Pulmonary hypertension (PHT) and cor pulmonale are important risk factors for post-operative death, and patients with severe lung disease should have PHT and right heart failure actively excluded by echocardiography.

Epidural analgesia may reduce post-operative respiratory morbidity and reduce length of ICU stay, but has implications for some drug therapies in the peri-operative period (see below).

(b) *Obesity*

Obesity is a multisystem disease with implications for both anaesthetic and surgical approaches. Patients with obstructive sleep apnoea may require post-operative respiratory support in critical care, rather than immediate transfer to a ward environment, since respiratory complications are more common in the obese. Local services will dictate where these patients are managed.

(c) *Diabetes*

In addition to predisposing to macro and microvascular disease, diabetes is a significant risk factor for many post-operative complications, including renal failure, myocardial infarction and death. The long-term benefits of good diabetic control are well established, but the optimal details of short-term peri-operative diabetic control are less clear. Comprehensive UK guidelines for managing all stages of a patient's admission were updated in 2015 [3]. Pre-operatively, HbA1c levels below 64–75 mmol/L are recommended, and peri-operative blood glucose levels of 4–12 mmol/L are safe and practical goals.

Traditionally, type 2 diabetics undergoing minor surgery are placed early on an operating list, and simply omit any morning hypoglycaemic agents. Type 1 diabetics may either take their normal insulin or have a glucose–potassium–insulin (GKI) infusion started, depending on the timing and nature of surgery and the local policies in use.

All diabetics having major surgery should have a GKI started pre-operatively and continued until enteral feeding is established again. There is an increasing emphasis on maintaining as near normal insulin regimes as possible, along with increased and early involvement of diabetic specialist teams.

(d) *Hypertension*

Systemic hypertension is a risk factor in the long term for cardiovascular and cerebrovascular complications, but the evidence that peri-operative outcomes are worse unless hypertension is severe (perhaps >180/100 mmHg) is weak. Local agreements about how an individual patient with hypertension is managed will depend on multiple other factors.

(e) *Permanent pacemakers (PPM) and implantable cardiac defibrillators (ICDs)*

An increasing number of patients present for surgery with pacemakers or ICDs. Aside from the traditional indications such as sick sinus syndrome and complete heart block, PPMs/ICDs may now be indicated as treatment of choice for diseases as diverse as refractory atrial fibrillation, vasovagal syncope and post-myocardial infarction ventricular dysfunction, as well as in survivors of first presentation life threatening arrhythmias.

It is important to know what type of device is in use prior to surgery. This allows planning both for deliberate actions and emergency management should device interference occur. Patients may be a source of useful information in this respect, and a 12 lead ECG is mandatory, but recent device interrogation by a pacemaker clinic is most helpful.

Although increasingly robust, some PPMs and ICDs may require reprogramming or deactivation prior to anaesthesia. Unipolar diathermy should be avoided if possible, as should prolonged periods of continuous diathermy during surgery. This reduces the electromagnetic interference that may reset the PPM to a backup mode, or trigger inappropriate defibrillation by an ICD. Post-operatively, the device may need reprogramming, and should be rechecked before the patient is discharged.

(f) *Percutaneous coronary interventions (PCI), coronary stents and cardiac surgery*

More than 90% of PCI involve insertion of at least one stent, the majority of which are drug eluting stents (DES). Although DES may have a short term advantage over bare metal stents (BMSs) regarding early stent thrombosis, they carry the disadvantage of requiring prolonged dual antiplatelet therapy (DAPT) to prevent late stent thrombsosis, which has a significant mortality rate.

PCI usually involves large doses of anticoagulant and antiplatelet agents. Intravenous heparin has a relatively short (dose dependant) half-life, but glycoprotein IIb/IIIa inhibitors such as abciximab or tirofiban may have activity up to 48 h (and can inhibit the activity of any transfused platelets). This, and the condition precipitating PCI, have obvious implications for the conduct of surgery and anaesthesia.

In the emergency situation, vascular emergencies may present around the time of a PCI, e.g., retroperitoneal haemorrhage due to vessel injury during angiography. Additionally, some patients requiring vascular interventions will have had a relatively recent PCI for intercurrent active CAD.

Although no specific rules apply to management, since the risk-benefit will depend on the nature and urgency of surgery, major elective surgery in patients with a DES in place may be best deferred for at least 12 months. Patients having PCI with BMS or PCI alone should have at least 6 weeks delay. Patients who have undergone coronary artery bypass grafting should have non-cardiac surgery delayed for at least 30 days if possible.

For emergency cases, or those where regional anaesthesia is considered essential, a platelet transfusion may reduce major bleeding without substantially increasing the risk of stent thrombosis. Recommended platelet target levels are between 50 and 80,000 μL^{-1}.

This is a rapidly evolving area of practice, and recommendations change frequently, so focussed discussion is essential when faced with such situations.

Specific Management of Drug Therapy

The scientific understanding of atherosclerosis has changed over recent years, from a simple mechanical obstructive model to one of a variable and ongoing inflammatory pathological process with central involvement of platelet activation and aggregation. This, and the observed hypercoagulable state following surgery, have implications for both drug management and surgical interventions.

(a) *Antiplatelet agents*

A significant indication for antiplatelet therapy is to prevent coronary stent thrombosis-untreated, around 20% of stents thrombose, with a 20% mortality. Premature cessation of antiplatelet therapy is a major concern, although it is difficult to precisely quantify the risk for most individual patients. At present, one month of DAPT is recommended for BMS, and 1 year for DES, followed by long-term aspirin for both types.

Generally, in cases where the risks of bleeding are small, and the risk of thrombosis high, dual antiplatelet therapy should be continued. For patients with a high risk of bleeding, discussion between anaesthetist, cardiologist and surgeon is essential. Although no unequivocal evidence exists, the emphasis is on continuing antiplatelet therapy whenever possible. This poses a potential problem for many procedures where epidural, central neuraxial blockade (CNB) or spinal drain insertion is planned.

(i) Aspirin

This inhibits thromboxane A2 to reduce platelet aggregation, although up to 40% of patients may be aspirin resistant. In general, the risk of excess peri-operative haemorrhage is sufficiently low to recommend that for most surgery, aspirin should be continued if possible. Prostate and intracranial operations may have a higher bleeding rate, so the use of aspirin should be discussed with the anaesthetist involved.

(ii) Clopidogrel

This pro-drug, when activated, inhibits fibrinogen binding to platelet glycoprotein IIb/IIIa receptors and reduces platelet aggregation. A small proportion of patients are clopidogrel resistant, but generally, a loading dose takes several days to exert its full effect, and the antiplatelet effect lasts for up to 7 days. During this time, any transfused platelets are also affected, although often to only a small degree. Frequently, clopidogrel is used as either combination therapy with aspirin or as monotherapy for patients intolerant or resistant to aspirin.

(iii) Prasugrel

This thienopyridine drug has a greater antithrombotic effect than clopidogrel, but also higher bleeding rates. A smaller proportion of patients are non-responders to this than to clopidogrel, and as with clopidogrel, the effect starts early (within hours), reaches a maximum over several days, and takes around 7 days to recede once treatment is stopped.

(b) *Oral Anticoagulants*

Many vascular patients take warfarin. Novel oral anticoagulant (NOAC) drugs, such as the direct thrombin inhibitor dabigatran and direct factor Xa inhibitors rivaroxaban and apixaban are now available, and are likely to replace warfarin. These drugs may be easier and safer to manage from a patients' perspective (predictable fixed dosing without intensive monitoring), but emergency reversal may be more problematic.

At present, only dabigatran has a specific antidote available, although similar reversal agents are under investigation for other NOACs.

Patients with mechanical heart valves should have an individual assessment of risk from surgical haemorrhage against risk of cardiac thrombotic complications. This will depend on the nature and location of the heart valve and the planned surgery. Traditional peri-operative management involves stopping warfarin 3 or 4 days before surgery, and using a continuous infusion of unfractionated heparin as bridging therapy until a few hours pre-operatively, then restarting post-operatively until adequate oral intake allows rewarfarinisation.

More recently, bridging therapy using low molecular weight heparin (LMWH) has been used. This is an evolving area of medicine, and the practical management will be dictated by the patient (risk group, co-morbidity, etc.) as well as local policies [2]. Increasingly, appropriate individual patient management will require discussion with an anaesthetist or haematologist.

(c) *Statins*

There is some evidence from retrospective and case control studies that statins reduce mortality following major surgery, possibly due in part to stabilisation of inflammatory atherosclerotic plaque. Small prospective trials have confirmed this observation, although high quality evidence is lacking, and any proposed mechanism of action is currently putative [4]. Nonetheless, patients with dyslipidaemias should have lipid lowering therapy started irrespective of their need for surgery.

(d) *β-blockers*

The evidence base regarding peri-operative β-blockade has been contaminated by fraudulent data, but even accounting for this, the role of β-blockade in the peri-operative period remains uncertain [5]. Initial small trials showed a reduction in all-cause mortality, but more recent evidence suggests that myocardial protection is more than balanced by all-cause mortality and stroke. Patients already taking β-blockers should probably continue these in the peri-operative period, but starting β-blockers in the immediate pre-operative phase for patients with uncomplicated CAD should not be considered routine practice at present.

(e) *ACE inhibitors and angiotensin II antagonists*

Angiotensin converting enzyme inhibitors (ACEI) are first-line therapy for heart failure. Angiotensin II receptor (AT II) antagonists may be used as an alternative or additional treatment. There is uncertainty regarding the optimal management of these drugs in the peri-operative period. Patients continuing these drugs may be more susceptible to refractory hypotension during anaesthesia, and to renal impairment and possibly even post-operative death. This is perhaps most marked in hypovolaemic patients. However, patients stopping ACEI or ATII antagonists may be at risk from non-fatal cardiac complications. If ACEI are withheld pre-operatively, this should be for at least 12 h. ATII antagonists should be withheld for at least 24 h due to their longer half life.

Management of Emergency or Acute Cases

Increasingly, carotid surgery should be carried out in acute setting, and many vascular patients present as emergencies. Time to investigate, treat or stabilise may be limited, and patient outcome then depends on the expertise and functioning of the whole team. Outcomes are better when experienced teams who have practiced and worked together over prolonged periods carry out these complex tasks, rather than random on-call teams of varying abilities. This has implications for centralisation of services and specialisation of staff, which are beyond the remit of this chapter.

Radiologic embolisation for control of bleeding is possible under local anaesthesia in selected emergency cases to avoid the risks of general anaesthesia and open surgery. Again, this has wider implications for service provision beyond the scope of this chapter.

Critical Care Considerations

Critical care issues cover a wide range of topics, both in exams and clinical practice, relevant to many surgical specialities. Some topics (e.g., brain death, organ donation) are covered elsewhere in this book. Others should be taken from source documents due to their regular revision. Examples include cardiac arrest management, treatment of common arrhythmias and anaphylaxis. These topics are clearly and concisely set out in the Resuscitation Council UK website (http://www.resus.org.uk, see the guidelines page for a link to the algorithms for a concise revision aid). A precise knowledge of current algorithms is vital not just for exam purposes, but for everyday clinical practice. It is reasonable to expect a senior surgical trainee to have a clear understanding of these areas of emergency management.

Practical procedures often associated with critical care are central venous line insertion, chest drain insertion and vascular access for haemodialysis. Indications for the procedure, common complications and the details of surface anatomy and actual insertion technique have all been asked in the exit exam and candidates should have a clear understanding of these. These areas are covered in the Care of the Critically Ill Surgical Patient (CCrISP) course and the handbook for that course sets them out well.

Definitions of levels of critical care

Critical care can be considered as a spectrum from enhanced ward care, including support from Critical Care Outreach services, up to the advanced multiple organ support provided in an Intensive Care Unit. In 2000, the Department of Health produced a document 'Comprehensive Critical Care' defining critical care into levels 0 to 3 (see Table 3).

In some hospitals, each level of care is provided for in distinct clinical areas. This is the traditional model of acute surgical ward (level 1), High

Table 3.   Levels of critical care.

Level 0	Patients whose needs can be met through normal ward care in an acute hospital.
Level 1	Patients at risk of their condition deteriorating, or those recently relocated from higher levels of care, whose needs can be met on an acute ward with additional advice and support from the critical care team.
Level 2	Patients requiring more detailed observation or intervention including support for a single failing organ system or post-operative care and those 'stepping down' from higher levels of care.
Level 3	Patients requiring advanced respiratory support alone or basic respiratory support together with support of at least two organ systems. This level includes all complex patients requiring support for multiorgan failure.

Dependency Unit (HDU, level 2) which may be directly supervised by the surgical directorates or managed as a step-down unit from Intensive Care by the intensivists, and Intensive Care or Intensive Therapy Units (ICU or ITU Level 3). Many hospitals are now moving to a system of Integrated Critical Care Units (ICCU) with all the enhanced level beds (2 and 3) in one location.

Definitions of organ failure

Most critical care therapy supports failing organ systems to allow time for other treatments, and the patients own defence mechanisms, to generate recovery. Multiple Organ Dysfunction Syndrome (MODS) describes what is often a secondary injury to tissues caused by a host inflammatory response to a primary insult. It is characterised by a progressive loss of function in several different organ systems and its treatment is the core of ICU care. Deterioration of any organ ranges from reduced to complete loss of function and there are many definitions of exactly what constitutes organ failure. The Sequential (Sepsis-related) Organ Failure Assessment (SOFA) score is a widely used measure of organ failure [6]. Calculated daily it can be used as a measure of severity of illness and response to treatment (see Table 4).

Monitoring and therapeutic measures for specific organ failure

All critical care measures must be built on a foundation of sound basic care.

Treatment of any organ failure needs to start with an assessment of airway, breathing and circulation (A, B, C) as per CCrISP or ATLS guidelines, and these should always be followed with immediate treatment of any deficit detected. A full physical examination including measurement of pulse, blood pressure, respiratory rate, pulse-oximetry and temperature is also mandatory. Critical care therapeutic options for specific organ system failure are set out below.

Respiratory failure

Immediate measures to treat respiratory failure begin with optimal positioning of the patient (e.g., sitting up in bed or in a chair to improve chest

Table 4. Indicators of organ dysfunction. Insert SOFA score table from Sepsis 3.

System		0	1	2	3	4
				Sequential [Sepsis-Related] Organ Failure Assessment Score[a]		
Respiration						
Pao_2/Fio_2, mmHg (kPa)		≥400 (53.3)	<400 (53.3)	<300 (40)	<200 (26.7) with respiratory support	<100 (13.3) with respiratory support
Coagulation						
Platelets, ×10³/μL		≥150	<150	<100	<50	<20
Liver						
Bilirubin, mg/dL (μmol/L)		<1.2 (20)	1.2–1.9 (20–32)	2.0–5.9 (33–101)	6.0–11.9 (102–204)	>12.0 (204)
Cardiovascular		MAP ≥70 mmHg	MAP <70 mmHg	Dopamine <5 or dobutamine (any dose)[b]	Dopamine 5.1–15 or epinephrine ≤0.1 or norepinephrine ≤0.1[b]	Dopamine >15 or epinephrine >0.1 or norepinephrine >0.1[b]
Central nervous system						
Glasgow Coma Scale score[c]		15	13–14	10–12	6–9	<6
Renal						
Creatinine, mg/dL (μmol/L)		<1.2 (110)	1.2–1.9 (110–170)	2.0–3.4 (171–299)	3.5–4.9 (300–440)	>5.0 (440)
Urine output, mL/d					<500	<200

Notes: Abbreviations: Fio_2, fraction of inspired oxygen; MAP, mean arterial pressure; Pao_2, Partial pressure of oxygen.
[a] Adapted from Ref. [27].
[b] Catecholamine doses are given as μg/kg/min for at least 1 h.
[c] Glasgow Coma Scale scores range from 3 to 15, higher score indicates better neurological function.
Source: The Third International Consensus Definitions for Sepsis and Septic Shock (Sepsis-3). *JAMA* 2016;315(8):801–810. DOI:10.1001/jama.2016.0287.

expansion). Oxygen should be used in all acutely breathless patients. If there is a strong suspicion of chronic lung disease likely to include carbon dioxide retention, then arterial blood gas analysis (ABG) to monitor this will be required soon after commencing oxygen. If sputum retention is suspected, then urgent physiotherapy may be required. When clinical signs suggest an active chest infection, then appropriate antibiotics should be started immediately, ideally after obtaining a sputum specimen. Other treatable causes for breathlessness should be sought and rectified, such as excessive pain or anxiety, pneumothorax, pleural effusion and cardiac arrhythmias.

For a patient who remains breathless or tachypnoeic, or whose peripheral oxygen saturations remain depressed in spite of supplemental oxygen, ABG analysis is appropriate. ABG results will provide information on pH, oxygen and carbon dioxide levels, base deficit, bicarbonate and often lactate. Respiratory failure can be differentiated into types 1 and 2, on the basis of reduced pO_2 alone (type 1) or in combination with elevated pCO_2 (type 2).

Standard mixed concentration (MC) oxygen face masks can deliver up to a maximum of around 60% oxygen, regardless of how high a flow rate of oxygen is used due to entrainment of air around the sides of the mask during rapid inspiration. The addition of a non-rebreathe bag to the mask allows more oxygen to be drawn from the bag during inspiration and may increase inspired oxygen concentration to approximately 80%. For CO_2 retaining patients needing tightly controlled oxygen, venturi masks will ensure a maximum inspired oxygen concentration is delivered independent of oxygen flow rate and inspiratory effort.

If levels of oxygen greater than 80% are required, then a tight fitting mask is needed to prevent entrainment. The use of continuous positive airway pressure (CPAP) may further enhance oxygen delivery. CPAP (delivered via a nasal or face mask or hood device) increases functional residual capacity (FRC) by preventing airway pressure falling to zero during expiration. A rise in FRC reduces ventilation-perfusion mismatch thereby improving gas exchange. CPAP requires a cooperative patient with a patent airway and intact airway reflexes. Above CPAP pressures of 20 cm H_2O insufflation of the stomach may occur with a risk of vomiting and aspiration. Oxygenation may be improved by CPAP, but CO_2 removal may not be improved with its use. In some cases, a reduced work of breathing may permit improved respiration and affect pCO_2, but this is not a predictable response.

For patients with rising pCO_2 or need for high oxygen concentrations in the presence of impaired airway protection or impending exhaustion, intubation and positive pressure ventilation may be indicated. A cuffed tube placed in the trachea will allow a degree of protection of the airway from aspiration and the application of airway pressure in excess of 20 cmH_2O without risk of gastric insufflation. Intermittent positive pressure ventilation (IPPV) can be delivered as a pressure controlled volume limited (i.e., bilevel positive airway pressure (BIPAP)) or as volume controlled pressure limited ventilation (conventional intermittent mandatory ventilation (IMV) which may be synchronised with patients' own respiratory efforts (SIMV)). Currently accepted methods include the use of high positive end expiratory pressure (PEEP) to enhance FRC, and thus oxygenation in conjunction with low tidal volumes (maximum 6 mL per kg body weight tidal volume) as per the ARDSNET study to reduce volutrauma damage to the lungs in acute lung injury (ALI). The use of demispan measurement (from sternum to fingertips of arm outstretched at 90 degrees from mid-line) allows estimation of patient height and ideal body weight for use in determining optimal tidal volume. Limiting tidal volumes may lead to rising pCO_2, but in the absence of marked acidaemia this is considered an acceptable side effect of this ventilatory strategy described as permissive hypercapnia.

Prolonged oral or nasal intubation may lead to long-term injury to vocal cords and to ischaemic mucosal damage of the trachea leading to stenosis. Tracheostomy has long been an established alternative. With the advent of percutaneous dilational techniques, there has been an increase in use of tracheostomy and also a tendency to perform them earlier in a patient's ITU stay. The TracMan study published in 2013 failed to show an improved mortality with early (less than 4 days) or late (more than 10 days) tracheostomy, but did not address longer term sequelae or other perceived benefits. Additional advantages include a reduced need for sedation, which in turn may reduce vasopressor requirements and direct access to the trachea for suctioning in a patient who is awake and able to cough, communicate and cooperate with physiotherapy. This may speed the process of weaning from ventilation.

Cardiac failure

Standard assessment of the cardiovascular system begins with clinical examination and non-invasive assessments including ECG and echocardiography, supplemented by invasive methods including arterial and central venous access and cardiac output estimation by one of several methods. Therapy builds from optimisation of cardiac filling and correction of rhythm abnormalities to inotropic and vasopressor regimes and perhaps cardiac assist devices such as intra-aortic balloon pumps. These therapies aim to ensure optimum oxygen delivery to end organs. Global oxygen delivery is a product of the haemoglobin concentration in the blood, the oxygen saturation of that haemoglobin and the cardiac output. Dissolved haemoglobin makes up a very small percentage of oxygen content of the blood. Therapeutic measures need to ensure each of these aspects is optimised. Less predictable or amenable to treatment is tissue level oxygen flux. Microcirculatory abnormalities and impaired enzyme function may reduce oxygen delivery at cellular level. This is particularly seen in severe sepsis.

The effectiveness of treatment of circulatory impairment at end-organ level can be assessed by simple means including GCS for adequacy of cerebral perfusion or urine output and creatinine levels for renal perfusion. Assessment of adequacy of global oxygen delivery can be estimated from lactate levels, although local ischaemia or liver failure may complicate this. Oxygen saturations of less than 70% on a central-line venous sample may indicate inadequate oxygen delivery.

To maximise cardiac function, left ventricular filling, myocardial contractility and afterload (resistances SVR) should be optimised. Starlings curve relates increased stretch on myofibrils to contractility of those fibres. It can be extrapolated to predict the effect of increasing left ventricular filling on myocardial contractility. With increased filling, myocardial contractility increases up to a certain point. Thereafter, further increases in volume lead to decrease in contractility and a failing heart. In a normal heart central venous pressure which estimates right atrial pressure will be a reasonable measure of left atrial pressure and therefore left ventricular filling. Where valves are damaged or pulmonary resistance increased, this may not be true. Pulse contour analysis of arterial pressure traces using complex algorithms are a surrogate measure of left ventricular filling, in particular showing what effect fluid boluses have on stroke volume (SV). If a bolus causes less than a 10% rise in SV, then further filling may not benefit contractility and may even have adverse effects.

A variety of methods are available to estimate cardiac output itself. The gold standard remains pulmonary artery flotation catheter methods using dilutional calculations, but risks associated with their use including death mean their use is declining. Less invasive methods include oesophageal Doppler (ODM), lithium dilution (LiDCO) and pulse contour cardiac output analysis (PiCCO). Each method has its own problems and none necessarily gives an exact measure of cardiac output. Most clinicians accept that the measure is an estimate and are more interested in the dynamic effects of interventions on the reading to demonstrate improvements or otherwise.

Once cardiac filling is optimised, contractility can be further assisted by ensuring a suitable electrolyte and pH balance in the myocardial tissues. Calcium, potassium, phosphate and magnesium are all essential factors for muscle contraction and should be closely monitored and optimised. Severe acidosis can have a detrimental effect on contractility and pH should be normalised whenever possible (see section Renal Failure). Effective contraction is also enhanced by sinus rhythm and any new onset arrhythmia should be corrected.

Thereafter, contractility can be augmented by the use of positive inotropic agents. The most commonly used are epinephrine (adrenaline) and dobutamine with strong agonist actions on beta 1 adrenoreceptors. Although cardiac output influences global oxygen delivery, the systolic blood pressure determines localised perfusion of tissues such that a very low systolic pressure is likely to be harmful. Drugs such as dopamine and dopexamine are known to be positive inotropes, but are often used in lower doses by clinicians who believe they can improve specific regional blood flow (in particular renal and splanchnic), but the evidence for this is not strong. Their other adverse side effects (tachyarrhythmia, dopaminergic receptor stimulation) make these two drugs less attractive as pure inotropes.

Profound vasodilation in severe sepsis may reduce systolic pressure to harmful levels even in the presence of a high cardiac output. Drugs acting as alpha adrenoreceptor agonists can produce vasoconstriction to improve overall tissue perfusion pressure and tissue oxygen delivery. Norepinephrine (noradrenaline) and phenylephrine are first line vasopressor agents. Vasopressin and terlipressin are second line agents that may supplement the actions of norepinephrine. In patients with severe sepsis and vasopressor resistant hypotension low dose steroids (50 mg hydrocortisone iv qds) may reduce vasopressor requirements, but effects on outcome are unclear.

Renal failure

Classically, causes of renal failure can be divided into pre-renal, renal and post-renal.

Pre-renal causes arise when an insufficient oxygen supply is available to the kidneys. Optimisation of the cardiovascular system as described above is key to preventing or limiting pre-renal renal injury. Clearly, ensuring patency of renal vessels is of primary importance. Thereafter, optimal filling, maintenance of cardiac output and adequate mean arterial pressure (with vasopressors if needed) are the only proven therapies that reduce the degree and duration of renal failure from this cause.

Treatable causes of renal-renal failure usually involve removal or avoidance of nephrotoxic agents. NSAIDS, aminoglycosides and iodinated contrast media are commonly encountered in critical care, but should be avoided when feasible.

In the specific case of renal failure following rhabdomyolysis, hydration and a forced alkaline diuresis may limit injury (myoglobin is precipitated in the collecting tubules at acid pH). Sodium bicarbonate infusion may be needed to achieve this. Furosemide should be used with caution if at all.

As a general rule, diuretics increase urine volumes and are useful in patients with volume overload, but do not reduce the occurrence of or duration of renal failure. Their use in patients with developing acute renal failure may worsen outcome by causing hypovolaemia.

Mannitol has been used particularly in the context of aortic surgery as a 'reno-protective' measure. It is an osmotic diuretic and may produce an increase in urine volume, but there is minimal evidence to support any effect on onset or severity of renal impairment.

Dopamine and dopexamine have both been used at 'renal' doses to try to enhance the perfusion of the reno-splanchnic vascular systems. Again, the evidence for efficacy is limited.

(a) *Contrast induced nephropathy* (*CIN*)

This usually occurs within 72 h of exposure to iodinated contrast media. It is usually transient, resolving in 7–10 days, but occasionally permanent and is associated with an increased morbidity and mortality. CIN is dose dependent and use of high osmolar contrast media carries an increased risk. Using the lowest possible dose of contrast media and adequate pre-procedure hydration are the key measures to reduce the incidence of nephrotoxicity. There is limited evidence to support use of N-acetyl-cysteine dosing pre-contrast in the ITU setting. Sodium bicarbonate infusion is used in some centres both pre- and post-contrast to reduce renal injury. There may be a subset of patients with pre-existing chronic renal impairment who may benefit from this strategy, but in other groups it may have little effect or cause harm. The evidence for specific treatment other than optimal hydration with either intravenous saline or oral fluids remains scarce.

Post-renal causes of renal failure consist of obstruction to outflow of urine, this may be due to an occluded ureter post-surgery, prostatic hypertrophy or tumour or other forms of bladder outflow obstruction. In most patients with impending renal failure an ultrasound of the renal tract is a mandatory part of investigation. Bladder catheterisation, both as a monitoring and also a therapeutic measure, is usual in patients with renal impairment.

(b) *Established acute renal failure*

Acute renal failure leads to raised levels of urea and creatinine, the potential for fluid overload and worsening acidosis and hyperkalemia. This combination if left untreated will result in arrhythmias and eventually death.

For treatment of severe hyperkalaemia calcium (gluconate or chloride 10 mmol iv), which acts as a membrane stabiliser to reduce the risk of life threatening VF, should be given immediately. Urgent reduction of serum potassium can be achieved by pushing the potassium ions into the intracellular space using dextrose and insulin (15 iu actrapid in 50 mL 50% dextrose over 15 min) and by correcting the acidosis. Salbutamol (either i.v. or nebulised) can also effectively reduce serum potassium in the emergency situation. Intravenous sodium bicarbonate infusion will increase serum pH as long as the patient maintains an ability to increase ventilation to remove the extra carbon dioxide this generates. Potassium is driven into the intracellular space by alkalosis. Chelating agents such as calcium resonium (for adults 30 g given as a PR enema) will further help to remove potassium from the serum.

Definitive treatment is still likely to be required. Intermittent haemo-dialysis (IHD) or continuous veno-venous haemofiltration (CVVH) can provide this.

In a haemodynamically stable patient, IHD over 3–4 h via a twin lumen venous access line (vascath) will clear acidosis, hyperkalaemia and uraemia rapidly. The rapid fluid shifts involved with this make it difficult to achieve in the more unstable patient. Many units prefer to use CVVH in this group.

In a CVVH circuit, venous, blood is pumped into a filter with a pore size suitable to allow water and small molecules to pass through whilst preventing passage of most proteins, cells and platelets. In this ultrafiltrate, waste such as urea and creatinine along with a mixture of electrolytes and water are separated out and diverted to a waste bag. The volume removed is carefully measured and then replaced with a balanced solution of water and electrolytes. Potassium is added sepa-rately as required. The replacement fluid is either lactate buffered (which remains stable for long periods) or 'lactate-free' bicarbonate buffered (which requires mixing immediately prior to use). Units treat-ing patients with liver impairment tend to use lactate free fluid, as the liver is the main site of lactate metabolism. If a greater degree of clearance is required, there is an option to apply a counter-current flow of the balanced solution through the filter with the aim of increasing the concentration gradient for solutes to exit into the waste flow (haemodiafiltration).

CVVH, as its name implies, is run as a 24 h a day process. By adjusting the amount of fluid replaced into the patient relative to the volume of ultrafiltrate removed, it is possible to remove water to achieve the desired daily fluid balance. In unstable patients the fluid shifts and haemodynamic effects of CVVH are better tolerated. There may also be less injury to the kidney during the filtration process due to the greater haemodynamic stability, than with IHD. In order to prevent clot formation within the CVVH circuit some form of anticoagulation is usually required. This may be in the form of systemic heparin, or citrate use targeting only the blood within the circuit itself to avoid systemic effect. For patients with pre-existing coagulopathy requirement for additional anticoagulant will need to be tailored to the individual.

Nutrition

Post-operative patients and those with sepsis and SIRS usually mount a highly catabolic response. Significant loss of muscle mass and strength may prolong ICU and hospital stay; inadequate nutrition may also affect wound healing. As such, nutrition is a vital part of their critical care therapy. The average catabolic patient in ITU will need a daily calorie intake of around 1600 kcal/day. Where possible the route of delivery should be via enteral feeding. Early enteral feeding, even at low levels (10 mL/h), has been shown to increase splanchnic blood flow, and there is better maintenance of gut mucosal anatomy.

In the unconscious patient this might be NG or PEG tube delivered. Many ICU patients develop gastroparesis for a variety of reasons, and post-pyloric feeding should be considered early in a patient with high gastric aspirates not responding to prokinetics. With foresight, nasojejunal tubes can be sited during a laparotomy using direct manipulation. Later insertion of post-pyloric tubes using blind techniques or with endoscopy causes delay in feeding and is not without risk.

A range of feeds is available, each with its own benefits, and the choice should be tailored to the individual. Osmolite is a standard feed with 1 kcal/mL. Nepro is a low volume feed with 2 kcal/mL, with low potassium, sodium and phosphate loads suitable for those with renal failure. Pulmocare and Oxepa have a high fat:carbohydrate ratio so generate less CO_2 on metabolism, which may be useful for those with severe respiratory failure. Impact has relatively high protein content with added arginine, fish oils and omega 3. It may be beneficial in immunocompromised patients with sepsis. Other feeds exist and the choice should be made in consultation with a dietician.

Where it is not possible to feed via the gut, then total parenteral nutrition (TPN) is used. A dedicated central venous access port and exemplary aseptic technique is needed when using TPN. Line related sepsis leading to septicaemia is a particular problem associated with TPN, as the solution provides ideal growth media for bacteria. The solution used for TPN should be tailored to the individual's biochemical and nutritional needs, although 'off-the-shelf' preparations are available. Due to the high lipid content of TPN fluids, fatty infiltration of the liver is relatively common, and liver function tests should be measured regularly.

Sepsis and septic shock

Definitions of systemic inflammatory response syndrome (SIRS), sepsis, septic shock and multiple organ dysfunction syndrome (MODS) are often a topic of discussion in the exam situation, and definitions are presented in Table 5. For a summary of the management of sepsis, the latest European surviving sepsis campaign editorial (2012) sets out an extensive discussion of treatment options [7]. Sepsis 3, The Third International Consensus Definitions for Sepsis and Septic Shock (JAMA 2016;315(8): 801–810) has redefined the parameters that represent 'Sepsis', 'Septic Shock' and 'Organ Dysfunction' giving a far greater emphasis to the use of the SOFA score to define these terms. The task force has suggested that the term 'severe-sepsis' is now obsolete. As a rapid assessment the quick SOFA (qSOFA) can be used for adult patients outside the critical care environment with suspected infection to identify those more likely to have poor outcomes typical of sepsis. This is positive if they have at least 2 of the following: respiratory rate greater than 22/min, altered mentation or a systolic blood pressure of less than or equal to 100 mmHg.

Care bundles for optimal treatment within 3–6 h windows from diagnosis have been defined (Table 6). Evidence of survival benefit from compliance with these care bundles was reported in the IMPreSS trial in 2015. Treatment revolves around source control to eradicate the infection site, with supportive therapy to maintain organ function during

Table 5.   Definitions in critical illness.

SIRS: Systemic inflammatory syndrome; requires 2 of:	• Pyrexia >38°C or hypothermia <36°C. • Tachycardia >90 bpm (in absence of beta-blocker). • Tachypnoea >20 breaths per min or $PaCO_2$ <4.3 kPa (32 mmHg) or a requirement for mechanical ventilation. • White cell count >12,000 cells/mm^3 or <4,000 cells/mm^3. • Continues to aid diagnosis of sepsis with specific signs of infection though SIRS can be considered a normal inflammatory response.
Sepsis	Life-threatening organ dysfunction caused by dysregulated host response to infection.
Severe sepsis	Now considered a redundant term (sepsis 3).
Septic shock	A subset of sepsis in which particularly profound circulatory, cellular and metabolic abnormalities are associated with a greater risk of mortality, than sepsis alone. Defined by a vasopressor need to maintain a MAP greater than or equal to 65 mmHg and serum lactate greater then 2 mmol/L (18 mg/dL) in the absence of hypovolaemia (associated mortality risk over 40%).
MODS: Multiple organ dysfunction syndrome	The presence of altered organ function in acutely ill patients such that homeostasis cannot be maintained without intervention. It usually involves two or more organ systems. Can be represented by an increase in SOFA score of 2 points or more (associated mortality risk of over 10%).

recovery. It is vital to liaise closely with the microbiology department and send regular culture specimens to screen for infection, identify pathogens and establish antibiotic sensitivities. Discussion of detailed antibiotic use is beyond the scope of this chapter.

Attempts to find specific treatments for the effects of severe sepsis have been frustratingly inconclusive. The failure of the PROWESS-SHOCK study to demonstrate any benefit from activated protein c (APC) led to the company who developed the APC formulation drotrecogin alfa (activated) to withdraw it from the worldwide market.

Tight glycaemic control (blood glucose 4.5–6.0 mmol/L) in patients with severe sepsis was thought to be beneficial following the Van den

Table 6.   Care bundles from international surviving sepsis campaign.

To be completed within 3 h	To be completed within 6 h
(1) Measure lactate level. (2) Obtain blood cultures prior to administration of antibiotics. (3) Administer broad spectrum antibiotics. (4) Administer 30 mL/kg crystalloid for hypotension or lactate ≥4 mmol/L. 'Time of presentation' is defined as the time of triage in the emergency department or, if presenting from another care venue, from the earliest chart annotation consistent with all elements of severe sepsis or septic shock ascertained through chart review.	(5) Apply vasopressors (for hypotension that does not respond to initial fluid resuscitation) to maintain a mean arterial pressure (MAP) ≥65 mmHg. (6) In the event of persistent hypotension after initial fluid administration (MAP <65 mmHg), or if initial lactate was ≥4 mmol/L, re-assess volume status and tissue perfusion and document findings according to Table 1. (7) Remeasure lactate if initial lactate elevated.

Berghe paper (NEMJ in 2001). However, an Australian study (NEMJ, 2009 NICE SUGAR study) suggested very tight control may be deleterious, in part due to hypoglycaemia. Current thinking supports blood glucose control between 6 and 10 mmol/L in septic patients.

In spite of all currently available treatment options for septic shock with MODS, the mortality rate remains high (approximately 25% ITU mortality, 40% hospital mortality).

Finally, it must always be remembered that the goal of any treatment is to allow the patient to return home with an acceptable quality and quantity of life. If the chances of achieving this become minimal, then consideration of the appropriateness of continuing that therapy is vital. This is certainly the case in ICU, where many life-prolonging treatments are available in the face of severe illness. National mortality figures for those admitted to ICU are that for all-cause admissions (approximately 150,000 per year for the UK) 15% die on the ICU with overall hospital mortality being 21%. For elective and emergency surgery, including an ICU stay, acute hospital mortality is 3.1% and 16.9%, respectively (Intensive Care National Audit and Research Centre Case Mix Programme (ICNARC CMP) Annual Quality Report 2014–2015). Where prognosis for survival becomes negligible, a change to palliation should be seen as an active decision in the course of ICU care. Appropriate use of palliative care has the primary aim of maintaining dignity for patients and ensuring relief from unnecessary suffering in the final hours or days of their lives. Proscriptive protocols for end-of-life care, such as the liverpool care pathway, although attempting to achieve these aims received widespread condemnation. Nonetheless, every healthcare institution must be able to provide effective and well planned end-of-life care.

References

1. Parasuraman S, Schwarz K, Gollop ND *et al*. Healthcare professional's guide to cardiopulmonary exercise testing. *Br J Cardiol* 2015;22:156.
2. Dhatariya K, Levy N, Flanagan D, Hilton L *et al*. Management of adults with diabetes undergoing surgery and elective procedures: Improving standards. Revised September 2015. HMSO.
3. Patel JP, Arya R. The current status of bridging anticoagulation. *Br J Haematol* 2014;164(5):619–629.
4. Berwanger O, Le Manach Y, Suzumura EA *et al*. Association between pre-operative statin use and major cardiovascular complications among patients undergoing non-cardiac surgery: The VISION study. *Eur Heart J* 2015;37(2): 177–185.
5. Wijeysundera DN, Duncan D, Nkonde-Price C *et al*. Peri-operative beta blockade in noncardiac surgery: A systematic review for the 2014 ACC/AHA guideline on perioperative cardiovascular evaluation and management of patients undergoing noncardiac surgery. *Circulation* 2014;130:2246–2264.
6. Vincent JL *et al*. The SOFA (sepsis-related organ failure assessment) score to describe organ dysfunction/failure. *Intensive Care Med* 1996;2:707–710.
7. Dellinger RP *et al*. Surviving sepsis campaign international guidelines for management of severe sepsis and septic shock:2012. *Crit Care Med* 2013;41:580–637.

Chapter 30

Basic Outline of Solid Organ Transplantation

Theo Tsiris, Jeremy French and Derek Manas

Key Points

- Solid organ transplantation is now commonplace and is the standard of care for patients with end-stage organ failure.
- Indications have changed over time and there are few absolute contraindications.
- Equity of access to transplant waiting lists is paramount and selecting the correct recipient and donor pair will optimise the outcome.
- The surgical techniques for all organ transplantation are now well established and standardised, and as a result there has been a year-on-year improvement in 1-year survival. Most recipients die because of comorbidity or poor organ function.
- Live donor transplantation for both kidney and liver recipients has become an extremely important source of donor organs.
- Complications are general to surgical patients, but indeed each organ has its own specific risks.
- Immunosuppression has advanced hugely over the past 10 years and, as a result, the overall attrition rate due to acute rejection has reduced considerably.

- The biggest problem facing transplantation today is the donor shortage. Over the next 5 years the organ donor taskforce set up by the Minister of Health has set out a plan to increase donation by 50%.
- Until this happens, transplantation will always have to deal with the ethical dilemmas of allocation, utilisation and fairness.

Introduction

Solid organ (liver, pancreas and kidney) transplantation is an important treatment modality for end-stage organ failure. Indeed, if a vital organ such as the liver fails, transplantation is the only management option currently available.

Organ transplantation increases life expectancy and quality of life (for the recipient and their family), but is not without risk. Since the pioneering days of solid organ transplantation (kidney 1950, liver 1963), there have been many advances, both surgical and medical, resulting in considerable reduction in overall risk.

While these advances clearly are beneficial in terms of graft and patient survival, these successes have lowered the threshold for acceptance of patients onto transplant waiting lists worldwide, thus significantly contributing to the observed increased demand.

The fact that the demand for donor organs outstrips supply creates ethical and medical considerations specific to transplantation, such as selection and deselection criteria, waiting list prioritisation, national organ sharing schemes, development of organ donation and retrieval methods, and the concept of transplant benefit.

This chapter will explore some of these issues as well as give an overview of the medical and surgical technical aspects of transplantation.

Indications

Liver transplantation (LT)

Following the death of a young woman with liver failure, a colloquium was set up in the UK in 1999 to establish guidelines for the selection of patients for LT. It was agreed that livers donated for transplantation should be considered a national resource. Patients should be considered for transplantation if they had an anticipated length of life (in the absence of transplantation) of less than 1 year or an unacceptable quality of life. It was also agreed that patients should be accepted for transplantation only if they had an estimated probability of being alive 5 years after transplantation of at least 50% with a quality of life acceptable to the patient. The British Society of Gastroenterology has published clinical guidelines on the indications for referral and assessment in adult liver transplantation [1].

The common indications for liver transplantation are shown in Table 1.

Special considerations

Alcohol-induced liver disease may be associated with significant damage to cardiovascular and neurological systems, as well as the risk of patients reverting back to alcohol abuse, resulting in them not complying with medication or follow-up schedules and thus damaging the new liver. A multidisciplinary approach is required to select those patients who are likely to comply; all potential recipients, once accepted onto the waiting list, have to enter into a written contract with the transplanting centre not to return to alcohol consumption after transplantation.

Table 1.   Disease-specific indications for liver transplantation.

Primary recipient disease	
Cirrhosis	Secondary sclerosing cholangitis
• Primary biliary cirrhosis	Alpha-1-antitrypsin deficiency
• Secondary biliary cirrhosis	Budd–Chiari syndrome
• Cryptogenic	Wilson's disease
• Alcoholic	Biliary atresia
Non-alcoholic fatty liver disease	Other congenital biliary abnormalities
Chronic active hepatitis (autoimmune)	Acute/subacute fulminant hepatic failure (FHF)
Chronic viral hepatitis B	Primary hepatocellular carcinoma in cirrhotic liver
Chronic viral hepatitis C	Primary hepatic malignancy
Congenital hepatic fibrosis	Inborn errors of metabolism not in CLF group
Primary sclerosing cholangitis	

Illegal drug use is not a contraindication to transplant if the patient will comply with the required schedules. However, continued intravenous drug use is considered a contraindication.

Age in itself is not a contraindication, although the survival rate after transplant of the over 65 s is significantly worse than that of younger patients.

Self-inflicted conditions such as overdose of paracetamol would only be contraindicated if there were good reasons to believe that the patient would, despite appropriate support, return to their premorbid lifestyle that would lead to liver failure or result in a quality of life unacceptable to the patient.

Comorbid medical or psychiatric conditions are relevant if they affect the patient's quality of life or prospect for survival post transplant. Patients in whom early graft damage from recurrent disease can be anticipated, such as recurrent hepatitis C virus (HCV) and hepatitis B virus (HBV) infections, should only be transplanted as part of an agreed protocol of treatment. There are well-developed protocols now for prevention of recurrence. With the advent of effective treatment, those coinfected with human immunodeficiency virus (HIV) may be suitable candidates for transplantation.

Regrafts will need special consideration depending on the circumstances that gave rise to the need for the regraft. This is because the results after early regraft are poor and of only limited benefit.

Where potential liver allograft recipients have suffered from previous extra-hepatic malignancy, the decision to proceed for liver transplantation depends on the probability of malignancy recurring following liver transplantation. Some immunosuppressive agents may encourage the growth of malignancy. In patients with primary hepatic malignancy (HCC), there are agreed criteria that predict a high probability of tumour persistence after transplantation: these include number and size of lesions. More than three liver tumours with a maximum diameter of 5 cm indicates that HCC is likely to persist following liver transplantation. However, these criteria are under regular review.

Currently in the UK, patients with cholangiocarcinoma are not appropriate candidates for transplantation.

It has also been agreed that if the condition of patients awaiting a liver transplantation deteriorates to the extent that the probability of a 5-year survival may fall below 50%, they will be removed from the waiting list, but only after full discussion with them. Such patients — although in greatest need — are at greatest risk of not benefiting after transplantation.

Kidney transplantation

With the tremendous improvements in transplant management, most patients with kidney failure can be considered for transplantation. Diseases that may be indications for renal transplantation are listed below:

- Glomerulonephritis
    1. Idiopathic and post-infectious crescentic
    2. Membranous
    3. Mesangiocapillary (type I)
    4. Mesangiocapillary (type II) (dense-deposit disease)
    5. IgA nephropathy
    6. Antiglomerular basement membrane
    7. Focal glomerulosclerosis
    8. Henoch–Schönlein

- Chronic pyelonephritis (reflux nephropathy)
- Hereditary
    1. Polycystic kidneys
    2. Nephronophthisis (medullary cystic disease)
    3. Nephritis (including Alport's syndrome)
    4. Tuberous sclerosis

- Metabolic
    1. Diabetes mellitus
    2. Hyperoxaluria
    3. Cystinosis
    4. Fabry's disease
    5. Amyloid
    6. Gout
    7. Porphyria

- Obstructive nephropathy
- Toxic
  1. Analgesic nephropathy
  2. Opiate abuse

- Multisystem diseases
  1. Systemic lupus erythematosus
  2. Vasculitis
  3. Progressive systemic sclerosis

- Haemolytic uraemic syndrome
- Tumours
  1. Wilms' tumour
  2. Renal cell carcinoma
  3. Incidental carcinoma
  4. Myeloma

- Congenital
  1. Hypoplasia
  2. Horseshoe kidney

- Irreversible acute renal failure
  1. Cortical necrosis
  2. Acute tubular necrosis

Trauma

All patients between the ages of 2 and 70, who require dialysis or expect to require dialysis within the next 12 months, will be considered for transplantation. It is important to satisfactorily resolve other comorbidities to increase the safety of the transplant. Patients must be evaluated early to allow them to consider their options for renal replacement therapy. This is particularly valuable since living donor kidney transplantation can be considered and timed appropriately to serve as renal replacement therapy, obviating the need for dialysis and access surgery. Live donation has increased significantly over the past 5 years with the advent of the laparoscopic donor operation. As a result, live donors now contribute up to 50% of the kidneys for transplantation in most large programmes in the UK.

Most patients are listed for a cadaver kidney when their creatinine clearance (Clcr), calculated by the Cockcroft–Gault formula, is less than 30 mL min^{-1}. The Cockcroft–Gault formula for calculation of the Clcr is now considered to be superior to actual measured creatinine clearance, as determined by 24-h urine collection, due to inherent inaccuracies and collection difficulties. The formula is as follows:

$$\text{Clcr (mL min}^{-1}) = ((140 - \text{age})(\text{weight in kg}))/(\text{creatinine (mg dL}^{-1}) \times 72)$$ For women, the result is multiplied by 0.85.

Although all causes for kidney failure can be considered for transplantation, some causes of kidney failure, such as certain types of glomerulonephritis, may occasionally recur in the new transplant. In most cases, transplantation is worthwhile since recurrence is usually very slow to develop. These risks are discussed with patients on a case-by-case basis. Patients with primary oxalosis require combined kidney-liver transplantation since without metabolic correction of oxalosis with liver transplantation, recurrent kidney disease would be very rapid.

Diseases that may recur in renal transplants are as follows:

- diabetes mellitus
- systemic lupus erythematosis
- IgA nephropathy
- focal segmental glomerulosclerosis
- membranous glomerulonephritis
- membranoproliferative glomerulonephritis
- amyloidosis
- cystinosis

Contraindications for kidney transplantation

There are certain absolute contraindications to renal transplantation:

1. Disseminated or untreated cancer
2. Severe psychiatric disease

3. Unresolvable psychosocial problems
4. Persistent substance abuse
5. Severe mental retardation
6. Unreconstructable coronary artery disease or refractory congestive heart failure

Relative contraindications:

- Treated malignancy — The cancer-free interval required will vary from 2 to 5 years, depending on the stage and type of cancer.
- Substance abuse history — Patients must be involved in drug-free rehabilitation. This includes negative random toxicology screens.
- Chronic liver disease — Patients with chronic hepatitis B or C or persistently abnormal liver function testing must be seen by a hepatologist prior to consideration.
- Cardiac disease — All patients over the age of 55 or those with a history of diabetes, hypertension or tobacco abuse must have dobutamine stress echocardiography, or exercise or pharmacologic stress cardiac scintigraphy. Any patient with a history of a positive stress test or history of congestive heart failure must have cardiology evaluation prior to consideration.
- Structural genito-urinary abnormality or recurrent urinary tract infection — Urologic consultation is required prior to consideration.
- Past psychosocial abnormality — Social work or psychiatry evaluation, as appropriate.
- Aortoiliac disease — Patients with abnormal femoral pulses or disabling claudication, rest pain or gangrene will require evaluation by a vascular surgeon prior to consideration. Patients with significant aortoiliac occlusive disease may require angioplasty or aortoiliac grafting prior to transplantation.

Special consideration needs to be given to

- Morbid obesity
- Antibody status
- Retransplantation
- HIV-positive recipients

Indications for simultaneous pancreas–kidney (SPK) transplantation patients with insulin-dependent (type 1, juvenile diabetes) diabetes who have end-stage renal disease (ESRD) and require dialysis or expect to require dialysis in the next 12 months may be considered for SPK transplantation. Special care is taken to exclude recipients with type 2 diabetes. Candidates with a strong family history, or late age or gestational onset, have a C-peptide level determined after glucose loading. Only those individuals with C-peptide levels of 0.2 ng mL^{-1} are further considered for transplantation. In addition, evidence of at least one type of progressive secondary diabetic complication including diabetic retinopathy, diabetic neuropathy, diabetic gastroparesis and accelerated atherosclerosis should be present.

Indications for pancreas transplantation (solitary pancreas transplant, pancreas transplant alone, pancreas after kidney)

Patients with insulin-dependent (type 1, juvenile diabetes) diabetes may be candidates for pancreas transplantation if they have secondary diabetic complications that are progressive despite the best medical management. This includes patients for whom the indication is brittle diabetes and hypoglycaemic unawareness with evidence of frequent hypoglycaemic events, despite an attempt at optimal medical management. Patients with brittle diabetes as the primary indication should have evidence of impairment of employability, hypoglycaemic-induced accidents involving themselves or small children in their care. Usually, there is evidence of frequent emergency care for hypoglycaemia or diabetic ketoacidosis. In some cases, these patients will have received a prior kidney transplant, usually from a living donor (living donor kidney transplant alone, LDKTA).

Absolute and relative contraindications for pancreas transplantation are similar to those for kidney transplantation.

Special consideration needs to be given to the cardiovascular system because of the high incidence of asymptomatic coronary artery disease in this population.

All type 1 diabetic patients require dobutamine stress echocardiography.

Allocation and Ethics of Organs for Transplantation

There is no doubt that there is a spectrum of ethical dilemmas within transplantation. These range from more straightforward issues, such as the allocation of scarce resources, to complex issues, such as financial reward for organ donation and xenotransplantation.

The system of allocation of organs for transplantation in the UK varies with the individual organ. Factors common to different organs, which are important in allocation, are ABO blood group compatibility (all organs) and the comparative sizes of donors and recipients (liver, heart, heart/lung and lung). Other important considerations when allocating specific organs include tissue matching (histocompatibility) in kidney transplantation, the model for end-stage liver disease (MELD) score for liver transplantation, the quality of the donor organ and how appropriately it matches a particular recipient, especially as it relates to marginal donors and recipients, and the concept of transplant benefit, currently being applied to lung transplantation in the USA.

All patients who are waiting for transplants in the UK are registered on the National Transplant Database held by UK Transplant — now part of an organisation linked with the National Blood Transfusion Service called National Blood and Transplant (NSBT).

Currently, UK Transplant run organ-specific national allocation schemes with an overarching principle of ensuring patients are treated equally. Donated organs are allocated in a fair and unbiased way, based on the patient's need and the importance of achieving the closest possible match between donor and recipient. Kidneys are allocated according to a national waiting list based on a weighted scoring system, which includes waiting time, time on dialysis, sensitisation levels and tissue match. Liver grafts are allocated to the centre, which prioritises locally based on the MELD/UKELD score (bilirubin, INR, creatinine and serum sodium) equating to how 'sick' the potential recipient is. This has been validated in the USA to predict survival up to 3 months post transplant. Currently, no potential recipient can be registered for a liver transplant unless they meet the minimum listing criteria, which is a UKELD score of 49 [2]. A national allocation system for liver transplantation operates for patients with acute liver failure deemed to have less than 72 h to live. These patients are categorised as 'super-urgent'. Pancreas grafts are currently allocated to the retrieving centre unless there is a potential recipient nationally who was previously sensitised, but has been shown to be suitable for a particular graft. These are patients who usually have transplanted previously and are awaiting a 'window of opportunity'.

Some patients have a greater clinical need, resulting in others waiting longer. Donation rates are greater in some ethnic groups, while in other ethnic groups the need for transplantation is greater. Utilitarian principles therefore compete against duty-based ones.

Organ donation and transplantation are covered by the Human Tissue Act 2004 in England, Wales and Northern Ireland and by the Human Tissue (Scotland) Act 2006. Consent, or authorisation in Scotland, is the fundamental principle of both acts and is required before organs can be removed from the deceased, stored and used. Consent is also required from live patients offering organs, but is covered by common law.

The number of people needing organ transplants in the UK is far greater than the number of donor organs available (Fig. 1). In the financial year 2007–2008, there were 2,385 organs transplanted from

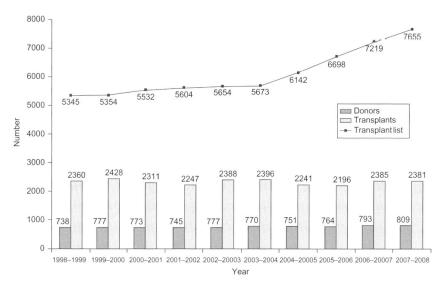

Figure 1. The number of deceased donors and transplants in the UK, 1 April 1998–31 March 2008, and patients on the active transplant list.

809 deceased donors with a further 839 live donor transplants, but there were 7,655 patients on the active waiting list. This list grows at 8% per year, with approximately 1,000 potential recipients dying each year while waiting or becoming too ill for a transplant.

This means there has to be a system in place to ensure that patients are treated equally and that donated organs are allocated in a fair and unbiased way, based on the patient's need and the importance of achieving the closest possible match between donor and recipient. The underlying ethical principles are straightforward in that organs should be allocated irrespective of age, gender, race, religion or social standing. But the reality is more complex because organs are a scarce resource and not every individual who needs an organ will receive one.

Many of the ethical issues that require consideration in decisions to offer transplantation to one patient in preference to another are shared in common, irrespective of the specific organ or tissue to be transplanted. Factors that must be taken into account in organ allocation include the following:

(1) Selection of the sickest patient — An offer of an organ to the patient most likely to die without it might appear the most reasonable basis for organ allocation. However, this method may also select the poorest outcome. This is not necessarily the 'best use' of a limited resource.

(2) Selection of the patient most likely to benefit based on medical or other criteria — If the major emphasis in organ allocation is placed on guaranteeing that the greatest number of transplanted organs are accepted and survive for the longest time, a preference should be for the best possible tissue match in the patient with the best outlook. Whilst this approach appears acceptable in isolation, it conflicts with a number of other criteria. This would disadvantage any potential recipient with advanced disease and result in an impaired chance of success. The best way of applying this criterion is, having identified patients with similar priority for allocation on other grounds, further choice might favour that case most likely to be successful.

(3) Selection of the patient on the waiting list for the longest period — The length of a prior waiting period appears fair. This criterion has

identifiability and defensibility. Against adopting this as the sole criteria is the fact that if a patient has survived for a long period after
meeting the requirements for entry to a waiting list this might indicate that he or she was in better condition than others on that list.
The question might then be whether his or her 'need' was less.

(4) All patients on the waiting list should have an equal chance of selection — It has the advantage of being seen to be free of any favourit-
ism. However, its application is impractical. The method could only
have a place in rare situations where several possible recipients are
judged to have equal priority on medical and other grounds (this
sometimes happens in the case of kidney transplantation).

(5) Selection of patients on the basis of their importance for the well-
being of others — Is it appropriate for a patient with a young family,
dependent upon him or her for support, or an individual with the
capacity to make a unique contribution to his or her community, to
be accorded priority? This criterion raises questions about the manner in which selection attributes are to be quantified and of who is
entitled to do so. During the early years of kidney transplantation
programmes in the USA, this was considered and subsequently
rejected.

(6) Preference or not in selection to patients who have previously had
one or more transplants — Patients who have already been transplanted, but who have had the misfortune of a failed graft, and so
received no benefit, might be seen to have a claim for priority for
another try or conversely 'have had their chance'. Here, the type of
organ graft is of importance. For example, recipients with failing liver
or heart grafts facing imminent death may achieve priority for this
reason. Renal recipients may return to dialysis following graft failure,
but the basis of loss of the first graft may persist (for example, high
antibody titres) and remain transplantable at a later date.

(7) Capacity of the patient to pay — equal access to medical care for all,
irrespective of capacity to pay, is a basic principle of the NHS.

(8) What about a potential recipient's lifestyle in selection for transplant
allocation — There are many who would argue that self-inflicted illnesses, such as alcoholism and drug abuse, necessitating liver transplantation due to alcoholic cirrhosis or HCV cirrhosis, should lessen a

patient's eligibility to be allocated a donor organ. The concern revolves around the extent to which recurrence of alcoholism or HCV in the new graft may compromise a successful outcome to transplantation. Any case for exclusion from organ transplantation because of a self-inflicted illness involves non-medical 'social' judgements. Whenever the issue of possible exclusion of patients with a particular lifestyle from access to any form of treatment that remains available to others is considered, it is essential that attention be given to the development of processes that will ensure adequate representation of the views and needs of marginalised groups, and this includes HIV coinfection in haemophiliac patients as well.

(9) Can we exclude patients on the basis of anticipated lack of compliance — Apart from recidivism leading to a recurrence of the disease that required treatment originally, grounds for exclusion might arise if there was considerable likelihood that a patient would not be prepared to participate in essential post-transplant treatment, for example, the use of immunosuppressive agents. The reliability of any prediction leading to exclusion creates a substantial ethical issue in most transplant units.

In *Transplantation Ethics*, Robert Veatch outlines an interesting way of assessing need. He calls it the 'over-a-lifetime perspective'. This approach takes into consideration a person's entire life when determining who is worst off. A 17-year-old and an 80-year-old both dying of liver failure are equally badly off, but this perspective allows that the person who has had 63 more years of life is better off, so the 17-year-old is neediest. Veatch writes, 'from this over-a-lifetime perspective, justice requires that we target organs for these younger persons who are so poorly off that they will not make it to old age without being given special priority — the younger the age of the person, the higher the claim.' This furthers the goal of utilising organs to their maximum potential. Presently, our system of allocation gives priority to those who are the sickest or most in need of a transplant. But sometimes, those who are the sickest and in the most immediate need will not receive the same benefit from the transplant as someone whose medical condition is currently more stable. They may be so sick that they have a higher chance of dying regardless of treatment. There is a moral obligation, due to the scarcity of organs, to maximise the potential longevity of donated organs and place them where they are most likely to do the most good (bring the most health) over the longest period of time.

Donors and the Donor Procedure

The widening gap between organ demand and supply has resulted in the relaxation of the criteria for organ donation as the clinician must weigh up the risk of transplanting the organ against dying on the waiting list. There are however, contraindications, all of which are relative (Table 2). It is highly unlikely however that an individual with an active extra-cranial malignancy would be considered as a donor.

It is important to note that organs used in transplantation can come from very different clinical scenarios (Table 3).

Table 2.   Organ donation (relative) contraindications.

- Human immunodeficiency virus (HIV)/active hepatitis B infection
- Extra-cranial malignancy (current) or cranial
- Glioblastoma/medulloblastoma
- Severe systemic sepsis
- Disease of unknown aetiology

Table 3.   Donor categories.

Category	Description	
Non-heart beating donors (Maastricht classification)		
I	Brought in dead	Uncontrolled
II	Unsuccessful resuscitation	Uncontrolled
III	Awaiting cardiac arrest	Controlled
IV	Cardiac arrest after brainstem death	Controlled
V	Cardiac arrest in a hospital inpatient	Uncontrolled
Heart beating donors (brainstem dead)	Usually patients in intensive care units having sustained irreversible brain damage (e.g., intracranial haemorrhage, cerebrovascular accident or head injury)	
Live donors	Increasingly common in kidney and liver donation	

Death confirmed by brainstem testing

The majority of donors in the UK come from heart-beating donors. Death is defined as irreversible loss of capacity for consciousness and the irreversible loss of the capacity to breath. Before organ procurement can commence, death by brainstem testing needs to be performed according to the UK code, which involves three steps.

(1) Preconditions — comatose patient with irreversible injury, on a ventilator (>6–24 h after last intervention aimed at reversing injury), with an identified underlying cause for coma.
(2) Exclusions — no drugs, alcohol, neuromuscular blocking agents or hypothermia.
(3) Clinical testing — these tests (two sets of tests at least 2–3 h apart performed by two senior medical personnel) demonstrate absent brainstem reflexes and total apnoea (Table 4).

All the major religions of the UK support the principles of organ donation and transplantation. However, within each religion, there are different schools of thought, which mean that views may differ. All the major religions accept that organ donation is an individual choice.

Table 4.   Brainstem death tests.

- Absent brainstem reflexes
- No pupillary response to light
- Absent corneal reflexes
- Absent vestibulo-ocular reflex
- No motor response to adequate stimuli in cranial nerve distribution
- No gag reflex to bronchial stimulation by suction catheter
- Apnoea testing
- No attempt to breathe despite a $P_aCo_2 > 6.5$ kPa. Hypoxia avoided by preoxygenation with 100% oxygen for 10 min

The donor operation

The principles are as follows:

- Preparation with antibiotics and neuromuscular blockade (to prevent spinal reflexes).
- Exposure is achieved through a midline laparotomy and sternotomy with pericardotomy. The colon and small bowel are reflected superiorly to expose the inferior mesenteric vein (IMV) and the aortic bifurcation. Hepatic vasculature is dissected to their origin (alternative arterial vasculature is identified), portal dissection and division of the bile duct is performed. The thoracic organs are then dissected.
- Perfusion cannula is placed in the aorta, the aorta is cross-clamped and 4 L of cold perfusate passed through the cannula. The inferior vena cava (IVC) is opened in the chest and the abdomen filled with ice.
- Procurement of the liver is done by dividing the arterial supply with an aortic patch, dividing the IVC just above the renal veins, the superior vena cava (SVC) during the cardiectomy and the portal vein preserving maximum length. Procurement of the kidneys is done by dividing the ureters as long as possible (with adequate tissue around them to preserve blood supply), and preserving the renal arteries on an aortic patch and the renal veins on an IVC patch. Important steps in procurement of the pancreas (in combination with liver procurement) involve identification and division of the splenic artery, preservation of the superior mesenteric artery and the length of the portal vein. After removal of the liver the duodenum is stapled at the pylorus and fourth part, and remaining attachments to the small bowel and transverse colon are divided. Following pericardotomy and mobilisation of the great vessels, the SVC is ligated and divided, the aorta cross-clamped and the heart perfused with a cardioplegic agent via an anterior aortic puncture. After cardiac arrest, the heart is emptied via incisions in the IVC and left pulmonary vein. The heart is excised by dividing all the remaining attachments. The procurement of the lungs follows as for the heart, except a perfusion cannula is placed in the pulmonary artery, and the left heart is vented via the tip of the atrial appendage as opposed to the pulmonary vein. Following manual

venting, the trachea is stapled and divided above to keep the lungs inflated during transport.

- Completion of the procurement involves removing a portion of spleen and mesenteric lymph nodes (tissue typing and cross-matching), iliac vessels (conduits) and removal of blood and neat abdominal closure.

Operative Technique

Liver transplantation

The operative technique can be classified based on the position of the graft in the recipient (orthotopic if graft is placed in the usual position and heterotropic if placed elsewhere in the body), whether all or part of the graft is transplanted (whole graft or partial graft transplantation) and whether the native liver (or part of it) is retained (auxiliary graft). Partial grafts can be a split liver, when the liver is divided for implantation into two recipients, or a reduced-size graft, when only one part is retained to be transplanted.

Living donor transplantation and rarely domino transplantations are other techniques used.

Standard liver transplantation technique

In this method, recipient hepatectomy is performed en bloc with the retrohepatic cava. Subsequently, the whole graft is implanted by end-to-end anastomosis of the supra and infra hepatic inferior vena cavae to the graft's vena cava. Then the donor portal vein is anastamosed end-to-end with the recipient's portal vein, following which the graft is revascularised. The arterial anastamosis is performed between the graft artery and the recipient hepatic artery. If the recipient hepatic artery is not suitable, then the graft artery can be anastamosed directly to the recipient's aorta or by using an arterial conduit. Lastly, biliary anastamosis is performed using a duct-to-duct technique or a Roux-en-Y biliary reconstruction. T-Tubes are not routinely used.

The operative technique has evolved with time and more and more surgeons perform liver transplantation using some, if not all, of the following modifications.

Veno-venous bypass

Cross-clamping of the vena cava, which is a requirement for the classical method, often results in haemodynamic instability and congestion of splanchnic circulation. Diverting the blood from the portal vein and inferior vena cava to either the jugular or axillary vein on one side (veno-venous bypass) overcomes this problem.

Preservation of vena cava

In this technique, the recipient's retrohepatic inferior vena cava is preserved during initial hepatectomy by dissecting the liver off the vena cava. This maintains the blood flow in the cava thus avoiding the need for systemic venous bypass. In addition, a transient portocaval shunt may also be constructed to maintain splanchnic flow.

With the recipient cava intact, the caval anastamosis can be performed with direct end-to-end anastamosis of the donor cava to the unified stump of the recipient's hepatic veins or alternatively performing a lateral cavo-cavostomy on the anterior wall of the recipient vena cava.

Kidney transplantation

The kidney transplant operation has been standardised over the last few decades. Unlike liver transplantation, the transplanted kidney is placed in a heterotropic extraperitoneal location, usually in the iliac fossa. A curvilinear incision in a lower quadrant of the abdomen (Gibson's incision) is made, with division of the muscles of the abdominal wall and dissection of the preperitoneal space to expose the iliac vessels and the bladder. The renal vein and artery are anastamosed to the recipient iliac vein and artery, respectively. Then an uretero-neocystostomy is created, with or without placement of a ureteric stent. If a stent is used, it is important to remove this in a few weeks to prevent complications of a non-removed stent (e.g., haematuria, renal stones, infection).

The kidney may be placed on either side, depending on history of previous transplantation, surgeon preference and the side of the donor kidney.

Pancreas transplantation

The pancreas may be transplanted simultaneously with a kidney (SPK), sometimes following a kidney transplant (pancreas after kidney, PAK) or as a pancreas alone (PTA).

The back table preparation of the pancreas is a crucial part of the procedure and can usually take 2 h. Following careful ligation of all peri-pancreatic tissue to prevent bleeding at reperfusion, an iliac Y graft from the donor is anastamosed to the superior mesenteric artery (SMA) and the splenic artery of the pancreas graft. The Y graft construction avoids the need for two separate arterial anastamoses between the donor and the recipient to vascularise the pancreas graft. Further important preparation of the graft involves meticulous attention to controlling the route of the small bowel mesentery, as well as preparing the portal vein.

In SPK transplantation, the pancreas is implanted first due to the lower ischaemia tolerance of the pancreas. The pancreas is usually placed in an intraperitoneal position, although extraperitoneal placement can also be done. The graft portal vein is commonly anastamosed to the recipient lower inferior vena cava. Alternatively, the venous drainage can be put into the portal circulation (graft superior mesenteric vein), giving the theoretical benefit of avoiding hyperinsulinaemia, which has been linked to atherogenesis. The Y graft is anastamosed to the lower aorta or the common iliac artery (CIA). The management of exocrine secretion is still a matter of considerable debate. The donor duodenum can be anastamosed to a Roux-en-Y loop of recipient small bowel (enteric drainage) or alternatively this can be anastamosed to the recipient urinary bladder (bladder drainage).

Post-operative Complications

Organ transplantation is susceptible to all the recognised complications of any major surgical procedure (e.g., bleeding, infection, hernia). There are, however, issues that can arise that are specific to organ transplanation. There are complications that are common to all transplants and some specific to individual organs. The manifestation of each complication can differ according to the organ involved. Complications are classified into early and late.

Liver

Early

1. Primary non-function — This can manifest as haemodynamic instability, hypoglycaemia, elevated transaminases, coagulopathy, minimal bile output, encephalopathy, systemic acidosis and renal failure. This is not compatible with life and most patients require re-grafting (incidence: 1–3%). More commonly one sees a less dramatic version of this scenario called initial poor function or delayed graft function. This is often related to graft ischaemia and will improve.
2. Vascular thrombosis — Arterial thrombosis can be early or late. This is more common in the paediatric population and can manifest as rapid or slow deterioration of graft function or as necrosis of bile ducts (incidence: adult liver transplant 2–4%; paediatric liver transplant 8–10%).
3. Bile leak — This occurs usually due to ischaemia of the donor duct or rarely an operative technical problem (incidence: 20%).
4. Infection — This remains the most significant complication in liver transplantation and is responsible for most of the early mortality with bacterial infections with resistant grampositive bacteria dominating in the first month. Multiresistant bacterial and fungal infections become a more prominent and life-threatening issue if infection persists.
5. Acute rejection — With the advent of the newer and more potent immunosuppressive drugs, this has become less of an issue in transplantation in general. It may present with fever, abdominal pain and elevated liver enzymes. The diagnosis is confirmed by a liver biopsy and most episodes are responsive to augmentation of immunosuppression with high dose corticosteroids.

Late

1. Arterial stenosis — Presentation is with slow deterioration of graft function.
2. Infection — Late infections are usually due to opportunistic pathogens such as cytomegalovirus, candida, aspergillosis, cryptococcus, legionella.

3. Chronic rejection — This is seen months or years after transplantation with poor synthetic liver function and hyperbilirubinemia.
4. Biliary stricture — Patients present with obstructive jaundice, usually due to an ischaemic stricture.
5. Recurrent disease — Recurrence of viral hepatitis is likely within a short time in infected patients, but this may be mild and in many cases will not result in graft loss.
6. Cancer — Recurrence if the patient was transplanted for HCC (outcome for small tumours: 75% 5-year survival). De Novo tumours, such as skin cancers, lymphomas and others, may occur in up to 3% of transplant recipients. This is most often secondary to immunosuppression.
7. Others — Diabetes, hyperlipidaemia, hypertension and metabolic bone disease – these are related to the immunosuppression agents.

Kidney

Early

1. Acute tubular necrosis (ATN) and delayed graft function — Some degree of ATN occurs in 5–30% of all heart-beating cadaveric donor transplantations. Delayed graft function may be associated with a reduction in the 5-year graft survival by up to 10% in some studies.
2. Primary non-function — The kidney never functions.
3. Arterial thrombosis — This Causes early post-operative oliguria or anuria. Immediate re-exploration is the only chance for salvaging such a graft.
4. Venous thrombosis — This can result from technical error or kinking or compression of the renal vein.
5. Acute rejection — Incidence varies, but with newer immunosuppression and pre-emptive treatment most centres report acute rejection rates of 10–20%. Diagnosis requires biopsy and treatment usually involves steroid boluses.
6. Ureteral obstruction — This could be due to blood clot in catheter, haematoma or oedema.
7. Urinary fistula — This occurs due to disruption of the ureteroneocystostomy or ureteral necrosis. Fluid biochemistry showing urea content several folds higher than that of serum is diagnostic.

8. Infection — 30–60% will suffer some type of infection during the first year. Conventional bacterial infections occur during the first month. Infections can be confused with rejection.

Late

1. Renal artery stenosis — Patients present with hypertension and diminished renal function. This presentation can be confused with that of rejection. The aetiology of renal artery stenosis is frequently technical. Most instances can be managed with percutaneous transluminal angioplasty.
2. Ureteral obstruction — Late presentation could be due to ureteral stenosis.
3. Lymphocele — This manifests weeks or months post-operatively with swelling of the wound, oedema of the scrotum or labia and lower extremity and urinary obstruction from pressure on the collecting system or ureter. The treatment of choice is fenestration of the cyst into the peritoneal cavity, and external drainage should be avoided as this puts the kidney at risk of infection.
4. Infection — The period between 30 and 180 days post-operative is the usual time for opportunistic infections as this coincides with the period of maximal immunosuppression. Viral infections are more important (e.g., cytomegalovirus). Other pathogens include aspergillosis, blastomycosis, nocardiosis, toxoplasmosis, cryptococcosis, candida and *Pneumocystis carinii*.
5. Hypergylcaemia — This is generally attributed to corticosteroid administration and previously normoglycaemic patients may become diabetic.
6. Hyperparathyroidism — Patients could suffer from tertiary hyperparathyroidism with significant hypercalcaemia and elevated parathyroid hormone levels despite a functioning graft. This is treated by total parathyroidectomy.
7. Cancers — In renal transplant recipients, an incidence of 6% is reported for de novo malignant neoplasms. This is related to the duration and degree of immunosuppression rather than to any particular agent. More prevalent tumours are skin cancers (squamous

cell carcinomas), lymphomas, renal cancers, Kaposi's sarcoma, carcinoma of the vulva and uterine cervix.

8. Post-transplant lymphoproliferative disease (PTLD) — This term is used to cover the spectrum of disease from benign hyperplasia to malignant lymphomas. Epstein–Barr virus is implicated as the most important factor in PTLD.

9. Chronic allograft nephropathy — This complication is characterised by a progressive decline in kidney function is not attributable to a specific cause. Chronic changes to the kidney allograft are mediated by both immune and non-immune factors.

10. Recurrent disease — Glomerulonephritides (e.g., mesangiocapillary glomerulonephritis type 1, IgA nephropathy) are most likely to recur; however, loss of the kidney generally occurs late, and, thus, these diseases are not contraindications to transplantation. Similarly, patients with diabetes mellitus have poorer outcomes following transplantation than do patients without diabetes; nearly all patients demonstrate histological evidence of diabetic nephropathy within 4 years. Hence the treatment of choice for diabetics with renal failure is combined kidney and pancreas transplantation.

Pancreas

Complications and issues specific to pancreas transplantation are discussed below.

Early

1. Vascular thrombosis — This is the most common non-immunological cause of graft loss.

2. Allograft pancreatitis — This occurs in 10–20% of all pancreas graft recipients. In its most severe form, it can result in graft necrosis and arterial thrombosis. This entity is difficult to detect and can be confused with rejection and pancreatic fistula.

3. Pancreatic fistula — This is more common in enteric-drained than in bladder-drained grafts.

4. Rejection — Hyperglycaemia is a late indicator of rejection, as islet damage results by the time such physiological evidence results.

Rejection of a kidney and pancreas transplanted simultaneously from the same donor often occurs at the same time. In such patients careful monitoring of serum creatinine level is a sensitive indicator of rejection.

Late

1. Urological complications — haematuria, urethritis, recurrent urinary tract infections and bicarbonate loss are common in bladder-drained recipients. This can necessitate enteric conversion if it does not respond to conservative treatments.
2. Autoimmune recurrence — the autoimmune response to native islets can be responsible for loss of transplanted pancreatic β-cells.

Graft Rejection and Immunosuppression

With the exception of identical twins, the organ donor and recipient are genetically different. Without medical manipulation a transplanted graft will be rejected within a number of days. Understanding the rejection process is a prerequisite to understanding the principles of immunosuppressive medication.

The rejection process

Organs are rejected as the recipient body recognises the graft as 'foreign'.

This recognition is based on the fact that the graft major histocompatibility complex (MHC) is different to that of the host cell. The role of the MHC is to present antigens for other immunological cells to screen. The antigens relevant to transplantation were first defined seriologically on leucocytes and are therefore called the human leucocyte antigens (HLAs). Minor histocompatibility systems (miHs) are of limited clinical importance in solid organ transplantation. Major histocompatibility class I proteins are found on most nucleated cells. They present antigens and are recognised by the T-cell receptor (TCR) on T-cells bearing the CD8 protein. CD8 T-cells cause lysis of the target (graft) cell. Major histocompatibility class II proteins are found on B lymphocytes and dendritic cells (antigen-presenting cells). They present antigens and are recognised by the T-cell receptor on T-cells bearing the CD4 protein. CD4 cells are referred to as 'helper' cells and have crucial specialised functions in the generation of the immune response (and therefore graft rejection) such as cytotoxic T-cell generation, B-cell maturation.

For immunological cells to be activated however, in addition to this MHC (with antigen)–T-cell receptor (TCR) interaction, various co-stimulatory signals are needed. Many have been detected (e.g., Il-2, the CD28-B7 and CD40 ligand-CD40 family), which is important when searching for immunosuppressive agents. It is noted that other cellular (natural killer cells) and humoral (antibodies) mechanisms of rejection exist.

Immunosuppressive agents

The main immunosuppressive groups and their mode of action are documented in Table 5. In solid organ transplantation, many immuno-suppressive protocols have been used, but, broadly speaking, most protocols are based on the principles outlined below. A calcineurin inhibitor, an antimetabolite and a reducing dose of steroid. In selected cases protein immunosuppressives are given. The calcineurin inhibitor is sometimes exchanged for sirolimus at 3 months post-transplantation (Table 5).

Outcome

Outcomes have steadily improved due to better surgical techniques and more effective immunosuppressive treatments and the development of transplant specialists and teams. Transplants are now so successful in the UK that a year after surgery:

- 94% of kidneys in living donor transplants are still functioning well,
- 88% of kidneys from people who have died are still functioning well,
- 86% of liver transplants are still functioning well,
- 84% of heart transplants are still functioning well,

Table 5.   Immunosuppressive agents.

Immunosuppressive agent group	Examples	Mode of action	Side effects (in addition to infection)
Drugs acting on immunophillins — calcineurin inhibitor (CNI)	Tacrolimus Cyclosporin	Forms a complex with immunophillins and inhibits calcineurin, which under normal circumstances induces the transcription of interleukin-2.	Nephrotoxicity Neurotoxicity diabetes Marrow suppression
It has been in use since 1983 and is one of the most widely used group of immunosuppressive drugs		The drug also inhibits lymphokine production and interleukin release, leading to a reduced function of effector T-cells.	
Corticosteroids	Prednisolone	Multiple immunomodulatory effects, e.g., reduces interleukin (IL) production and hence activation of B- and T-cells, reduces immune cells protein transcription.	Multiple including hyperglycaemia, obesity, osteoporosis, skin fragility
Antimetabolites	Azothioprine Mycophenolate Mofetil	Inhibits synthesis pathway of B- and T-cells.	Gastrointestinal (nausea, vomiting, diarrhoea, ulcers, gastritis) Bone marrow suppression

(Continued)

Table 5.   (*Continued*)

Immunosuppressive agent group	Examples	Mode of action	Side effects (in addition to infection)
mTOR inhibitor (mammalian target of rapamycin)	Sirolimus	Inhibits response to IL-2 and hence blocks activation of B-and T-cells.	Hyperlipidaemia Leukopenia Thrombocytopenia Poor tissue healing
Protein immunosuppressives	Antithymocyte globulin	Contains cytotoxic/blocking antibodies (anti-CD2, 3, 4, 8, 11a, 18 25, 44, 52, HLA classes I and II) to circulating lymphocytes.	
	Anti-IL-2 (CD25) receptor Daclizumab Basiliximab	Blocks IL-2 and the resulting activation of B and T-cells.	
	Anti-CD52 Alemtuzumab	Causes apoptosis of circulating lymphocytes, monocytes, macrophages and natural killer cells.	

- 77% of lung transplants are still functioning well,
- 73% of heart/lung transplants are still functioning well.

Longer-term outcomes are similarly improving although most organs, with the exception of liver grafts, suffer from 'chronic fatigue', otherwise known as 'chronic rejection'. Most transplanted organs are still functioning at 5 and 10 years, but the percentage attrition rate varies from 10% at 5 years for livers through to 25% for lungs. A recent analysis based on 3,673 adult liver recipients for whom the 15-year patient survival rate was 58% (95% confidence interval 54–62%) suggests that adult liver transplant recipients have an average life expectancy of 22 years. The average life expectancy of the equivalent UK adult population is 30 years, and so on average 8 years of life are lost. Furthermore, female recipients lose fewer life-years than male recipients, and younger recipients lose more life-years than older recipients.

References

1. Devlin J, O'Grady J. Indications for referral and assessment in adult liver transplantation: A clinical guideline. British society of gastroenterology. *Gut* 1999;45(6):VI1–VI22.
2. Neuberger J, Gimson A, Davies M, Akyol M, O'Grady J, Burroughs A, Hudson M, Liver Advisory Group; UK Blood and Transplant. Selection of patients for liver transplantation and allocation of donated livers in the UK. *Gut* 2008;57: 252–257.

Further Reading

1. British Transplant Society. Standards for solid organ transplantation, 2003. http://www.bts.org.uk/Forms/standards%20document%20edition%202%20 20-%20final.pdf.
2. *Transplantation — A Companion to Specialist Surgical Practice*, 3rd edn. Philadelphia, PA: Elsevier Saunders, 2005.
3. United network for organ sharing. http://www.unos.org/.
4. *The Practice of Liver Transplantation*. Oxford: W.B. Saunders, 1995.
5. *Organ Donation and Transplantation after Cardiac Death*. New York: Oxford University Press, 2009.

6. Strategies for safer liver surgery and partial liver transplantation. *NEJM* 2007;356:1545–1559.
7. Guidelines for selection of patients for liver transplantation in the era of donor-organ shortage. *Lancet* 1999;354:206–214.
8. Adult liver transplantation: What non-specialists need to know. *BMJ* 2009;338:b1670.

Index